THE ASIAN DIET SECRET
for
PERMANENT WEIGHT LOSS
and
VIBRANT HEALTH

FEED YOUR TIGER

LETHA HADADY, DAc

RODALE

© 2007 by Letha Hadady

All rights reserved. No part of this publication may be reproduced or transmitted in any form or by any means, electronic or mechanical, including photocopying, recording, or any other information storage and retrieval system, without the written permission of the publisher.

Rodale books may be purchased for business or promotional use or for special sales. For information, please write to: Special Markets Department, Rodale Inc., 733 Third Avenue, New York, NY 10017.

Printed in the United States of America
Rodale Inc. makes every effort to use acid-free ∞, recycled paper ♲.

Illustrations by Letha Elizabeth Hadady and Letha Hadady.

Library of Congress Cataloging-in-Publication Data

Hadady, Letha, date
    Feed your tiger : the asian diet secret for permanent weight loss and vibrant health / by Letha Hadady.
       p.   cm.
    Includes index.
    ISBN-13 978–1–59486–414–8   hardcover
    ISBN-10 1–59486–414–4 hardcover
    1. Energy metabolism.   2. Reducing diets.   3. Medicine, Chinese.   I. Title.
    RM222.2.H216   2007
    613.2'5—dc22   2006029368

Distributed to the book trade by Holtzbrinck Publishers

2   4   6   8   10   9   7   5   3   1   hardcover

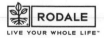

For you—bright, beautiful, and hungry

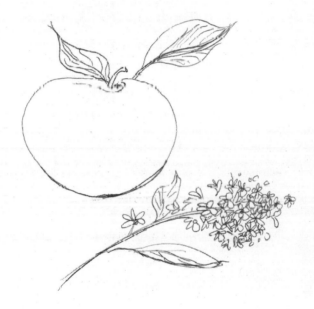

Contents

Acknowledgments

I thank the New York Open Center; the Renfield Center for Nursing, a division of Beth Israel Medical Center; Anna E. Story, RN, MS, MSN, director of continuing education at Continuum Health Services; and Karen Fuller, director of programs at DOROT senior center in New York, for hosting my "Feed Your Tiger" weight loss workshops. I thank my many students, health clients, and friends who participated in my classes and weight loss observations. Their encouragement and information made this book possible.

I thank Andrew Weil, MD, respected author and director of the department of integrative medicine at the University of Arizona, for his encouragement in writing this book. I thank Michel Czehatowski, director of East Earth Trade Winds in California; Andrew Gaeddert, director of Health Concerns in Oakland, California; Susan and Frank Lin of Lin Sister Herb Shop in New York; Robert McCaleb, president of the Herb Research Foundation in Boulder, Colorado; and my brother, Dr. Eric S. Hadady, for their medical advice. Suggestions by Cambridge University genetics researcher Aubrey de Grey and articles on the antiaging potential of phytochemicals published in his journal, *Rejuvenation Research*, were also enlightening.

I thank my partner at Karma Unlimited Inc., Michael Foster, for his unfailing, Bearish financial support and unending love. I thank Joachim Stroh, Xiaoning Wang, and Paul Paulson of ChinaSprout for their encouragement and technical support for my Web site, www. asianhealthsecrets.com. I thank Wal-Mart marketing managers Curt Jones and Mike Taylor for their interest in this book. I thank Pia Garcia, executive vice president of Porter Novelli, for her support and encouragement. I thank celebrated author Jack Engelhard and Amazon.com for their enthusiastic support.

I thank my darling mother, Letha Elizabeth Hadady, in Albuquerque, for her lovely illustrations of foods and herbs. I thank my expert editor, Alice Feinstein, for her valuable suggestions in structuring and writing the book; and Rachelle Laliberte for her careful copyediting. I thank Lisa Silverman and Peter Miller, the literary lion of the Peter Miller Agency, for their introduction to Rodale. Finally, I thank you—Tigers, Dragons, Bears, and Cranes everywhere—for your priceless input and efforts to advance this book.

Preface

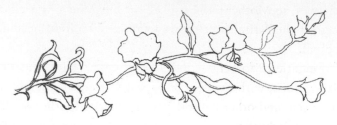

We spoke Hungarian at home. My maternal grandmother, Erszebet, took care of the house and garden—a profusion of purple dahlias, blue irises, red and yellow tulips, and roses mixed with stock, petunias, marigolds, and snapdragons. My first herbal concoctions came from Gramma's garden.

My family's cuisine has been marked by an expanding cultural reach increasingly focused on Asia. It took generations because the flavors of our eastern European cooking and close-knit lifestyle made us reluctant to change. Gramma, from Hungary's Tokay wine region, followed the conventions of that rich cuisine. Her dishes, some made with bacon drippings, included pickled pigs' feet; chicken paprika in cream sauce with egg noodles; cabbages rolls stuffed with pork, beef, and rice; and elaborate homemade pastries. She lived into her nineties, dangerously overweight and with an enlarged heart. She suffered severe pain and swollen joints from arthritis, migraine headaches, and cataracts. We all suffered from her tyrannical temper. Gramma had health problems that anyone would develop given her energy type, rich diet, and personal frustrations.

A Victorian, she was obsessed with protecting herself and her girls from strange men who, she was convinced, lurked in the shadows. She tried to beat me with a wooden spoon if I came home late from school, but I ducked under a bed. At age 8, I plotted my escape, planning to live in neighborhood backyards and eat the fruits of their gardens. Fortunately, Mother caught wind of my scheme.

Since I could not leave home, I declared my independence with cooking. My first creation was an elegant, slightly lopsided applesauce cake with blue frosting. The summer that I was 12, Gramma visited other relatives, so Mother and I cooked for the family. Mothers and daughters set the eating style in most families, so food becomes a lifelong bond.

In her eighties, Mother is youthful, optimistic, slim, and active. During the 1960s, with the help of books written by Adelle Davis, Bernard Jensen, and other natural health experts, Mother modified her cooking, switching from shortening and bacon fat to olive oil and from red meat to chicken and fish. She increased our fruits, vegetables, salads, and light, low-fat baking. This book includes several healthy European-inspired dishes.

My cooking was also influenced by my college years in France. While studying opera and completing a master's degree in psychology at the University of Paris, I lived across from Les Halles when it was the farmers' market that served the city's chic restaurants.

Culinary ingredients sold in Paris streets are among the finest in the world. What counts is how you prepare them. My slimming dishes have been refined by master chef Pierre Checchi, a professor/chef at Kendall College in Chicago and a gourmet who has lost more than 100 pounds and regulated his diabetes by eating well. Robert Barral, executive director and head chef of New England Culinary Institute for 16 years and owner of Café Provence in Brandon, Vermont, has also inspired my light, healthy European dishes by substituting olive oil for butter, a custom from his native town of Montpelier, France.

My interest in acupuncture and Asian herbal studies, as well as world travel during the 1980s and 1990s, greatly influenced my diet and health practices. For one thing, I learned to cook dishes appropriate for rapid weight loss by avoiding unhealthy fats and proteins. Whether taking the train or bus through China, India, and Tibet; traveling through Thailand by chauffeured royal limousine or elephant; or sampling dishes at lively sushi parlors in Tokyo, I rarely saw obese people. Asians tend to eat less than one-third the protein that Americans consume, yet they are energetic and robust.

I marveled listening to the boisterous street noise at night in Shanghai. People were out playing with their kids, yelling, gossiping, and full of zip into the late hours, then awake at dawn doing tai chi and qigong exercises in the street. Watching Asian people eating rice, fish, and vegetables or garlic dumplings at outdoor shops in Shanghai or enjoying a late-night papaya salad at a market in Bangkok, I realized that Asian people live longer and better. They have more fun with food. They do not eat to lose weight; they eat to enjoy life.

The traditional Asian diet, which stresses tea, fresh fruits and vegetables, select whole grains, exotic mushrooms, whole soy products, seaweeds, and fish, is energizing because it is easily digested. It takes the body much less time and effort to reap the benefits of plant fiber and nutrients. This book can enhance life: The Asian weight loss diet leads to less cancer, heart trouble, diabetes, and obesity.

If you know you should eat better but are not ready for a completely plant-based diet, this book can help you to head in the right direction. Asians have been eating smart for a long time.

It has been my karma to learn from my own and others' illnesses and to transform that knowledge into healing. I have explored traditional Asian medicines because they worked well for me when modern health care offered no alternatives but a lifetime of addictive drugs, surgery, or despair. I loved discovering my Eastern roots. Traveling in Asian jungles and villages has been a great adventure, sometimes made perilous by poor food and sanitary conditions. My resulting discomforts required revamping my diet at home with Asian superfoods and herbs. I learned that building vitality is essential for maintaining good digestion, emotional well-being, and a healthy weight.

My professional health practice in New York, along with my world travel, led to writing. My first book, *Asian Health Secrets*, called a classic in complementary and alternative medicine, is required reading for holistically minded nurses and doctors, but my long hours spent crunched over a desk led to cellulite and arthritic pain. This new book has given me the opportunity for a personal overhaul. It contains proven recipes for light, cleansing, and nourishing meals. Using them, my friends, clients, readers, and I lost extra weight and firmed flab while eating a wide variety of foods.

As you will learn from this book, improving digestive energy improves life. The fact is, our individual dietary needs and mental outlook can improve as we improve our diet. At the very least, to answer the emotional needs for comfort foods, this book offers convenient, easily available natural remedies for nervous snackers and emotional bingers.

Good cooking enhances all areas of life. Master chef Pierre Checchi incorporates into his menus foods that control his diabetes, such as noncaffeinated rooibos tea and the herbal sweetener stevia, and occasionally enjoys a glass of red wine with dinner. Meals bring the family together to reestablish bonds cut by a high-speed, junk-food culture. With wholesome foods lovingly prepared, people may again be able to sit down together and talk.

This book came about because I wanted to share with my readers some of the family togetherness I enjoy at home. During my Asian studies, I became interested in the Five Animal Form exercises of qigong, an ancient Chinese martial art and system of health maintenance. The animal exercises enhance agility and vitality. I realized they might be adapted into energy types useful and amusing enough to interest adults and children. After all, don't some of our friends resemble bears, dragons, tigers, and graceful birds? They crave different foods and expend energy in differing ways. Each type has health and weight problems related to diet.

The Asian-inspired Baseline Diet for rapid weight loss, described in Part 1 of this book, worked well for me and most of my overweight students and clients. I noticed that it also eliminated many of their problems related to menopause and arthritis by reducing the effects of stress and excess acids from the body. Losing flab and feeling physically fit for the first time in years, I attempted things I never dared before—like swimming!

With this book, you will certainly find a slimming diet and health routine to suit your energy type, lifestyle, culinary tastes, and budget. Your kids will enjoy being compared to Bears, Dragons, Tigers, and beautiful Cranes. I am happy to share with you my heartening experiences with Asian food-medicines, the dieting success stories of my students and clients, and my deep appreciation of nature.

Introduction

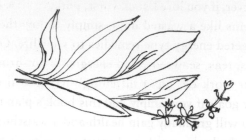

I magine yourself sleek, strong, and agile as a cat. Imagine you can achieve vibrant health at any age. This is a life-changing book. It shows you ways to achieve your ideal weight and stay attractive and healthy with delicious foods, teas, herbs, and body treatments enjoyed by millions of slim, active Asians. The essential message of this book is: Gain vitality to lose weight. Feed your tiger!

This may be the last diet book you will ever need. (If you find that hard to believe, you are addicted to dieting.) It can help you conquer unhealthy cravings for sweets, salty foods, and harmful fats, as well as overcome chronic stress and yo-yo dieting, which challenge your weight and well-being. Our comprehensive program is organized to gradually introduce empowering foods and slimming techniques so that you can avoid unpleasant side effects. It includes an Asian-inspired low-protein, high-fiber Baseline Diet and convenient foods to jump-start weight loss when you hit a plateau.

In addition, this unique approach, based on your energy type adapted from Chinese medicine, enables you to overcome common food addictions and fatigue as you enhance your metabolism and increase your willpower to succeed. To ensure continued success, several chapters describe how to stay slim while eating in Asian restaurants and during the holidays. Other chapters cover weight loss plans appropriate for people at risk of developing chronic illnesses associated with their energy types. This book proves once and for all that the same-diet-for-everyone approach simply does not work. You can say *no* to harmful diet fads!

You will not suffer with this diet. Most people enjoy Chinese,

Japanese, Korean, Tibetan, or Thai cooking or other spicy health foods. However, if you love knockwurst, pork, or fries—if a day without cake seems like a wasted day—simply follow the Baseline Diet and add targeted energy type remedies to your life. Our tasty Asian foods, spices, teas, seaweeds, and energizing mushrooms and herbs will do their work despite a fattening diet. It will take longer to achieve your goals if you simply add this book's plan to your regular diet, but you will gradually gain health and a waistline.

Because the body, mind, and spirit shape one's figure and lifestyle, a change in diet alone is never enough for weight loss. Tuva, who managed a beauty salon, followed a diet that consisted of fresh fruits and 1 liter of water during the day. Her dinner at home included meat, potatoes, and wine. She hated vegetables. Her shape resembled a large pear. She complained of severe fatigue, backache, and terrible menopausal hot flashes. Her fruit diet did not serve her, despite all the fresh, high-fiber foods.

Tuva added our balanced Baseline Diet, which controls the ratio of fruits to vegetables and greatly simplifies meals, to what she was already eating. After 3 weeks, she lost 10 to 15 pounds (her weight varied, depending on her mood).

Unfortunately, Tuva drank wine nightly to soothe her depression over family matters, so she quickly regained lost weight. Her mood and sweet cravings dampened her metabolism. She could not maintain a healthy weight until she used gymnema, an East Indian herb suited to her energy type. It curbed her sweet tooth and fortified her stressed pancreas. This book, which treats food addictions and weight loss problems resulting from energy imbalances, uses an Asian medical approach: Improve your energy to live better and longer.

Nancy, like a number of my New York clients, could neither sleep nor digest her food properly after September 11, 2001. No matter what diet she tried, she remained 50 pounds overweight and addicted to junk food, which she said quieted her nerves. Neither following a high-protein diet nor eating every 3 hours solved Nancy's weight problem; she needed an approach that worked for *her*, not for everyone under the sun. She was finally helped by a deep-acting homeopathic remedy for anxiety described later in this book. She gradually lost weight as she gained emotional balance.

In this book, I explain how some remedies are useful for an energy type, while others benefit anyone who wants to lose weight. The Baseline Diet is in agreement with the largest, most important weight loss studies to date, as well as the research-based food guidance system developed by the USDA and supported by the U.S. Department of Health and Human Services (HHS), which recommend fresh fruits, vegetables, whole grains, select proteins, and regular exercise for weight loss.

Lessons from China

The China Study, which the *New York Times* has called the most comprehensive nutrition study ever conducted—it represents a 20-year partnership of Cornell and Oxford Universities and the Chinese Academy of Preventive Medicine in Beijing—provides support for this approach. According to researchers who studied dietary habits and health throughout China, Americans consume approximately 10 grams of dietary fiber daily, whereas the Chinese take in 34 to 77 grams each day. The typical Chinese diet contains less fat than the typical U.S. diet. In a comparison of blood cholesterol levels, Chinese people average 85 to 170, while American adults rarely have cholesterol under 180. Only about 15 percent of the total calories of the Chinese diet comes from fat, compared with 40 percent for the American diet.

It may surprise you to hear that although Chinese people consume less calcium than we do and mainly from vegetable sources, they rarely have osteoporosis. The China Study proved that the body loses calcium in proportion to the animal protein consumed. The more animal protein we eat, the less calcium we absorb. Extensive research has shown that a plant-based diet can prevent and reverse illness and obesity. The *New York Times* termed the combined efforts of this study the Grand Prix of epidemiology.

As wonderful and useful as science is, you cannot *eat* science. This book offers practical guidance on slimming Asian foods, herbs, teas, energy tonics, and recipes that brings this important research work as well as the successful health traditions of Asia into our kitchens.

Lessons from My Students and Clients

To create a workable diet plan, I gathered my own data quite informally with the participation of my students, clients, and readers on the Internet via my Web site: www.asianhealthsecrets.com. I studied the relationship of diet, weight loss, and quality of life. My inquiry included these questions: How does losing weight improve our daily life? What physical and emotional factors prevent weight loss? Under what conditions—PMS, fatigue, boredom, depression, or something else—do you most often experience your food addictions?

T. Colin Campbell, PhD, the top researcher from Cornell University who guided the 20-year China Study, gained insights about Chinese health, longevity, and diet by studying mortality statistics. His group charted the diseases that people in China developed in a prescribed geographical area—how long the village people lived and at what age they died. Then the researchers compared those mortality facts with the typical diet followed by people in that area of China. That was possible because diets are more uniform in Chinese villages than are ours in the West.

Using a very different approach, I wanted to discover not only how diet and weight loss are related but also how they both affect the quality of life. I wanted to observe factors other than genetic predisposition to weight gain and traditional diet involved in our American obesity epidemic. You might say there is no one American cuisine but a mixture of regional cooking styles and several universal food addictions. We love sweets, fried foods, overprocessed starchy foods, and junk foods.

This book is about a lot more than losing 10 pounds in 2 weeks. We eat to satisfy needs beyond food hunger: Our addictions, personality, and energy levels are most important in determining weight and health. Such factors are the basis of the energy types described in this book.

It does not matter whether you live in New York, San Francisco,

Auckland, Milan, or Hong Kong. You may binge on cookies, plain pasta, white rice, white bread, or alcohol. It is energy type, not just geographic location, that rules food choices. With that in mind, this book addresses the problems of overweight people everywhere.

During my research for this book, in each case that resulted in significant weight loss, the person following my suggestions reported that she had better control of her life. She felt centered, happier, and healthier. The individualized diet addressed her emotional as well as dietary needs. Over the years, I have observed how people affected with specific imbalances stemming from their energy type craved specific foods. The examples in this book are drawn from real people, including their struggles and triumphs with food, not numbers indicating statistical probability. You will share their enthusiasm for a new dietary lifestyle.

Eileen is a typical example of how healthy improvements in the body and metabolism liberate the spirit. While following our protocol, she left her job of many years as a television producer to become a yoga instructor. After using the Baseline Diet and a few individualized remedies for her energy type for several months in New York, she traveled through India. She e-mailed me from California: "I have made peace with my body, which has slimmed down and is experiencing a much more comfortable perimenopausal time after the proper nutrition you suggested. I can continue with your diet anywhere I live. I am looking at turning 50 next year and truly feel it will be a great time as I move forward in the second half of my life."

Customizing a Diet Just for You

One major reason diet books fail is that they do not address our fundamental emotional involvement with food. Of the 54 million people currently dieting in America, only 5 percent can keep weight off.

Helping people lose weight and gain health has taught me that food privation only clouds the mind and troubles the emotions. I have known people who, after losing 100 pounds or more by dieting, regained their weight after suffering an emotional setback or an illness. Cravings for fattening foods, faulty digestion, and major illnesses cannot be eliminated without health improvements stemming from dietary changes.

Part 2 of this book specifically addresses common food addictions with healthy alternatives. The book includes many recipes, such as middle-slimming foods; a no-calorie Japanese noodle; Chinese teas for reducing cellulite and edema; Asian miracle foods, such as reishi mushrooms, that boost energy and immunity; and natural treatments for addictions aggravated by stress.

Have you tried dieting and given up disappointed? The fault is not yours. We easily gain unwanted weight when bored, sick, exhausted, or depressed. Low vitality dampens our mood, slows metabolism, clouds concentration, and keeps us overweight. Having an open mind and increasing stamina are essential for reducing fat and cellulite and enhancing physical and mental fitness. However, energy, willpower, and the ways they affect dietary addictions are rarely addressed in weight loss books. This book helps you transform harmful cravings to achieve lasting vitality.

My years of work as a holistic health professional specializing in traditional Asian healing arts, including herbs and acupuncture, have convinced me: We must increase vitality to lose weight. The best foods in the world turn to waste and disease if digestion and absorption are inadequate. This book offers targeted digestive remedies and health foods.

There are more centenarians living in Japan than anywhere else in the world. Many people attribute their longevity to their traditional diet, which includes exotic mushrooms, bitter melon, and turmeric root. Unfortunately, most Asian health elixirs remain a mystery to Westerners, with the exception of athletes and martial artists who use Panax or Eleutherococcus ginseng to sustain stamina. Chinese herbs described in this book help you slenderize, firm muscles, and energize for work and play. High-energy herbs also fuel willpower for weight loss. Ayurveda, the traditional natural medicine from India, offers herbal foods and teas, pleasing beauty massages, and special baths with organic essential oils to boost metabolism and erase cellulite.

Most Americans are addicted to yo-yo dieting; they lose a few pounds, hit a plateau, and switch to a new diet. These diets do not adequately address our energy, digestion, and mood-related addictions. If they did, we would be slim, active, and healthy. Rudolph Leibel, MD, a respected authority from Columbia University's Obesity Clinic who is known for research on hereditary weight gain and brain chemistry, believes any diet that reduces calories and increases exercise can work—if only temporarily. He believes that a high-protein, high-fat diet works only for a couple of weeks because no one can stand to eat so much meat for long. The result is that people eat less. However, a serious health problem remains: Eating less junk food sustains neither vitality nor lasting weight loss.

Our Asian-inspired diet is spicy, light, and delicious. Jackie, one of my formerly overweight clients, lost 90 pounds within 6 months using this plan and the following motto, which she posted in her kitchen: Eat well, eat less, enjoy your food, and exercise.

This book offers practical ways for everyone to improve energy, digestion, physical fitness, and mental clarity. You can begin today. Your success, one day at a time, increases willpower and allows for healthy weight loss.

How to Use This Book

The directions for using this book are simple. Follow the order of information presented from beginning to end in consecutive chapters. In that way, you can add new foods and remedies as you read about them. While broadening your diet and healthy lifestyle, you will learn to monitor your digestive capacity and weight loss progress with diagnostic techniques used by Asian herbalists.

Part 1 explores your relationship to foods—what I call your food karma. I offer, among other treatments, homeopathic remedies to correct depression bingeing. To get everyone's diet started on square one, we have a low-fat, low-protein diet called the Baseline Diet. In addition, I suggest foods to jump-start stalled weight loss. Some are Asian superfoods, including teas and seaweeds known to boost metabolism.

In Part 2, individually tailored menus and herbs, selected according to your energy type, are added to suit your ongoing dietary and emotional needs as a Tiger, Dragon, Bear, or Crane. To help you maintain your ideal weight and health, Part 3 details a maintenance program called Weight Loss Insurance. In Part 4, I offer targeted simple exercise, slimming dishes from Asian restaurants, and natural ways to lose weight and avoid bingeing during the holidays.

Most people want an edge for quick, lasting weight loss. They can neither rearrange their schedules for elaborate cooking nor feel deprived of pleasure foods. This book is essential for anyone living an active life while eating on the run. With this book, you remain free to travel, celebrate life, and experiment with new foods—it's all part of the adventure.

Finding Your Energy Type

Do your dietary habits resemble a Dragon, Bear, Tiger, or Crane? Each is distinctive; each eats and lives in different ways. One or perhaps two energy types will strike your fancy because they more closely resemble you. Each animal energy type in this book has specific weight loss and health issues that can be improved with the appropriate slimming routine. A few examples will illustrate. See which energy type most applies to you. (If all four seem to apply, you'll start with recommendations tailored for the Dragon.)

BEARS love sweets, are heavy in the middle, and often feel sleepy after meals. Healthy, slimming Bear foods include sugarless pies, cherries, berries, parsnips, pumpkin, and an Asian superfiber called shirataki. Eating healthful sweets improves a Bear's mental clarity and mood. The chapter for Bears offers natural ways to prevent and treat diabetes.

TIGERS love to move swiftly and conquer. But too often poor circulation restricts their activities and increases cellulite. If they overindulge in fried or oily foods or alcohol and live under stress, they often become irritable and frustrated or have headaches, allergies, and stiff, aching muscles and joints. Green herbs such as alfalfa and chlorella cleanse the body and promote clarity on many levels.

DRAGONS lay low and develop edema and obesity but become fiery when aroused. Their hot flashes, anxiety, or heart palpitations are like fire rising out of a swamp of polluted water. They need foods and tonics to build endurance and reduce water retention and salt cravings.

CRANES may eat poorly or not at all and still gain weight and cellulite. They can feel isolated or depressed and seek comfort from fattening foods, alcohol, or smoking until they are stymied by an illness. Antidepressants and certain psychiatric drugs are notorious for putting on excess pounds. Cranes, or anyone who has excess mucus congestion, can improve breathing, elimination, and mental clarity by increasing antimucus foods and teas.

By applying Asian foods and diet secrets to your life, you will notice that your body, mind, and spirit achieve a more harmonious balance. At the very least, it will be easier for you to resist former habits, exercise more regularly, and take better care of yourself and family. You will feel and look better than you have in years. The tigress in you will gain a renewed sense of wonder and ease of movement as she glides effortlessly through the forest.

Part 1

Your Food Karma

You have an intimate relationship with foods: They may be friends or enemies. This book helps you transform your food karma to gain health and happiness as you lose weight. That makes food a means to victory.

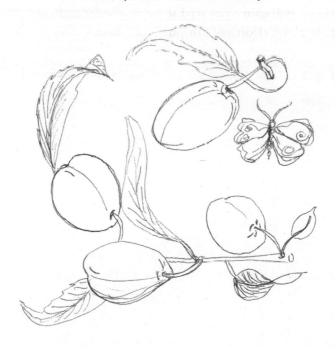

Chapter 1

Foods and You

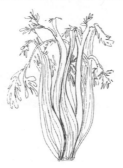

You can't remember snuggling into Mother's arms while nursing, but that memory has left a trace. The warm hug and the aroma, taste, and texture of comfort foods reach into our collective consciousness. Our love of food echoes other vital relationships because, without realizing it, we eat to fulfill emotional needs. Human beings are not merely digesting machines that register calories taken in and work put out; your favorite sweet snack may be a needed pause from work for stress relief. Spicy dishes may stimulate social chatter with friends. Your eating habits have created ongoing relationships with foods, places, events, and people. To improve dietary habits, over the course of reading this book, you will alter your relationship to fattening foods.

Do you consume fast foods on the run, purchase bargains at the supermarket, or prepare ethnic dishes from family recipes? Convenience, price, and tradition are important aspects of our socialization. However, there are other more fundamental reasons that we select one food over another. This chapter addresses our emotional and energetic needs for fattening foods. How adventurous are you when trying new dishes? What catches your attention—color, shape, aroma, taste, or texture? They are the sensory aspects of foods. Hopefully, you will expand your appreciation of them while discovering your optimal diet. Home, job, and friends often change over time. With a little help, your diet, too, will broaden and eventually improve.

Feed Your Senses

Many overweight people express fears and desires when talking about foods. Food and figure play an important role in self-image. When you clarify your language, you change your experience. As much as possible, eliminate words of blame or guilt concerning diets. Foods are neither "good" nor "bad." You can rethink your relationship to food by paying close attention to your words. All habits become reinforced over time.

Slimming foods like celery, cucumber, apple, watermelon, pear, and salad greens are refreshing and cooling. Dense whole grain breads and steel-cut oats are chewy and tasty, compared with bland white breads and mushy cereal. Fries and bacon are salty and greasy. Taste and texture adjectives engage the senses.

I think healthy, slim people often perceive digestive comfort more acutely than overweight people do. To remain slender, we should neither abuse nor ignore digestion. For example, when was the last time you were lost in thought, worry, or work and stuffed yourself with your addictions?

Part of the fun of weight loss is enjoying a variety of tastes and textures in foods. Overweight people may be weakened from illness or hormonal imbalances or feel emotionally preoccupied. Food addictions arise from eating without tasting. If you snack while working, watching television, or driving, you are bound to gain weight because you are not paying attention to the flavors and textures of the foods you are consuming.

An Asian energetic approach to diet frees discovery and experimentation. You will discover that food qualities such as taste and texture often indicate their effects. For example, Chinese herbalists consider overly sweet, heavy, and oily foods to be sedating for body and mind. Salty foods are drying; they increase thirst and dry the complexion. Eat popcorn to prove it. Bitter and pungent foods like tea and ginger are considered digestive.

Enhancing Appreciation

As a rule, try to vary the flavors, colors, and textures of your ingredients. A meal can be a feast for the senses. A fine chef knows that delicious foods are savored in small portions. Wise health experts know that foods requiring chewing, such as whole grains (coarse breads and al dente pastas), cooked dried beans, crisp fruits and vegetables, nuts, and seeds, require less insulin from the pancreas. They digest more slowly, satisfy us longer, and protect us better against overweight, high blood pressure, and diabetes than foods high in simple sugars, such as potatoes and breads made with finely milled flour. Chewy foods are healthy foods that taste better.

It may surprise you that some of our healthiest fats are found in nuts such as walnuts, almonds, and cashews; in seeds such as sesame, pumpkin, flax, and hemp; and in olives and avocados. Other healthy oils come from fatty fishes such as eel, salmon, mackerel, herring, and sardines. Extra-virgin olive oil and canola, grapeseed, and flaxseed oils are fine in salads. Grapeseed and peanut oils tolerate high heat without smoking, an important consideration for preventing cancer.

Asian populations who eat plant-based diets, cold-water fish, and seaweeds live longer and enjoy better health than most Americans who overeat meats, margarine, salad dressings and mayonnaise, whole-milk products, cakes, cookies, refined foods, and simple sugars found in most starches and sweet drinks. Most nutritionists recommend cutting calories as the best method for weight loss. Unfortunately, despite the popularity of fat-free foods, we have grown fatter from eating more calories found in simple refined carbohydrates.

Counting calories will never alter your addictions—or, if you'd rather, your food preferences. You don't have to be a math major to lose weight. By increasing your intake of teas, fresh fruits and vegetables, and salad dishes (bitter, sour, alkaline, cleansing, and crunchy foods) with the Baseline Diet in the following chapter, you will naturally ease digestion and elimination and, therefore, enhance slimming. Traditional Chinese herbal doctors express the relationship between healthy foods and good digestion this way: Stimulating herbs and spices (such as ginger, cardamom, and pepper) and cooked whole grains (such as barley and cornmeal) enhance digestive energy—known in traditional Chinese medicine as digestive *qi* (or *chi*, pronounced "chee"). These foods and spices make digestion work better.

Why Is Digestive Qi Important?

This book contains many ways to enhance digestive qi, the absorption of nutrients, and weight loss. However, before we can make any progress at all, we must discover the fundamental source of your food cravings. In other words, we need to look at the factors that can weaken your digestive qi.

To a great extent, our cravings are *emotional*. You might not realize it, but when your general vitality (qi) is low, you are more likely to crave fattening comfort foods. The more low-value comfort foods you consume, the more troubled your digestive qi becomes. Here is the progression: Low vitality from overwork, illness, hormonal issues, or emotional factors leads to depression and stress, which lead to comfort foods, which lead to poor digestion, which leads to addictive cravings and overweight. People do not experience low qi directly, only its effects. What interests me is how you feel when you overeat—that is, what makes you need comfort foods in the first place. If you can stop the low qi vitality cycle anywhere along the line, you are ahead of the game.

Many people overeat to reduce stress. Chronic stress and anxiety greatly weaken qi. Unfortunately, a desire for comfort and safety can never be satisfied with food because we always require more food. There begins an addictive craving. You can't make progress with dieting or reducing addictions or excess hunger until you address your emotional needs and their relationship to your food choices. We are going to pay close attention to the kinds of comfort that foods can give.

Vary Your Experience

Transforming food cravings takes more than nerves of steel because your addictions have been with you a long time. You may need to dine at new restaurants or set the table differently to create a new context for meals. Using smaller plates may help you to eat less but will not improve health unless you eat better foods. Eating small meals and snacks throughout the day and drinking plenty of liquids between meals tones and balances digestion. Some experts say that small meals shrink the stomach so that you feel full sooner. In any case, you need a new awareness of your own body.

When you recognize the *energy* in foods, you can select slimming, satisfying dishes instead of fattening ones. For example, some foods are stimulating and cleansing; others, sedating or depressing for body and mind. Consider your current diet for a moment. Which foods, among those that you regularly consume, make you feel:

- Light
- Clean
- Limber
- Centered
- Nourished
- Satisfied (but not heavy)

By emphasizing those slenderizing foods, you reinforce positive habits. That liberates you to achieve things that seemed impossible.

Weight Management Goals and Cravings

You may set yourself a realistic weight loss goal and follow a sensible diet and exercise program but still continue to crave junk food. Throughout this book, we will find ways to improve energy and

A VISUALIZATION EXERCISE

Deep relaxation satisfies like a tasty meal followed by a nap. You can create a sense of inner harmony by practicing the following Chinese *qigong* visualization exercise as needed throughout the day or evening. Qigong has long been revered by martial artists, athletes, students, and elderly or sick people who need to enhance circulation, digestion, mental tranquillity, and physical vigor. Such exercise aims not to build muscles but to focus the body's attention in order to free deep channels of energy circulation that acupuncturists call meridians.

Sit comfortably with your back touching your chair and your feet on the floor, toes pointing straight ahead. Your neck, shoulders, and chest remain relaxed as you breathe deeply and slowly into your lower abdomen.

Place your hands gently at your navel and slowly inhale to inflate the abdomen. Slowly exhale as though through your thighs, knees, ankles, and feet. Repeat this for up to 10 minutes. You will begin to feel calm as you rhythmically breathe through your nose.

Close your eyes and visualize the bright, beautiful tiger within. Her muscles are sleek and long. Her bones are straight and strong. Her coat is shiny; her eyes, brilliant. She is sitting on her haunches, gazing at you. Acknowledge that her untamed power and courage make you eager for life's adventure.

---

digestion and reduce those addictions. For now, let's examine your weight loss goals and compare them with your cravings.

My current weight management goals are:

___I want to lose 10, 50, or more pounds.

___I want to lose some weight but mainly tone muscles and reduce cellulite.

___I want to lose water weight (edema) because I feel puffy all over.

___I want to slim my abdomen and thighs.

_____I want a total makeover to find my ideal weight.

_____I want to improve my health, vitality, and mood.

_____I want to gain weight and improve energy following an illness.

It is possible to achieve any and all of the above results because a healthy, balanced diet eventually leads to an ideal weight, fitness, and vitality. The hard part is to adjust your food cravings to match your present needs. Each person's body is different. The comprehensive Baseline Diet plan in Chapter 2 accomplishes many of the above goals. You can also zero in on your particular needs in upcoming chapters on energy types.

Asian health experts believe that your qi (energy and vitality)— expressed by your general health, digestion, breathing, circulation, and mood—affects your food cravings. They use diet, herbs, and body treatments to influence qi (yogis call it *prana*) and thereby improve body functions, including digestion, elimination, and breathing. Our dietary habits are both a result of stress and a cause of stress. Most often we crave foods that maintain our level of energy—whether for better or worse. In other words, when exhausted or sad, you may crave foods that keep you down in the dumps.

Getting a Handle on Food Cravings

When considering the items below, ignore your dieting ideology and pay attention to the foods you actually crave. In other words, you may be a vegetarian but currently crave meat or cream sauce.

I most often crave foods or beverages that:

_____Make me feel relaxed and happy

_____Quench my thirst

_____Satisfy my sweet tooth

_____Taste salty

_____Taste sour or bitter

___ Taste spicy and hot

___ Are cold or raw

___ Are creamy and rich

___ Are crispy and crunchy

___ Are high in protein, especially meats, chicken, or fish

Nervous eaters can be addicted to any of the above flavors and foods. Starving yourself cannot reduce addictions because your physical and emotional attachment to foods always remains intact, despite almost any diet. Your particular cravings for bitter, sweet, hot, salty, or sour foods, meats, and alcohol are influenced by your qi energy— not your diet philosophy. As we shall see, this notion is encompassed by the traditional Chinese five elements (discussed at length starting on page 65).

If you eat to make yourself feel relaxed and happy, you may be eating to avoid stress, anxiety, or depression. In that case, it is better to treat your emotions directly with a natural remedy. Some diet experts suggest that you can avoid hunger by distracting your attention with an activity such as reading, watching television, or telephoning a friend. If that works for you, great. Reducing stress has many health benefits. However, to get to the *source* of your diet problems and make permanent improvements, you need to enhance your energy and digestion.

The Five Flavors

One concept that you can institute right away is that of balancing flavors to enhance digestion and feelings of well-being. This concept has been around for a long time. After Chinese medicine had been practiced for nearly 1,000 years, a book called *The Yellow Emperor's Classic of Internal Medicine (Nei Jing)* appeared as a shorthand guide to assist practitioners. Without giving detailed reasons or proofs, the text offers rules to live by in order to be in harmony with the seasons. Chinese doctors still refer to the book because it provides an energetic understanding of the body. We can apply its dietary advice to food addictions.

According to these ancient principles, the five flavors of foods—bitter, sweet, pungent hot, salty, and sour—affect body, mind, and spirit. They regulate metabolism, circulation, breathing, and other subtle expressions of well-being. In other words, we crave specific flavors that indicate our state of health. Did you think that craving junk was healthy? An addiction indicates that we crave too much of a certain flavor that, eaten to excess, causes health problems. To summarize the energetic effects of the five flavors:

- **BITTER** stimulates the heart and small intestine to regulate circulation, body temperature, and elimination. People who overconsume coffee, tea, or salad become jittery and nervous or develop diarrhea.
- **SWEET** fruits are nourishing and harmonize digestion and mood. Licorice improves digestion by reducing cramps. However, sugar and sweet or oily foods increase water retention and fat. Cookies and yeast bread increase cellulite and indigestion.
- **HOT OR PUNGENT** foods such as ginger increase appetite and vigor and sometimes cause perspiration. A little goes a long way. An appetizer made with a dash of chile pepper can reduce appetite. Dousing foods with hot sauce burns the tongue, increases thirst, and dries mucous membranes.
- **SALTY** foods overstimulate the kidneys and increase water retention. Table salt is an enemy to weight loss, although some high-sodium foods like celery are useful because they improve calcium absorption and reduce cellulite. To avoid edema (water retention), cut out table salt and use a substitute.
- **SOUR** foods such as lemon drain the liver and blood of wastes, but too much sour weakens muscle tone and mental focus. The next time you make lemonade, add a dash of hot sauce to simultaneously stimulate and drain the body.

Barring special considerations for treating illness, a combination of all five flavors works best for meals. It is balanced. Think of a big salad—bitter greens, celery, and cucumber; pungent radishes; sweet carrots and tomatoes; a little canola or olive oil; and lemon juice.

To lose weight, we will stress bitter, pungent, and sour foods and reduce or find substitutes for certain sweet, oily, and salty foods.

You may crave one flavor more than others out of habit. For example, Italian cooks use tomato as an ingredient. It is traditional, and we enjoy its tart, sweet flavor. If you like one sweet food, you will more likely crave other sweet flavors as well. Later in this book, when you determine your energy type, you will observe the relationship between your cravings and vitality. Some people tend to crave sweets if their digestion is weak or blood sugars unstable. Others crave salty foods and retain water (causing edema and cellulite) if adrenal energy is low. And salt is a stimulant.

To begin weight loss, pay attention to the taste, texture, and aroma of your dishes to sensitize your palate. Notice how different foods affect your drive and enthusiasm. Avoid foods that invariably

---

ACHIEVING BALANCE

Keep in mind this simple rule: Always balance a fattening food with its opposite. Combine a cheese dish with a salad. Combine gooey, sweet, and oily foods with drying popcorn, barley soup, or cooked yellow cornmeal. Follow a spicy hot meal with cooling cucumber and yogurt with a dash of cumin powder, a twist of lemon, or a little coconut. Follow a hard-to-digest meal with fresh ginger, mint, or lemongrass tea. Here are more examples of how to balance food flavors to reduce bloating and toxins trapped in the digestive tract.

BALANCE	EXAMPLES
Bitter with pungent	Green tea and a dash of turmeric powder
Sweet with drying	Applesauce and whole grain toast
Oily with spicy, digestive	Fish steamed in pineapple juice and onion
Sweet with spicy	Prunes cooked with clove or cardamom
Salty with diuretic	Chicken, cheese, or celery with parsley

lead to a nap. Successful weight loss always requires more than an act of will. Use stimulating flavors and foods to reinforce your positive efforts.

Food combining is very important for digestive comfort and proper absorption of nutrients. Let's consider the energetic effects of combined foods as though we were making an herbal mixture. If you enjoy fattening chocolate or cheese, eat it along with cleansing (laxative and diuretic) foods such as tea, grapes, cherries, or berries. The stimulating caffeine in chocolate or tea will enhance the slimming effects of cleansing foods. (For an overview of this important concept of balancing foods, see "Achieving Balance.")

The difference between a healthy habit and an addiction depends upon the results. If you knew for sure that your meals lead to weight gain, sluggish energy, mental depression, nervous tension, and body odor, you would probably change your diet. I hope so.

A Clinical Observation

During the time I collected data and wrote this book, I conducted an informal clinical observation. Over a period of approximately 2 years, diet volunteers came from among my students at the Institute of Integrative Nutrition and the Acedemy of Healing Nutrition; nurses from the Renfield Center for Nursing, Beth Israel Medical Center; medical doctors attending my walking tours of Chinatown herbal markets during the annual conference on Complementary and Alternative Medicine at Columbia University; and my private clients.

Then something incredible happened. I posted information about my weight loss approach on my Web site www.asianhealthsecrets. com, and the observational study took off like wildfire around the world. Each person filled out the questionnaire found on page 73, and I recommended specific diet guidelines for them based on the energy types covered in this book. People from New Zealand to California, from Canada and the Americas to Israel, were using advice from this plan to lose weight and gain health. You will benefit from their ongoing input and support.

I realized something important. Some people do not care a whit about food theory, Asian medicines, or lifestyle changes. They just want to lose 20 or more pounds. Comments from my readers and to my Web site also confirmed that before significant, lasting progress can be made in weight loss, individual emotional factors concerning diet have to be addressed.

Marcia, a full-time student, illustrates how nervous eating habits dig a rut of intractable stress-related addictions. She answered my questionnaire frankly, without realizing that her food cravings continued her addictions and depression.

> I am 28 years old, and I have had serious issues with food and body image since I was a child. I have been in a cycle of binge/starvation for some time. I have a tendency toward depression and definitely eat when I am depressed. I have cellulite on my thighs and butt. I have an addictive personality; I'm an all-or-nothing person. I have struggled with alcoholism but live drug and alcohol free now. I get depressed and irritable, have migraines and nausea pretty regularly. When I crave food, it is usually sweets or bread.

Faced with complicated, long-term eating problems such as these, what sort of remedy should you choose—one for depression, sweets and bread cravings, irritability, or headaches? They all play a part in addictions. Trying to find comfort, we eat the wrong things. The right remedy for now depends partly on what troubles you the most. *When in doubt, treat one addiction at a time.*

I suggested a homeopathic remedy for Marcia because, as I explain below, it would improve a number of problems simultaneously. Homeopathic Pulsatilla 30C, often recommended for sadness and shortness of breath, improved her digestive bloating, excess mucus conditions, and a melancholic craving for sweets, carbohydrates, and bread.

After using Pulsatilla along with the Baseline Diet for 1 week, she e-mailed that she felt "MUCH better—more in power of myself!" and that her "water weight also seems to be going away!!" After her emotions were moderated with the homeopathic remedy, Marcia was free to enjoy new slimming foods and a happier lifestyle.

Three Homeopathic Remedies

Let's take a look at homeopathic remedies right now. It's just possible that one will provide the breakthrough you need to get your food cravings and additions under control and make weight loss happen for you.

Recognized around the world for their effectiveness, safety, and wide availability, homeopathic remedies treat physical and emotional problems in a simple, straightforward way. They affect our energy and well-being by giving the body a subtle suggestion. Made by diluting many times a tiny trace of a substance such as a flower, mineral, or animal product in a medium such as milk or alcohol, the remedies are given in standardized doses that provoke a healing reaction. Sometimes a homeopathic remedy is made from an irritant such as poison ivy so that the body's immune response to the irritant provokes the desired reaction. The remedy is chosen according to symptoms and treats many health issues simultaneously.

A number such as 6X following the name of the remedy refers to the number of times the remedy has been diluted—the strength or potency. The higher the number, the more times the remedy has been diluted. A higher dilution enters the body more easily and works faster than a lower number. A 6X strength works like a food. It is fine for most physical problems, such as gnawing hunger. A 30C strength is recommended for an acute treatment such as a sudden, violent headache, anxiety, or hysteria.

How and when you take a homeopathic remedy is important. Here are the basics.

PAY ATTENTION TO STRENGTH. For our purposes, 6X up to no more than 30C works best. Use higher strengths only under the advice and supervision of a health care professional.

ALLOW IT TO ENTER QUICKLY. Melting the tiny white pills

under your tongue or dissolving three of them in a 4-ounce glass of water as a beverage allows them to enter the bloodstream immediately. For convenience, you can add five pills to a glass of water and sip throughout the day between meals, so the remedy has a chance to work as needed.

LET IT DO ITS JOB. Never combine a homeopathic remedy with food, beverages (other than water), toothpaste, or anything else, because the remedy enters your blood from under your tongue. Wait 2 hours after taking a remedy to eat a meal, and wait 30 minutes after eating or drinking coffee (either regular or decaf cancels homeopathic remedies) to take a remedy.

REPEAT AS NEEDED. After its work is done, no trace of the remedy remains in the body. For that reason, you may need to use the remedy more than once daily until you achieve its desired effects. Usually one or two doses in total will be enough.

KNOW WHEN TO STOP. When the remedy has improved your symptoms, *stop using it.* Overuse of a homeopathic remedy may sooner or later cause symptoms. Homeopathic Gelsemium, Pulsatilla, and Nux vomica are three remedies that I think apply to dieting.

DON'T COMBINE REMEDIES. Choose just one remedy and use it one to three times daily for 1 week to find if it makes a difference in your energy, mood, and cravings. If you decide to use a different remedy, wait a day or so before switching. You can cancel the remedy at any time with a sip or two of coffee.

You will very likely feel your energy improve within in a day or two. You may stop craving fattening foods because your nervous or emotional dependence will be reduced. At least, you will feel stronger and more confident about making improvements.

Which homeopathic remedy is best for you?

Do you overeat or eat fattening foods when you:

___Feel tired, weak, anxious, or worried? **Gelsemium**

___ Feel sad or depressed or have weepy PMS? **Pulsatilla**

___Celebrate, overwork, or blow off steam? **Nux vomica**

HOMEOPATHIC GELSEMIUM 6X, made from yellow jasmine, is recommended for anxiety. It also works great for chronic weakness with low spirits. You know how worry weakens: You have to deal with a tough situation or a difficult person, but it is easier to clean house or watch television.

Gelsemium is a good antiprocrastination remedy. It settles nervous jitters and shortness of breath that arise from anxiety. If you overeat to avoid conflict or cope with daily stress, Gelsemium may work for you. It settles a nervous stomach. Actors and singers have used it successfully for stage fright.

Are you tense about being in public or taking an exam? Does eating a meal, a slice of pie, or a loaf of bread make you feel like you are withdrawing to a comfortable hiding place? Do you feel shaky inside? Does your tongue shake or quiver? Do you sometimes have insomnia or nightmares?

Homeopathic Gelsemium helps you to feel calmer and stronger without food. Many of the people who filled out the questionnaire for our weight loss observation said they ate fattening foods when bored. They may have snacked to settle their nerves. One woman e-mailed her reply to my questionnaire: "I started taking Gelsemium, and *I am much more focused!!!* I'm still craving sugar (not nearly as much) but then again, I've only been taking it for a few days. It also seems to give me energy, too."

HOMEOPATHIC PULSATILLA 6X, made from the flower of that name, is an excellent remedy for people who seek comfort and consolation. I recommend it for timid, overweight children or adults who often whine or complain; women with weepy PMS; and people who eat when sad. Often the Pulsatilla patient craves creamy, rich, or doughy foods as a solace. This leads to abdominal bloating, stomachaches, and sometimes hypoglycemia and candida yeast problems.

Homeopathic Pulsatilla feels like a soothing "tummy rub" and a relaxing moment when you can take a deep breath and let your cares float away. Pulsatilla is drying and therefore recommended for people who have asthma with thick, bland phlegm; a heavy feeling in the chest, with shortness of breath; and/or a sensation of being shut in a confined space. I would use it also for chronic depression that some-times accompanies phlegmy conditions like wheezing. The person who might benefit from Pulsatilla may have an oversize pale, coated tongue, which indicates poor digestion and water retention in the digestive tract.

HOMEOPATHIC NUX VOMICA 6X, made from a bitter nut, is the best remedy for hangover, overeating and overdrinking, overwork, and related crabbiness. It brings the body back into balance with a cleansing action, working equally well for people who drink or eat alone when angry or upset and those who paint the town red with friends. It helps clear the foggy, out-of-focus feeling that accompanies headaches and stuffed sinuses. Keep it in the medicine cabinet for use after feasts and celebrations or for beginning a natural cleansing rou-tine such as a fast. Usually, one or two doses can uncross your eyes after drinking. (However, let someone else drive home.) We will address common addictions and the use of Nux vomica in Chapter 8.

Food Karma

You might believe that your environment, heredity, education, fam-ily, or work experiences have made you what you are. But the tiger in you awaits new possibilities. You are what you do, think, and say. Experience makes you unique, and a big part of your experience is your diet.

Karma is usually defined as the relationship of cause and effect, like the old saying "You can't get away with anything." Whatever you do will have a reaction—achieve an effect. That effect then causes something else to occur. Food karma is cause and effect applied to dieting. The results of any diet are nearly immediate. For example, overloading digestion affects more than your waistline; mental clarity and a sense of well-being also suffer.

The other extreme is also damaging. One friend of mine tried to eliminate years of fat by fasting on wheatgrass juice. She felt fine for a day or two, then the impurities flushed from her body lodged in her weakest area. She (a Dragon) developed symptoms of an inflammatory urinary and vaginal yeast infection. Her body was simply not strong enough to eliminate all the toxins.

To avoid exhaustion, most people need to combine strongly cleansing foods and herbs with supportive ones such as reishi mushroom extract. Unsalted barley and parsley soup, another cleansing food, reduces mucus and water retention without weakening effects.

There is more to dieting than losing weight. Once a troubled student asked a Tibetan doctor for help to improve his karma. The young man explained, "Feeling sad, I ate a cake." The doctor replied, "Try using kindness. When you are sad, imagine that you are the cake." Beyond being kind to cakes, be kind to yourself. If you eat the Baseline Diet consisting of small meals and healthy snacks, add the juices and herbal teas recommended for your type, and practice the simple qigong movements that I describe in this book, you will certainly lose weight while increasing vitality.

To start even more simply: Increase your fruits and vegetables because they contain valuable vitamins, minerals, and water. They are not fattening. Be content to start slowly and lose weight gradually. Soon you will begin to feel wonderful. That is the easy part. However, to improve your lifestyle, you need to change your cravings, which always entails more than your diet.

At best, we consume food as an intimate, life-sustaining relationship, the same way we incorporate close friends and lovers into our lives. Our relationship to food deserves as much attention as those relationships that form our personalites, work habits, and marriages. Foods can cure or kill us.

Seeking Solace (Inappropriately) from Food

Julia, in her late forties, gained 50 pounds during the year following her divorce. She informed me that she binged when bored and lonely, and, during weepy and angry PMS, and she had frequent nervous headaches. After her husband left her, she took antidepressants and gained weight from the medicines. She consulted a nutritionist and psychotherapist, but she could neither nourish herself without bingeing on sweets nor consider the possibility of a new love relationship. Her vitality and self-image were stuck in reverse.

The trauma of her marriage breakup was like a toxin inside that made her sick. To cleanse her body and mind of the emotional trauma and the drugs she had taken, I recommended homeopathic Nux vomica 30C, a potent detoxifying remedy. After taking it for less than a week, she said her mental clarity, concentration, and overall energy improved. She felt she could start fresh. Sometimes, overcoming a destructive life pattern requires only a step in the right direction, using a simple cleansing and rejuvenating remedy.

Many of the women who participated in my clinical observation reported that they binged on bread, chocolate, and sweets during PMS. They had had weight problems and a poor self-image since childhood. In a sense, they turned to food for comfort in an attempt to overcome boredom, pain, and female discomforts. Seeking comfort became their basic relationship to food and, therefore, much of their time and activity. On a broader level, it is a pity to substitute food for love, considering what excess food turns into and how love has the ability to transform our lives.

The High Cost of Excess

Tough guys and sportsmen have nervous habits, too. An article in the April 2005 *Wall Street Journal* reported that General Motors health care spending during 2004 amounted to $1,525 for every vehicle GM produced in the United States. GM employees, most of them men, smoke on the job. During breaks, many head to a nearby tavern and drink liquor with a beer chaser and discuss hunting. GM has initiated employee programs to discourage unhealthy habits, adding gyms to some plants, helping workers prepare for hunting season, and warning those with heart trouble not to try dragging a dead deer back to the pickup. According to GM LifeSteps program consultant Charlie Estey, "These guys go out, sleep late, drink beer, climb into a tree stand, then see a deer and get heart palpitations."

Current employees and their families account for about 31 percent of the total GM health bill. Retirees make up the remainder. The company is hoping to make a dent in the hundreds of millions of dollars a year it spends on drugs to combat the ill effects of smoking, obesity, and stress. GM says 26 percent of its 1.1 million beneficiaries are considered obese under federal guidelines—slightly below the national average—and cost the company between $1,000 and $3,000 more, on average, in health services than beneficiaries who aren't obese. In other words, obesity costs GM at least $286 million a year.

Robert Moroni, who runs GM's health plans, says drugs for cholesterol, high blood pressure, and diabetes are among the highest-costing items for the carmaker. Another health expense for GM and other large companies is cancer treatments for people who develop the disease from secondhand smoke. The bottom line: GM is laying off workers because it cannot afford its health bill. Our health habits affect medical costs, basic comforts, and social services for everyone.

An older couple once sat across from me in an airport. The man pulled out a pack of cigarettes, smiled, and said, "Guess I'll smoke a cancer stick." He looked shocked when I jumped up and crossed the room to get out of the way. His wife sadly grimaced.

It's Time to Pay Attention

My intellectual friends can be especially insensitive to how they nourish themselves. It is as though they lack body awareness. Ruth, a dedicated teacher and author friend, told me that her students first noticed she was overweight. "What happened to you?" they asked. "Your body has blown up too big."

Ruth realized something was wrong because she cried often and had writer's block. She may have become weak from "digesting" her next book. I recommended homeopathic Pulsatilla. After a week, she told me, "That Pulsatilla is really working! My puffiness is gone. I can fit into my clothes again. I feel wonderful and look gorgeous!" It is remarkable that a remedy recommended for sadness and a sense of heaviness can so strongly affect shape. Although the remedy can be used by either sex, I have heard of cases where Pulsatilla has improved hormone irregularities and corrected infertility by normalizing menstruation. Our water balance affects so many aspects of life.

Here's another example: Lorna lived among scattered papers and books, mounds of old clothes, and work in progress; you could not move anywhere in her small New York apartment. She stashed foods in the refrigerator for weeks and ate them after they had spoiled. She was not overweight. She exercised regularly and took many vitamins, but her cellulite was noticeable. She looked pale, weak, and puffy as a marshmallow.

Her story began with a mother who failed to nourish her. Consequently, Lorna could neither nourish nor comfort herself. She felt overwhelmed by her surroundings. I wondered if a few cleansing foods and herbs might have a positive effect. She might even rethink her personal relationships, which were backed up in forgotten corners. She had the most success reducing her doldrums and cellulite by following the antiyeast diet routine found on page 273.

There are more powerful actions in herbs than nourishment. They are catalysts that promote vital changes. Sometimes, I have to caution my students about using cleansing herbs, especially antiparasite or anticancer herbs. Clarifying, mucus-reducing herbs tend to stimulate our vitality and psyche, which may have repercussions upon relationships when we become motivated to clean up every aspect of our lives. I caution my clients to use a comfortable dose when trying new foods and herbs. The rewards of using natural remedies are often remarkable, not only because they promote well-being but also because they encourage us to assume responsibility for body and mind.

One e-mail I received from a woman I never met but who answered my questionnaire is typical of the transformational benefits gained from using targeted foods and natural remedies. She wrote: "You are *sooo* right!! The basic diet and homeopathic remedy you suggested are working so well, I feel so empowered by it all. I have dropped 5 pounds already, am so much less bloated, feel my blood sugar getting more in balance, have stopped overeating—*wow*—it is like magic!" The magic comes from feeling your body express its natural vitality.

The Liberation of Eating Wisely

Eating well can actually help reduce stress because there is safety in a slimming diet. Several firefighters in Texas will stand up and cheer to that. Firefighters are known for chomping steaks, fries, and pizza when not chasing fires. Not so at Austin Fire Station No. 2 on West Martin Luther King Jr. Boulevard, where five firefighters—Rip Esselstyn, James Rae, Matt Moore, Derick Zwerneman, and Scott Walters—now eat vegan meals (vegetarian, omitting all animal products).

They take turns whipping up plant-based meatless and cheese-less pizza, pasta primavera, and spinach enchiladas. This change in cuisine was prompted when several firefighters bloated with meat diets tested their cholesterol levels and found that they bounced off the wall.

According to the American Heart Association, a cholesterol reading of 200 or over signals that a man is at high risk of a heart attack. Firefighter Rae, age 36, found out his was 335, an especially dangerous level for a man who has had only one male relative live beyond his fifties because of heart attacks. Rae is married with two children. His cholesterol reading prompted a diet revolution in Station No. 2.

Firefighter Esselstyn's father, Caldwell B. Esselstyn Jr., MD, had been a general surgeon at the Cleveland Clinic and still conducts diet research there. Dr. Esselstyn's 12-year trial with patients with terminal heart disease showed that a very low-fat, plant-based (vegan) diet with cholesterol-lowering medicine could bring striking improvement. Heart disease "never need exist," Dr. Esselstyn said, but if it does, "it never need progress."

To reach the boys at Station No. 2, you can call up their Web site at www.engine2.org and find their photos and recipes. Posing with fruits and vegetables, they look like they are having a wonderful time.

Chapter 2

The Baseline Diet

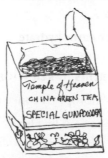

Anyone can slenderize with our low-fat, high-fiber, Asian-inspired diet. This chapter explains food choices, which foods to emphasize, and when to consume them. Recipes pay special attention to deep cleansing foods for dramatic weight loss. Many more recipes are included later in the book.

The Baseline Diet can be used for rapid weight loss and for cleansing and slimming after holiday celebrations. It can also be used long term for optimal health. There's no limit to how long you can stay on this diet. It's your choice. This chapter ends with special cleansing and fasting principles that jump-start weight loss in case you get stuck along the way.

You don't really need to know what your energy type is in order to benefit from the Baseline Diet. That's because this diet works for everyone.

In the next chapter, you'll find out just what your energy type is. And in Part 2, you'll learn about a number of diet tips that apply to your energy type. You can add those to the Baseline Diet, as well as use them with your regular diet. As you can see, there's a lot of flexibility here.

Baseline Diet Overview

Here's what the Baseline Diet looks like.

Daily

2 fruits

6 to 9 vegetables

1 protein source

1 serving of a complex carbohydrate

Weight Loss Supplements Taken with Meals

3 alfalfa tablets or 2 chlorophyll concentrate capsules

1 to 3 tablets of Laminaria 4 by Health Concerns or another source of mixed minerals, including iodine for proper thyroid function (such as a handful of dried dulse or toasted green kelp seaweed)

Quiet Digestion pills or other digestive remedy, as needed, for smooth digestion and absorption (for example, a cup of ginger, mint, and lemongrass green tea)

Between Meals

Slimming beverages and energy-boosting snacks

That's the big picture. We'll go into some detail about each of these items, but you can refer to this overview for quick reference.

If, while on the Baseline Diet, you feel deprived of pleasure foods, eat as many fruits as you wish during the morning and three times as many vegetables during the afternoon and evening.

Fruits, especially when they are acidic, dislodge fat and impurities. Vegetables, because they are alkaline, eliminate toxins and water retention. Make noon your changeover time from acidic to alkaline foods. Otherwise, to avoid bloating and indigestion, have fruits first, wait for 2 hours, then consume other foods. People who feel temporarily weak or spacey from diet changes can enhance digestive *qi* with fresh ginger added to hot green tea, which is laxative.

Please do not drive yourself crazy with the Baseline Diet. There is no need to count berries on your plate, calculate calories, or measure portions with a scale. The proportions of fruits, vegetables, grains, and proteins are the important aspect of the diet. Fiber foods satisfy without adding weight. They cleanse the body and tone digestion while providing valuable nutrients. Once you understand that, you can apply the Baseline Diet recommendations to your own menus.

Because weight loss diets can result in cramps, diarrhea, and mood swings, I advise adding new foods in small portions one at a time. The Baseline Diet is alkalinizing—therefore, cleansing. It avoids the usual side effects associated with high-protein diets, including nervousness, insomnia, bad breath, acne, constipation, headaches, and unpleasant body odors. In addition, our recommended cleansing and balancing remedies reverse withdrawal symptoms.

Some people feel that the Baseline Diet is a big change from their usual habit of mixing every kind of food together during meals. But the Baseline Diet merely separates food groups and limits portions to ease digestion and increase elimination. You can do that with any type of diet. Here are some examples of what that looks like in practice.

In Homestead, south of Miami, I love Mexican and Cuban restaurants like Mario's. A delicious chicken fricassee is served there with rice, beans, and potatoes. To remain slim, I have the chicken, avoid two of the starches, and add a salad. I often take home half the meal. Smaller portions are enough when the cooking is good and you are used to eating less. I never have dessert after a meal. It slows digestion. Think of dessert as a separate meal to be enjoyed at leisure with tea during midafternoon. (This book has recipes for slimming sugarless pies you can whip up for breakfast or a snack at home.)

In Georgia and the Carolinas, I love southern vegetables made without pork, a salad, and tea as a slimming meal. Think of starchy white potatoes, white rice, and regular pasta as poor-quality nutrition because they are sticky. When you consume them, your pancreas releases insulin to excess and eventually wears out.

A WORD ABOUT PROTEINS AND STARCHES

The Baseline Diet calls for limited consumption of proteins and starches. Since you may require more than one serving of protein daily, choose just one *source* of protein daily until your body adjusts. For example, you might consume only eggs for your protein source one day, only seafood the next, only dairy the third day, and so on. That way, you can gradually reduce your overall protein and fat intake for weight loss. Mixing animal proteins causes indigestion and overweight, because it taxes digestion and energy.

Here are some of the best choices.

Protein: tofu; tempeh; low-mercury-content fish, such as salmon, tuna, or Japanese eel; organic chicken or duck eggs; dry, breakable cheese; nuts and seeds; and seaweeds. When it comes to dairy products, I recommend goat and sheep products over those from cows. Dairy products from cows seem to be more irritating and more likely to cause inflammation and trigger allergies and autoimmune illnesses.

Starch: whole grain bread, legumes, sweet potatoes, potatoes (not fried), parsnips, and whole wheat or multigrain pasta. Shirataki noodles (made from a no-calorie Japanese yam), bean thread noodles, and other slimming noodles can help reduce both fat and cholesterol.

Baseline Basics

The Baseline Diet is organized to suit your busy schedule and features cleansing and rejuvenating meals, slimming snacks, and energy-packed beverages. It is also organized to avoid digestive troubles. Cleansing teas and acidic fruits are stressed during the morning, while alkaline, energy-enhancing vegetables and beverages are stressed during the afternoon and evening. There are a number of herbal supplements and remedies that you can add to the diet to address food addictions. I'll be discussing those throughout the book.

Essential mineral supplements may accompany select foods to assure maximum absorption. For example, I recommend that calcium, magnesium, and joint- and bone-supporting supplements such as vitamin D_3, goat whey capsules, SAMe, and, when necessary, anti-edema herbs be taken along with the morning fruit and tea to reduce digestive bloating and joint discomforts. Each meal includes herbs essential for weight loss and internal cleansing, such as alfalfa tablets and seaweed kelp. I'll tell you about those further on.

This diet is slimming because it is energizing, relieves indigestion, and maximizes absorption of quality nutrients. In this way, it supports endurance and mental acuity. You can also incorporate Asian superfoods, such as Reishi+ mushroom extract, that stimulate metabolism, energy, and willpower. We'll learn more about those as well.

Now let's take a closer look at some of the foods and supplements you should be emphasizing in the Baseline Diet.

Think Greens

Fresh, leafy green foods and concentrated green foods supplements make the body more alkaline and, therefore, begin the cleansing, healing, and slimming process. I recommend some with each meal.

ALFALFA is full of chlorophyll that encourages the bacteria necessary for digestion. It eliminates gas and sluggish bowel action. Alfalfa is an inexpensive, nearly perfect cleansing, nourishing, high-fiber food. Crack three pills in your mouth and swallow them with water during meals, and add alfalfa sprouts to salads and raw juices.

GREEN FOODS SUPPLEMENT, another useful option at mealtime, is a vitamin and mineral supplement made with green foods, such as Green Source from Puritan's Pride. Each pill provides a large array of absorbable nutrients that cleanse the body and support health.

SEAWEEDS are an excellent source of trace minerals in the daily diet if their ocean source is free of pollutants. The minerals in seaweeds help maintain an alkaline environment in the bloodstream. An alkaline environment is a healthy one, resistant to fatigue and stress.

You can eat it as is, use it in cooking, ot toast seaweed in a 200°F oven until it is crisp and crunchy. This makes a tasty snack that you and the kids can enjoy anytime. See the Natural Products Information and Resource Guide on page 348 for sources.

Among the particular kinds of seaweed that you might come across:

- Kelp (*Laminaria longicruris*) contains iodine 127, which improves metabolism and protects the body against radiation.
- Alaria (*Alaria esculenta*) is a good source of calcium. It is similar to wakame, the standard sea vegetable for miso soup.
- Dulse is a stimulating, salty-tasting snack that detoxifies the body and tones metabolism. It is a good source of vegetable protein, iron, potassium, magnesium, iodine, chlorophyll, enzymes, vitamin A, B vitamins, and dietary fiber.
- Hijiki is rich in calcium. Lightly simmered with tamari, grated carrot, and scallions, it makes a nourishing salad.
- Nori offers a combination of minerals and is one-third protein. Kids love to crunch it.
- Laminaria, or kombu, is a fluffy, light-green Japanese dried seaweed that can be cooked as a side dish along with rice and fish. Simmer a handful of the thoroughly rinsed seaweed in 1 cup of water for about ½ hour.

You might prefer to get your seaweed in supplement form, which is easy to do. Many supplement companies make seaweed pills and powders.

For further information about the nutritional benefits of seaweed, as well as additional recipes, visit www.alcasoft.com/seaweed or www.seaveg.com.

LAMINARIA 4 PILLS made by Health Concerns combine laminaria and sargassum seaweeds and two powdered seashells to provide a source of calcium, potassium, and iodine. The ingredients tone thyroid action for sluggish digestion, water retention, and low vitality. Hypothyroid problems often lead to poor eating habits and chronic depression. Your thyroid may be sluggish if you feel heavy and water-logged, your digestion is slow, and you tend to sleep a lot. Laminaria 4 reduces cellulite and mucus congestion throughout the body. The recommended dose is usually three pills with meals, but start with a dose that is comfortable, and slowly increase it to the recommended amount. Overstimulating the thyroid may lead to nervous insomnia.

Leafy Greens and Colon Cancer

Numerous studies link the vitamin folate with reducing the risk for colon cancer—and that is just one of many reasons to make sure you get your greens. Greens help make any meal light and cleansing. Folate is found in high amounts in dark, leafy green vegetables; orange juice; and fortified grains and cereals. Of course, it's also found in folic acid supplements. If for some reason you're not eating greens or taking a greens supplement every day, you need to make sure you're getting enough folate.

A Harvard study of more than 80,000 female nurses found that for the greatest protection against colon cancer (and possibly heart disease), you need to supplement folate intake with a multivitamin.

Fruits and Vegetables

Fruits and vegetables are at the heart of the Baseline Diet, and for good reason. Besides being ideal weight loss foods, fruits and vegetables are rich in essential vitamins, minerals, fiber, carbohydrates, and phytochemicals that lower your risk of developing certain cancers, stroke, heart disease, and high blood pressure.

A Harvard Study of nearly 80,000 women and 40,000 men found that people who ate five servings of fruits and vegetables every day had a 30 percent lower risk of one kind of stroke (ischemic). Cruciferous vegetables like broccoli; green, leafy vegetables like spinach; and citrus fruits and juices seemed to provide the greatest benefit. Ischemic stroke is by far the most common type of stroke and, like coronary heart disease, is caused by the blockage of blood vessels.

That in itself should be reason enough to eat more fruits and vegetables, but there's more: Despite Japan's large number of smokers, the incidence of lung cancer there is very low. Experts attribute this to fresh fish, fruits, and vegetables in the typical Japanese diet. Professor J. Gordon McVie, MD, director general of England's Cancer Research Campaign, told BBCnews.com that adenocarcinoma lung cancer—about 5 percent of all cancer cases in Japan—is the one most affected by diet.

Clinical nutritionist Jim Ehmke, PhD, founder of Complete Health Services in Milwaukee, said in the same report that during the 1940s and '50s, when per capita consumption of tobacco peaked in the United States, the incidence of lung cancer was less than half of what it is currently. Despite a significant decrease in smoking, lung cancer has increased substantially and is now America's number one cancer.

Dr. Charles E. Butterworth Jr. at the University of Alabama discovered over a decade ago that two-pack-a-day smokers who consumed 10 milligrams of folic acid (10,000 micrograms) daily for 60 days had complete healing of lung lesions, even while they continued to smoke. Folic acid, a B vitamin derived from fresh fruits and vegetables, has a remarkable healing effect on lung tissue.

The Japanese diet is 10 to 20 times higher in folic acid than the American diet. By comparison, American per capita consumption of

---

GET RID OF PESTICIDE RESIDUE

Unfortunately, most produce, especially that originating from other countries, is sprayed with harmful pesticides. For that reason, use the following rinse on every piece of fresh fruit or vegetable before eating it raw or cooking it.

1   quart or more of water
1   drop of nontoxic dish or glycerine soap
1   tablespoon apple cider vinegar

Mix all ingredients together. Gently rub the mixture onto the produce with your hands, then flush it off with lots of water.

---

fresh fruits and vegetables, our best sources of folic acid, has decreased 400 percent from 1945 to 2000. Americans eat four times less fresh fruits and vegetables per capita than they did 55 years ago. According to Dr. Ehmke, this decrease directly parallels the rise in lung cancer.

Research has uncovered links between specific fruits, vegetables, and disease prevention. Throughout this book, I cover foods that treat specific weight loss issues for our energy types, but the following foods are important for everyone to keep in mind. (Also see Stock These Healthy Foods on page 343.)

Cooked Tomatoes and Cancer

A Harvard study of more than 40,000 health professionals found that men who ate the most cooked tomato-based foods (cooked tomatoes, tomato sauce, and dishes made with red sauce) had a 35 percent lower risk of developing prostate cancer than those who ate the least amount of these foods. Tomatoes are rich in the carotenoid lycopene. Carotenoids are the pigments that color dark green and orange vegetables. Many are precursors to vitamin A and act as powerful antioxidants that protect cells from damage by free radicals, which leads to many health problems, including cancer, heart disease, and cataracts. Antioxidants protect us against such diseases. Try to have some cooked tomato with each meat protein meal. Its acid improves digestion. If you have diabetes, you can lower your blood sugar with stewed tomato sweetened with stevia powder.

FRUITS AND VEGETABLES: THE BOTTOM LINE

Try to increase the fresh fruits and vegetables you eat daily. Many nutrition experts recommend at least nine servings a day, and that lines up perfectly with the Baseline Diet.

Choose a wide variety, being sure to include dark green, leafy vegetables; yellow, orange, and red fruits and vegetables; cooked tomatoes; and very ripe citrus fruits.

Nuts, Seeds, and Sprouts

Most people find it difficult to change eating habits all at once. You
might starve yourself to lose weight, but pounds always creep back
after an extreme diet ends. Instead, be moderate: Try adding nuts,
seeds, and sprouts to your salads.

NUTS AND SEEDS provide protein. Oil and lecithin from raw
nuts are foods for the brain, nerves, and glands. Among nuts, the
most nourishing are hard-shelled almonds, walnuts, cashews, and
coconuts. Sunflower seeds put on weight, but sesame seeds, a great
source of protein, do not add pounds. Sunflower sprouts are nourishing and less fattening.

SPROUTS are an excellent source of vitamins, minerals, and
enzymes. They make a nice addition to salads and sandwiches and
can be whipped into juices.

   To make sprouts at home, soak a handful of raw organic sunflower seeds, adzuki beans, lentils, or other seeds overnight in a glass
jar of water. The next morning, pour off the water and cover the top
of the jar with cheesecloth fastened with a rubber band. Place the jar
on its side in a dark cupboard or cold oven. Four or five times daily,
rinse the seeds with fresh water and put the jar back in the cupboard.
Sprouts grow in 2 to 3 days, depending on moisture and heat. Sprouts

that are longer than half an inch taste bitter. In Chapter 7, you will learn to make a delicious sprout bread from whole grains.

OILS best used for salads are walnut, grapeseed, canola, and extra-virgin olive. For protein, add walnuts or grated raw coconut meat to your salads. For added fiber, grate raw beets on salads. In fact, the oils and fats you use on a regular basis are tremendously important, not only for keeping off the pounds, but also for your health in general. Let's take a look at those next.

Good Fat, Bad Fat

Some fats are great for health and beauty. They reduce harmful cholesterol; feed muscles and the brain; and nourish the skin, hair, and internal organs. Other fats clog the body with waste and increase uric acid, which leads to skin rashes, inflammation, body odors, and irritability. It's also important to know how fats and oils affect your cholesterol.

Cholesterol comes in two kinds: LDL and HDL. Low-density lipoproteins (LDL) carry cholesterol from the liver to the rest of the body. When there is too much LDL cholesterol in the blood, it can be deposited on the walls of the coronary arteries. Because of this, LDL cholesterol is often referred to as the "bad" cholesterol.

High-density lipoproteins (HDL), on the other hand, carry cholesterol from the blood back to the liver, which processes the cholesterol for elimination from the body. HDL makes it less likely that excess cholesterol in the blood will be deposited in the coronary arteries, which is why HDL cholesterol is often referred to as the "good" cholesterol.

Here's how to keep your cholesterol levels under control while following the Baseline Diet or any other diet.

CHOOSE MONOSATURATED OR POLYUNSATURATED OILS. These lower harmful LDL cholesterol. Monounsaturated fats include raw grapeseed, walnut, olive, canola, and peanut oils. They are found in olives; cashews, almonds, peanuts, and most other nuts; and avocados. Polyunsaturated fats include soybean, safflower, and cottonseed oils. Fatty fish also contains healthy fat and should be eaten three times a week.

REDUCE SATURATED FAT. This kind of fat raises both LDL and HDL. Saturated fat is found in whole dairy products, including milk, butter, cheese, and ice cream; red meat; chocolate; and coconut meat, milk, and oil.

ELIMINATE TRANS FATS. These are just bad news all the way around. They raise LDL. Trans fats are founds in most margarines, vegetable shortening, partially hydrogenated vegetable oil, deep-fried foods, many fast foods, and most commercial baked goods.

READ LABELS. Be sure to choose monounsaturated or polyunsaturated fats.

DO NOT HEAT OILS. Heating to the point where cooking oils smoke makes them carcinogenic. Instead, steam fish or vegetables in a small amount of water in a covered pot. If you like, pour on some healthy oil when steamed vegetables are slightly cooled. When possible, recycle the vegetable cooking liquid.

STORE OILS CAREFULLY. Refrigerate oils, especially those made from seeds, such as canola oil. Discard any oil that develops a strong odor.

High Fiber, Low Fats, and Animal Proteins

A great deal of research has been done by major universities, including Harvard Department of Public Health, Cornell Medical School, and Oxford University, concerning the many benefits of a low-protein diet. In addition to better weight control, a low-protein diet (no more than one protein meal per day) leads to:

- Slower aging
- Lower fat and cholesterol intake (lower LDL and total cholesterol levels)
- Decreased liver and kidney stress
- A stronger immune system response
- Decreased loss of body minerals, particularly calcium, through excretion
- Decreased hunger
- Lower risk of heart disease and cancer

In a 2004 *New York Times* article entitled "Sane Weight Loss in a Carb-Obsessed World: High Fiber and Low Fat," Jane Brody describes how her friend lost 72 pounds by working out at the gym for 1 hour a day and changing to a heart-healthy diet of whole grains, low-fat cottage cheese, fruit, soup, fish, salad, and regular dinners. In that same article, Brody reports on a 12-week study of 34 men and women in their sixties done at the University of Arkansas at Little Rock. The study found those who consumed a diet high in fiber-rich carbohydrates, low in fat, and moderate in protein lost more weight and a higher percentage of body fat than did those who ate a typical high-fat, low-carb American diet. Whole grains and high-fiber foods are slimming because some of their calories are eliminated unabsorbed. (Japanese cooks take full advantage of this fact with high-fiber konnyaku noodles, also known as shirataki noodles. Internet sources for ordering shirataki and several recipes are included later in this book.)

If you are going to eat animal protein at all, limit it to one source daily or one serving for lunch or dinner (preferably dinner). If it is an egg day, avoid beef, chicken, and cheese. Fish with eggs or fish with dairy are bad combinations. A famous Tibetan physician, Dr. Yeshi Donden, has called them *fatal* combinations.

Take a tip from my Hungarian grandmother, who had beautiful skin at age 90: If you love milk, don't drink it—splash some on your face. It is less troubling to digestion. Think of animal flesh and cow dairy products as being heavy, oily, rich, and fattening. Therefore, combine animal protein with its opposites—pungent digestive foods, stimulating spices, and slimming teas. Bernard Jensen, PhD, recommends eating a cooked or very ripe tomato or grapefruit wedges along with your evening protein meal because they are acidic.

You will lose weight if you increase your fiber. It washes fat out of the body and prevents disease. The following high-fiber vegetables are only 5 percent carbohydrate: artichokes, asparagus, beet greens, broccoli, Brussels sprouts, cabbage, cauliflower, celery, chard, chicory, cucumber, dandelion, eggplant, endive, escarole, leeks, lettuce, mushrooms, mustard greens, okra, radish, rhubarb, sauerkraut (fresh, not canned), sea kale, sorrel, spinach, sprouts, string beans, Swiss chard, tomatoes, turnip greens, and watercress.

Did you notice how many of these taste somewhat bitter? Bitter foods are cleansing. Eat them daily, both raw and cooked. One easy way to immediately increase fiber foods is to grate 1 tablespoon of raw beet into your salads.

Mushroom Magic

It's also a good idea to learn to love mushrooms and add them to your diet on a regular basis. Asian shiitake, enoki, and oyster mushrooms are nature's wonder medicines, available in your supermarket. They grow on or near trees. (Avoid white button mushrooms because they are grown in the dark, which attracts pests, so they are routinely treated with pesticides. See the recipe note on page 45.)

Always cook mushrooms. Never eat them raw. Rinse them with water and squeeze out excess moisture before cooking.

Here's one simple way to enjoy an important health remedy.

Tiger Mushroom Wine

This wine will amaze your friends. Alcohol is not slimming. However, if you already enjoy the grape as a heart protector, an Asian mushroom extract adds a tart, earthy flavor to any full-bodied red wine. Reishi (*Ganoderma lucidum*; in Chinese, *ling zhi*), a medicinal fungus known to Chinese people as the immortality mushroom, protects the heart and lowers harmful cholesterol. Reishi also protects against cancer and aging and eases inflammatory pain in arthritis. Used daily, reishi builds vitality and eventually diminishes a sweet tooth. Add 20 drops of Reishi+ liquid extract to a glass of red wine.

The mushroom extract, available from www.eastearthtrade.com, can be taken in 40 to 60 drops daily by mouth or in soup stocks. However, this wine is convenient and fun to make.

Baseline Diet Summary

This section may clear up many of your questions. You may want to make a copy of the box on pages 38 and 39 and post it in the kitchen as a reminder. (It repeats the Baseline Diet as outlined at the beginning

(continued on page 40)

THE BASELINE DIET

Daily Foods

2 fruits, 6 to 9 vegetables, 1 protein source, and 1 complex carbohydrate serving

Supplements taken with meals:

- 3 alfalfa tablets or 2 chlorophyll concentrate capsules
- 1 to 3 tablets Laminara 4 or a handful of diced seaweed for enhanced thyroid function
- Quiet Digestion pills or other digestive remedy for smooth digestion and absorption

Between Meals: Slimming beverages and energy-boosting snacks

The following are suggestions for the kinds of foods you might choose for each meal.

Note: In the examples below, proteins and starch suggestions are included for breakfast, lunch, and dinner. Please remember that you're having only one source of protein and one serving of starch daily. So, if you elect to have a complex carbohydrate such as bread or cereal for breakfast or lunch, you'll need to select other options for dinner.

There may be foods or supplements that you're not yet familiar with among these examples. They will be covered elsewhere in the book. You can look them up on my Web site www.asianhealthsecrets.com.

Morning and Breakfast

- 1 to 2 (8-ounce) glasses half fruit juice, half water (for cancer prevention or for prostate, urinary, blood pressure, or hormonal problems, see the Broccoli Water recipe on page 190)
- 1 to 3 cups Yin/Yang Sisters Get Svelte instant beverage or tea
- 1 to 2 cups of maté tea or 10 to 20 drops of maté liquid extract for energy
- 2 to 3 servings fresh fruit along with calcium, magnesium, and vitamin D$_3$ supplements

From ½ to 1 hour later, one or two of the following:

- 4-ounce serving breakable goat or sheep cheese
- A whole soy food (a block of soft tofu with a dash each of light soy sauce and vinegar)
- 1 hard-cooked omega-3–enriched organic egg
- ½ cup cooked yellow cornmeal, steel-cut oatmeal, or dry breakfast cereal and fat-free milk

- 1 slice whole grain toast and sliced avocado, a few drops of walnut or canola oil and dried herbs, or sugarless jelly; or 2 ounces Essene Bread (page 198).

Afternoon and Evening

- 6 to 8 servings raw and cooked vegetables and 1 serving mixed vegetable juice
- A protein: tofu; tempeh; low-mercury-content fish such as salmon, tuna, or Japanese eel; organic chicken or duck eggs; or goat cheese
- Whole grains, whole grain bread, or legumes: Choose among home-made mushroom/barley soup (which reduces mucus congestion and edema) or sweet potato, parsnips, pumpkin, squash, one small potato, or ½ cup al dente whole wheat pasta. Shirataki (Japanese yam), bean threads, and other slimming noodles reduce fat and cholesterol.
- Sprouted seeds in salads or smoothies
- 1 cup of dried or toasted seaweed (dulse, kelp, or nori) or the supplement below
- Nuts and seeds eaten raw, toasted, or in drinks
- Oils: walnut, grapeseed, extra-virgin olive oil, canola, or a healthy butter substitute
- Snacks and low-fat, sugarless sweets and desserts (see recipes in Part 2)
- Beverages, at least 3 quarts daily: mineral water; seltzer; Shiitake/Fu Ling Tea (page 45); Garden Greens juice and other herbal beverages; natural juices; white, green, pu-erh, oolong, black, and rooibos teas; and Yin/Yang Sisters Instant beverages (Get Svelte, Gorgeous You, and Happy Garden Tea)
- 1 to 2 cups of maté tea or 10 to 20 drops of maté liquid extract for energy

Daily Food Supplements and Seasonings

- At least ¼ to ½ cup of dried dulse seaweed or kelp seaweed sheets as a crunchy snack
- 40 to 60 drops reishi mushroom extract, alone or in a little water, for energy, immunity, and willpower necessary for slimming
- Potassium salt substitute, powdered seaweed, or Spike and herbs and spices useful for slimming: cumin, coriander, fennel seeds, tarragon, mint, dill, clove, pepper, turmeric, paprika, savory, herbes fines, Italian seasoning, garlic, and onions

of this chapter and then gives additional information about what each meal throughout the day might look like.)

Recipes and recommended servings provided throughout this book may vary, depending upon your age, lifestyle, and health condition. We will cover such individual differences later.

To keep metabolism revved, it is best to eat small portions of meals and slimming snacks every several hours during the day. One yogi recommended eating no more in one meal than can easily be held in your hands. Small portions prevent indigestion. If that thought is depressing, try spacing courses of one meal throughout the day. Have a green salad and low-calorie gelatin as one meal, a protein with salad or vegetables for another meal, a bowl of spicy popcorn along with a slice of cheese as a snack, and your dessert with tea in the afternoon instead of following a meal. You'll actually enjoy the flavors of foods more when they are not all mixed together in one meal.

In the Baseline Diet, we stress vegetables because they are alkaline and enhance the slimming, healing process. If you have a sensitive stomach, choose fruits only during the morning and vegetables during the rest of the day and evening. Also, use noncaffeine rooibos tea (African red bush tea) instead of regular tea (*Camellia sinensis*). If you are currently taking thyroid medication, adjust the dose of laminaria seaweed supplements to suit your comfort. (They contain iodine, which stimulates the thyroid.)

A Sample Daily Menu

As you get used to this way of eating—and the weight loss and better health that comes with it—you'll enjoy the flexibility and food choices allowed in this diet. Here's an example of what just 1 day might look like. You'll find many additional sample menus in each of the chapters in Part 2.

Before Breakfast (at least ½ hour before eating)
8 ounces water or half water and half fruit juice—prune,
    grape, cherry, berry, pineapple, papaya, apple,
    watermelon, green coconut, or orange—taken along with

calcium and other supplements (low-sodium tomato juice diluted by half with water, broccoli cooking water, or white or green tea if unable to eat fruit)

Breakfast
3 alfalfa tablets, chewed; acidophilus as needed
Hot white, green, oolong, or red bush tea, or Get Svelte instant beverage
1 to 2 servings fresh fruits or stewed prunes
1 slice whole grain bread, melba toast, or rye crisp with (optional) nut or seed butter, spiced pumpkin pie filling, applesauce, or cooked cranberries

One of the following:
- 1 slice of homemade sugarless pie or 2 ounces Essene Bread (page 198)
- 1 serving of cooked yellow cornmeal or steel-cut oatmeal
- 1 hard-cooked or poached egg
- 2 ounces goat or hard Cheddar cheese
- 4 ounces steamed or baked fish made without fat; dried seaweed

Note: Because vitamins and minerals taken with coffee are eliminated from the body, wait 1 hour after drinking coffee, then take mixed trace minerals or minerals.

Midmorning (10:00 a.m.) Energy Boost
8 ounces water, tea, or Get Svelte or Gorgeous You instant beverage
1 to 2 cups of maté tea or 10 to 20 drops of maté liquid extract for energy
Optional: fruit or mixed vegetable juice, nuts or seeds, 8 ounces whey protein drink using half juice and water, crunchy seaweed, or bee pollen

Before Lunch (½ hour before eating, if possible)
Acidophilus capsule
Slimming supplements
8 ounces water or Shiitake/Fu Ling Tea (page 45)

Lunch
A big salad with one of the following:
- Eggs
- Chicken or fish, including sushi or canned tuna
- Cold shirataki sesame noodles and seaweed
- Vegetable barley soup
- Tofu vegetable pie

Shiitake/Fu Ling Tea or Get Svelte instant beverage

Afternoon Snack (4:00 p.m.)
Gorgeous You instant beverage, Garden Greens juice,
Shiitake/Fu Ling Tea, or broccoli green tea
One of the following:
- Raw vegetables and dried seaweed
- Watermelon
- 1 square semisweet cooking chocolate and a rice cake
- Air-popped popcorn with olive oil, salt substitute, and pepper

During Daily Half-Hour Exercise
12 ounces water with homeopathic minerals (tissue salts) or
Shiitake/Fu Ling Tea

Dinner
Salad and cooked vegetables
1 protein (whole soy food, fish, eggs, or cheese), along with
stewed tomatoes or grapefruit wedges
Optional: homemade Digestive Bitters made with gin and
herbs (page 130) or 1 glass red wine with 20 drops of
Reishi+ mushroom extract
Shiitake/Fu Ling Tea

In Evening or Between Meals
Shou Wu Chih tonic beverage as needed, Shiitake/Fu Ling
Tea, Happy Garden Tea, or other herbal tea
Optional: homemade low-fat cookies or sugarless pie or, on
a goat dairy day, a glass of milk or serving of yogurt,
with digestive spices or goat cheese

Before Bed

Optional: 1 cup low-fat yogurt with ½ teaspoon
    turmeric powder; baked pumpkin, squash, or
    apple with a dash of nutmeg; or a very ripe orange

Happy Garden Tea or mint, chamomile, or vervain tea

For Special Problems: Optional Supplements

Some of the supplements I recommend will be new for you. The following information will help you to use them effectively. A natural products resource guide on page 348 offers contact information for products mentioned in this book.

Slow Digestion, Bloating, and Cramps

DIGESTIVE BITTERS are fun to make at home. (See the recipe on page 130.) Very bitter herbs such as gentian and dandelion release the digestive bile necessary for elimination. Gentian is a main ingredient (along with food coloring) in Angostura bitters.

QUIET DIGESTION PILLS made by Health Concerns combine herbs to reduce bloating, cramps, irregular elimination, and some food allergies. It contains poria (a diuretic), barley seed, *shen qu*, magnolia bark, angelica root, pueraria, red atractylodes, jurinea, pogostemon, oryza sprout, trichosanthes, chrysanthemum flower, mint, halloysite, and citrus peel. The formula is a derivative of popular Chinese digestive pills such as Xiao Yao Wan and Curing Pills. If they are not available, you can make a digestive tea by seeping sliced fresh ginger and mint leaves in hot water.

Water Retention (Edema)

DRAIN DAMPNESS Chinese herbal pills contain alisma, poria, *zhu ling* medicinal mushroom, cinnamon, and white atractylodes. They are made by Health Concerns in Oakland, California, whose high-quality products are tested for purity according to FDA regulations. A recommended dose is on the bottle, but highly sensitive people should start with the lowest dose or one pill to observe the reaction.

Drain Dampness is diuretic and diaphoretic—it encourages sweating—to reduce edema. This action helps reduce puffy cellulite around the middle and thighs. You might also try diuretic teas, such as Shiitake/Fu Ling Tea or Juniper Berry Tea, which are described on the following pages. The Broccoli Green Tea not only reduces edema but also protects against cancer.

A Few Quick Recipes

Throughout this book, you will learn many recipes that have been successfully used by my many readers, students, and friends. Some are children of the moment—a joyous celebration of natural flavors. Make them your own. Adding them to your regular diet—any diet—will greatly improve your chances of weight loss because wholesome foods satisfy the appetite without adding body fat.

Some of the following recipes include fresh fruits and vegetables known to reduce pounds and inches.

Juniper Berry Tea

Easy to make, tangy, and delicious, this tea keeps your kidneys in good working order.

MAKES 2 CUPS | PREPARATION TIME: 20 MINUTES
Handful of dried juniper berries
1 teaspoon vinegar
3 cups water

Soak a handful of dried juniper berries in 1 cup of water and the vinegar for a few minutes. Rinse the berries with fresh water and crush them. In a ceramic-coated pot, combine 1 tablespoon crushed berries and water. Bring this to a boil and turn off the heat. When the tea is cooled to a warm temperature, enjoy 1 to 3 cups daily until your urine is light, clear, and odorless. Overuse of juniper, like any diuretic, may be weakening.

Shiitake/Fu Ling Tea

Shiitake mushrooms reduce your chances of cancer, while they eliminate extra weight and water retention. Used throughout Asia, shiitake mushrooms can be bought fresh or dried in many supermarkets and online. Fu ling (Poria cocus), a diuretic medicinal fungi, comes in dried, thin white sheets rolled up to resemble cigarettes.

This medicinal brew, made with inexpensive dried mushrooms, can be prepared in large quantities in a slow cooker and stored for up to 3 days in the refrigerator. Drink 1 quart per day to prevent fatigue and reduce a sweet tooth. If you start the day with tea, coffee, or Juniper Berry Tea, wait until the afternoon to drink this mushroom brew, because those beverages will wash its valuable nutrients out of the body. You will enjoy its subtle, stimulating effects.

MAKES 1 LITER | PREPARATION TIME: 8 HOURS

½ cup dried shiitake mushroom
½ cup dried, sliced fu ling
Stevia extract to taste (optional)

Add the mushrooms to your slow cooker, fill the pot with water, and cook at low heat overnight or for 8 hours. Strain the liquid and store it in a sealed plastic container or wine bottle in the refrigerator. Add the stevia, if using, when you're ready to drink it.

You can recook the mushrooms a second time with fresh water.

Note: A few people are allergic to mushrooms. Symptoms of an allergic reaction include sudden facial swelling, shortness of breath, or dangerous hyperventilation. If you have eaten mushroom dishes before and do not have a yeast candida infection, you can safely drink this tea.

BROCCOLI GREEN TEA

Dr. Ibrahim Saracoglu recommends broccoli to prevent and treat cancers, including breast and prostate cancers. This easy-to-make tea uses broccoli and hides the taste. You can make a large quantity if you use it all during the same day. You can eat some of the broccoli if you like, but do start with a fresh batch daily to make the tea.

MAKES 1 QUART | PREPARATION TIME: 15 MINUTES
1 quart water
1 cup chopped fresh organic broccoli

Pour the water into a saucepan. Add the broccoli. Simmer for 15 minutes. Pour the water over your favorite tea—preferably green, white, or red bush tea.

FRUIT-BASED SALAD DRESSING

Here is a quick, tangy, low-calorie taste boost for your salads.

MAKES 1 CUP | PREPARATION TIME: 10 MINUTES
1 clove garlic, chopped
1 handful chopped, fresh parsley
Potassium salt substitute, lemon pepper, turmeric powder, and
cumin powder to taste
½ cup fresh orange juice
½ cup tomato juice
Juice of ½ fresh lime
1 tablespoon finely milled flaxseed meal (optional)
1 tablespoon low-fat yogurt (optional)

Mash together the garlic, parsley, salt substitute, lemon pepper, turmeric, and cumin with the back of a spoon. Place the mixture in a blender, add the orange, tomato and lime juices, and the flaxseed and yogurt (if using). Blend until it is smooth. Store the dressing in a glass jar in your refrigerator. The flavors blend and taste smoother on the second day.

Apple Celery Pie

If you love sweets, you are most likely a Bear. Bears can read about their particular habits and weight problems and find many healthy sweets in Chapter 7. This spicy breakfast pie will start your day with a zing. It can be made the night before and kept in the refrigerator.

MAKES AN 8-INCH PIE | PREPARATION TIME: 60 MINUTES

> *1 tablespoon quick tapioca pudding*
> *1 tablespoon unsweetened prune or grape juice*
> *3 large tart apples, chopped into bite-size pieces*
> *1 cup sliced celery, chopped into bite-size pieces*
> *⅛ cup raisins*
> *¼ cup walnuts*
>   *Potassium or seaweed salt substitute, clove powder, and lemon*
>   *pepper to taste*
> *1 prepared sugarless graham cracker piecrust*

Preheat the oven to 425°F.

In a large nonmetal bowl, mix the tapioca and prune juice. Toss the apples and celery in the tapioca mixture. Blanch the raisins and walnuts in boiling water to awaken their flavor. Add to the apple mixture. Mix in the salt substitute, clove powder, and lemon pepper. If necessary, moisten with another few drops of prune juice and add it to your unbaked piecrust.

Cover the piecrust with aluminum foil that has been pierced with a knife 3 times to let steam escape. Bake the pie for 1 hour. Remove the foil top and cool the pie for at least 30 minutes before cutting.

Onion–Tree Ear Soup

Modest when compared with its rich French cousin, this onion broth makes a tasty, satisfying dish nonetheless. It contains no added fat or sugar. Onion is useful for all catarrhal, bronchial, and lung disorders. Its sulfur and potassium content also make it an anticellulite food. Sulfur foods stimulate the action of the amino acids to the brain and nervous system. Cook or eat onions along with parsley to ease the effects of sulfur in the intestines. Chinese tree ear fungi (Auricularia) are natural blood thinners useful for reducing cholesterol. Buy them dried in Chinese groceries or online.

MAKES 10 SERVINGS (2 QUARTS) | PREPARATION TIME: 3 OR 4 HOURS

> 4 *medium yellow onions*
> 1–2 *cloves garlic, peeled*
> ¼ *cup dried tree ear fungi*
> 2 *bags rooibos tea*
> 1 *cube low-sodium instant chicken bouillon*
> ¼ *cup fresh parsley or cilantro leaves*
> *Seaweed salt substitute, black pepper, or paprika to taste*
> *Cooked baby lima beans (optional)*

Wash and chop the onions. Combine them with the garlic in a 2½-quart slow cooker. Meanwhile, soak the tree ears in water for 10 minutes to make them soft. Rinse and add the tree ears to the pot. Add 2 quarts of water, the tea bags, and the bouillon to the slow cooker and cook on high heat for 3 hours. Add the parsley during the last ½ hour of cooking. When it is done, adjust the seasoning with a salt substitute, black pepper, or paprika. You might wish to add cooked limas for added nutrition. To fast, eat only this soup for a couple of afternoons.

If you prefer to use your oven, slice the onions and put them in a glass dish with the garlic and a little water. Cover and bake for 4 hours at 400°F, or until the onions are mushy and golden brown. Separately simmer the tree ears and other ingredients in water for 1 hour. After the onions are done, place them with the tree ear liquid in a blender and blend until smooth.

This soup is not as innocent as it tastes. Onions and garlic are powerfully cleansing to the kidneys and intestines. They are also stimulating aphrodisiacs. Their pungent odor comes out of your pores to perfume the room! Have no more than ½ cup of warm soup once or twice daily and no later than 6 o'clock in the evening, or you may be cleansing at night and visiting the bathroom so often that it will disrupt your sleep. To reduce digestive gurgling that may result from this or other cleansing soups, add a pinch of hingvashtaka powder per serving.

TOMATO AND GREENS SOUP

This easy-to-make soup will allay the empty feeling between meals. Its healthy, slimming ingredients—squash, watercress, and garlic—reduce cholesterol. Turmeric has powerful anticancer properties. Cayenne stimulates circulation.

MAKES 2 QUARTS | PREPARATION TIME: 20 MINUTES

   1 can (8 ounces) stewed tomatoes or 5 ripe tomatoes, sliced,
        and ½ cup water
   2 cups chopped green leafy vegetables; for example, spinach, kale,
        dandelion, watercress, or cabbage
1–2 zucchini, sliced
        Peelings from 3 large Idaho potatoes
   1 can (8 ounces) unsweetened pumpkin pie filling or 2 cups peeled,
        sliced raw pumpkin
   1 clove garlic, crushed
        Freshly chopped herbs, such as parsley, tarragon, mint, or
        lemongrass
  ¼ teaspoon (or more) each cumin powder, fennel powder, mild
        paprika, and turmeric powder
        Pinch of cayenne powder (optional)
        Fresh lemon juice

In an airtight ceramic-coated or stainless steel pot, simmer all the ingredients at low heat for up to 15 minutes. When steamed but still slightly firm, blend with the cooking water until the soup is smooth. Enjoy it hot or cold—3 to 4 cups daily between meals.

NO-CARB NOODLES

Quick-fix, high-fiber Japanese shirataki noodles, available at Chinese and Japanese food markets and many national chain stores, are fully cooked and packed in plastic bags filled with water in the refrigerator sections. Shirataki noodles reduce cholesterol, body fat, cellulite, mucus congestion, and edema and are used for cleansing, fasting, and reducing weight and cholesterol. They satisfy a carbohydrate hunger and boost fiber in meals without adding pounds. (More shirataki recipes are offered in Chapter 6.) Here is a fast, tasty recipe.

   1 *package shirataki noodles*
   1 *teaspoon low-fat peanut butter*
   3 *drops sesame oil*
   1 *tablespoon water*
      Raw sesame seeds to taste
      Fresh watercress to taste

Rinse the noodles with water, then warm them in boiling water for less than 1 minute and drain. In a bowl, mix the peanut butter with the oil and water. Add this to the noodles along with sesame seeds to make slimming cold sesame noodles. Garnish with watercress.

TIGER LOW-CAL GELATIN

Remember the overly sweet gelatin we loved as kids? Gelatin, made without sugar, supports healthy cartilage, joints, bones, and fingernails and improves arthritis. Enjoy this dish with a big green salad for lunch. Each envelope of gelatin provides 6 grams of protein with no fat, cholesterol, or carbohydrates.

MAKES 4 SERVINGS | PREPARATION TIME: 3 HOURS

   3 *packs unflavored gelatin*
   2 *cups fruit juice*
   1 *cup water*
   1 *pack Get Svelte instant beverage*
      Fresh fruits or vegetables, sliced

Mix the gelatin with 1 cup of the juice. (I like pineapple, apple, berry, papaya, or grape.) In a saucepan over high heat, mix the remaining 1 cup of juice with the water and bring to a boil. Stir in the Get Svelte.

Pour the hot liquid over the cold gelatin mixture and stir well.

Refrigerate for 1 hour, then add the fruits or veggies. (Slightly chilling keeps the produce from floating on the surface.) Refrigerate at least 2 more hours, or until set.

Note: Get Svelte powdered drink, available from Lin Sister Herb Store in New York's Chinatown or online at www.eastearthtrade.com, contains hawthorn, a heart protector herb, and other safe slimming herbs.

I hope you enjoy incorporating these new foods into your diet. Consuming fruits, vegetables, whole grains, Asian mushrooms, nuts, seeds, legumes, slimming teas, and safe proteins will keep you slim, healthy, and wise. God's creatures—from the giant bear to the elegant crane, from the powerful tiger to the compassionate dragon—seek health and harmony through a wise diet, clean air, and pure water.

Jump-Start Weight Loss

Most people hit a plateau after losing a few pounds and remain at the same weight for weeks or months. And some people just can't get started with weight loss. Let's make things easy: Cut your favorite addiction in half or combine it with its opposite, and watch how the ill effects are reduced. That will sound heretical to some, but try it.

One of the women who took part in my clinical observation study admitted sheepishly that she adored dairy products, but they increased her sinus congestion and fat intake. I suggested that she spend one afternoon a week consuming only fat-free milk with a dash of cardamom powder and fresh berries. Why not enjoy weight loss? Fat-free milk has fewer calories than whole milk, and the cardamom and berries reduce mucus congestion, a common problem with dairy products.

Applying our principle of balancing a food with its opposite: Fresh, crisp pineapple, strawberries, blackberries, blueberries, or cherries cut through milk's richness. She could consume as much of those two foods as she wished and observe the results. I heard she continued what she called her Queen of Sheba Diet 1 day a week for several weeks and enjoyed losing 10 pounds.

There are a number of other techniques you might find helpful to jump-start weight loss or get it moving once again if it has stalled.

START THE DAY WITH CITRUS. Have orange, lime, or lemon juice diluted in water. Use half juice and half water. If citrus fruits are irritating for you, or if you have intestinal parasites or a yeast infection, start with hot broccoli water instead. Simmer a handful of fresh broccoli in 2 cups of water for 10 minutes, then drink the resulting liquid at a comfortably warm temperature. You may eat a few pieces of broccoli to increase your fiber intake, but most of the nutrients are in the water.

GO GREENER. For convenience, you can also take chlorophyll concentrate or chlorella capsules with meals. Greens encourage cleansing and reduce acid discomforts from skin rashes, stomach upset, constipation, or bad breath.

STAY HYDRATED. Drink plenty of water or half water and half juice between meals.

FOCUS ON FOODS THAT ENCOURAGE WEIGHT LOSS. You'll find a number of star performers in "Foods for Fast-Action Weight Loss" on page 261.

Cleanse with Juices and Fasting Foods

Focusing on one or two cleansing foods during one afternoon or one entire day a week can get your weight loss rolling again. It allows your digestive qi to rest and recuperate from rich meals. Use fresh fruits and vegetables as much as possible because they are more stimulating than bottled juice. In a blender, you might combine 1 cup of sliced ripe fruit with 2 cups of water, whip 5 to 15 minutes, or use a juicer, and strain the liquid.

USE RAW FOODS CAREFULLY. While raw fruits and vegetables are certainly good for you, don't start with an all-raw diet immediately, unless you have excellent digestion, and you live in a warm climate. Raw foods require digestive qi, which can gradually be enhanced with herbs. Most traditional Asian doctors believe that cold, raw foods reduce digestive qi. Try adding no more than 1 cup of raw juice during the afternoon to see how you tolerate it. I suggest aiming for a ratio of no more than 60 percent raw foods and at least 40 percent cooked foods. This will help maintain a healthy acid/alkaline balance in the digestive tract. The difference between our method and the typical fast is that we recommend many (acidic) tropical foods and warming spices and closely monitor digestive qi to avoid unpleasant side effects expected from cleansing.

DON'T FAST IF IT WILL UNDERMINE YOUR HEALTH. People who are sick or pregnant or have blood sugar problems, such as diabetes or hypoglycemia, or mental or emotional problems become too weak from a water or juice diet. They should avoid fasting and overusing cleansing foods. People with strong digestion and good health can proceed with caution using my recommended herbs and spices.

Never start the day with a cold, raw juice because it may result in a migraine in the afternoon. If you prefer, have a cup of hot water with a twist of lemon or a cup of hot ginger, green, or mint tea. You need to avoid as much as possible extreme diarrhea, chills, dizziness, and fatigue.

CLEANSE WITH WATER AND GREENS. The strongest method of cleansing is to drink a glass of distilled water every 2 hours, adding 1 teaspoon of liquid chlorophyll or taking a chlorophyll capsule with each glass. Liquid chlorophyll is usually made from concentrated alfalfa, one of the best-known supplements to tone bowel muscles and overcome slow elimination. Rich in minerals, including magnesium and silicon, chlorophyll helps nourish intestinal flora, including acidophilus bacteria, and reduces bloating.

If you have no time to fast, take two chlorophyll capsules with meals to purify and deodorize the body and improve blood quality. Over time, chlorophyll clears complexion blemishes and bad breath and strengthens weak hair fiber and fingernails. Because it purifies the blood and tones digestion, it can help to eliminate fat and cellulite.

Chlorophyll is not sweet, so you should not feel spacey from using it. However, if you become chilled or weak during a water and chlorophyll fast, alternate with a cup of warm tea made with fresh mint; peeled, sliced raw ginger; and a dash of cardamom powder.

If you have chronic diarrhea, drink no more than 1 ounce a day of green juice, or avoid it completely. Broccoli green tea (see the recipe on page 46) can be helpful for weak digestion or chronic illness.

CHECK YOUR TONGUE. If you use a liquid diet for a day or more, be sure to check your tongue for guidance. A pale, puffy tongue requires warming spices such as raw or powdered ginger or cardamom added to fresh juices. Your tongue naturally becomes more coated with cleansing foods.

USE CAUTION. You may wish to continue fasting for longer than a single afternoon. If you do choose to fast for a full day or longer, however, it is very important to stop all work, use a daily enema, and get lots of rest. Otherwise, cleansing becomes weakening.

BREAK YOUR FASTS WITH CARE. No matter how you fast—with water or cleansing fruits, vegetables, and juices—be very careful returning to a normal diet. If you drink water and liquid chlorophyll, you can break the fast by drinking one 8-ounce glass of either fruit or vegetable juice every 3 hours. Do this 1 day for every 5 days you fasted. Then, after a day or two of juice, start the day with sliced, peeled oranges or shredded, steamed carrots. Have a small salad and steamed vegetables for lunch. Continuing adding steamed vegetables and salad for dinner. You might continue with juice between meals, but gradually increase cooked foods—for example, yellow cornmeal or oatmeal—until your digestion is normal.

If you are taking enemas during an extended cleansing diet, stop them 3 days before you start eating solid foods. It is important to return to healthy bowel movements.

Advanced Cleansing

At some point, you will want to speed things along with additional cleansing methods. During a raw food or juice diet, because of decreased bulk, you may need a laxative tea or stimulating spices.

HAWTHORN BERRY is an ingredient often used in Chinese weight loss teas. The bush grows wild in New England and old England, where it is sometimes made into a semisweet jam. The Chinese use sweetened hawthorn as a candy called haw fruit, which looks and tastes a bit like pink chewing gum. The berry is a tonic herb that enhances muscle tone, especially for the heart. It is recommended to reduce cholesterol and moderate an uneven, nervous heartbeat.

Hawthorn is added to Chinese white or oolong teas to make slimming beverages, such as Bojenmi Tea, to protect circulation. Hawthorn prevents the slimming tea from becoming too energy draining.

The first time that you try a slimming tea, have only 1 cup and observe the results. Hawthorn can overstimulate people prone to headaches or dizziness. Avoid teas containing senna, because the herb can cause cramps.

GET SVELTE is an instant beverage made from fine-quality powdered Chinese herbs by Yin/Yang Sisters. Their picture is on the box.

GARLIC AND PARSLEY OIL CAPSULES can be either swallowed or used as a suppository—perhaps swallow one and insert another by rectum. Coat it with a little aloe vera gel to insert it with ease, then wash your hands with an antibacterial soap. Garlic kills germs, parasites, and yeast. Used as a suppository, garlic has no odor. Aside from detoxifying the colon, garlic firms abdominal and thigh muscles and stimulates circulation to reduce cellulite. Parsley is purifying and deodorizing.

SKIN BRUSHING allows the skin to breathe. Some people recommend a morning skin brushing with a soft fine-bristle brush sold in pharmacies or health food stores for the purpose of exfoliation. Nothing keeps me from my morning pot of hot green tea, and I prefer to have the tea's laxative action take effect before I brush, which brings impurities to the surface of the skin.

LESSONS FROM TIBET

Traditional Tibetan doctors, trained at the Tibetan Institute of Medicine and Astrology in Dharamsala, India, are taught the ways of ancient healers. Each August they gather herbs in India's Manali Valley during the full moon. The physician/monks chant many Buddhist prayers over the herbs, infusing them with the spiritual reverence and tranquillity of a peaceful Earth.

You can order their herbal teas online at www.tibetan-medicine. org. They include teabags of Sorig Loong Tea, Sorig Tripa Tea, and Sorig Bad-Kan Tea. Sorig Loong Tea is used to relax and refresh the body, reduce chronic anxiety, and ease arthritis, back pain, nervous habits, and bingeing. A cup in the evening or after a hectic day brings well-being. Sorig Tripa Tea cools inflammation and anger. It restores healthy blood pressure as it eases liver, gallbladder, and prostate problems. It is suitable for hot days or during a fever. Sorig Bad-Kan Tea restores healthy digestion and is useful for weight loss. It stimulates vibrant health and energy. It is especially useful during cold weather and for depression, hypothyroid conditions, and cancer prevention.

Because these remedies affect the body, mind, and spirit simultaneously, they greatly enhance your quest for balance and total health. Sophisticated diagnosis is not necessary to use them because they are formulated for the general public. You can enjoy the dosage that suits you best. Foods or herbal treatments such as these, which harmonize the entire person, allow us to adapt to daily stress and greatly reduce illness and overweight. Please make any changes to your diet gradually and try to avoid very cleansing foods during working hours.

You are on your way to becoming slim, fit, and squeaky clean. Free your body of poisons and be safe from disease and depression. It is also the best and fastest way to lose weight. The Baseline Diet can work quickly and efficiently for anyone. Next, we will find the best approach for you to stay slender, healthy, long-lived, and wise according to your energy type.

Chapter 3

What's Your Energy Type?

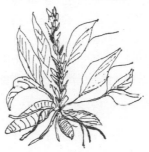

You may be a 180-pound smoker or a 35-year-old mother of two. You may be an athletic woman of 56 troubled by cellulite. You may be a young woman in your twenties who has gained weight during pregnancy. You may be an athletic man who wants to improve energy and endurance. Or you may be none of these. Why should everyone follow the same diet?

Some people hold extra fat in the middle and others in the buttocks or thighs. A one-diet-for-all approach, neither practical nor healthy, is perfect for squeezing the most consumers into the latest weight loss craze. It may be tempting, but applying data from weight loss studies is at best confusing. British philosopher Benjamin Disraeli said, "There are lies, damn lies, and statistics." The fact is, there is a tremendous amount of confusing and misleading misinformation about diet out there, some of it from seemingly reputable sources.

An article in a May 2005 *New York Times*, for example, misinterpreted a study published in the *Journal of the American Medical Association (JAMA)*. Under the headline "With Potbellies Back In, Buffet Pots Are Humming," the *Times* reporter wrote: "The study suggested that people who are somewhat overweight are at less risk of early death than people who are thin. . . . While the government continues to warn that excess weight and related concerns are a major threat to 65 percent of adult Americans, the message that many people are getting from the study is: 'Supersize me, without guilt.'"

The study in *JAMA*, "Excess Deaths Associated with Underweight, Overweight, and Obesity," concludes that both extremes—underweight and high levels of obesity—are associated with increased mortality relative to a normal weight. The study is by no means an invitation to a banquet. The *Times* later printed an apology. If slightly overweight Americans are living slightly longer than before, it may be from a decline in smoking.

That same month, in several major newspapers, a new disease hit the top 10 in popular weight loss research. Variously named syndrome X, metabolic syndrome, and insulin resistance syndrome, the disease was defined as a cluster of risk factors, including mild hypertension; elevated glucose (blood sugar) levels; high triglycerides; low levels of HDL cholesterol (the good kind); and high levels of C-reactive protein (CRP), a substance linked to heart disease. The disease supposedly affects 55 million Americans, but scientists disagree about its cause, how to diagnose it, how to treat it, and what to call it. You can bet that when they name it, a company will patent an expensive treatment.

Some endocrinologists blame belly fat and others, insulin resistance; but whatever its cause, researchers agree that losing weight reduces all components of metabolic syndrome. That means all sorts of expensive tests and treatments can be replaced by paying attention to your bathroom scale! Plenty of people, no matter what their size, want to look and feel better, fit into nice clothes, and live longer by eating a sensible, if not sparse, diet.

Here's Looking at You

As a practical source of personalized weight loss information, let's observe your own body, dietary needs, food cravings, energy level, habits, and moods as they relate to your eating. When—or under what circumstances—do you crave fattening foods? What do you crave most often? Where do you hold excess fat? Such questions reveal your weight loss–energy potential, which is more informative than age, sex, and any standardized weight measurement. This kind of information is really useful in customizing a diet appropriate to meet your needs. And that's exactly what I've done in this book.

In January 2004, I began an informal weight loss observational study among my students at the New York Open Center; the Renfield Center for Nursing Education and Research, a division of Beth Israel Medical Center; the Institute of Integrative Nutrition; and my private health clients. In 2005 and 2006, I added Internet clients from around the world. At my Web site, www.asianhealthsecrets.com, you can plug into the recipes that I created from that study and others updated to contain the most recent diet information.

Participants in my weight loss observation completed a questionnaire, similar to the one that you'll find on page 73, to determine their energy type. I sent them diet suggestions according to their types, and they e-mailed back their results. Based upon that information, I further refined the energy types.

You can jump ahead and complete that questionnaire right now to determine which type you are. But if you do, please make sure you come back and read about how I created the four animal types—Tiger, Dragon, Bear, and Crane—and how they relate to traditional Chinese medicine (TCM) and martial arts. You'll need this information to understand the reasoning behind the specific dietary recommendations for each type that you'll find in Part 2.

Four Animals and Five Elements

I hope your curiosity is aroused by the energy types. This section covers the artistic, philosophical, and medical origins of our four types.

The use of animal icons in painting and teaching is not revolutionary. Chinese and Tibetan Buddhist art have shared symbols such as rocks to connote longevity. Such borrowing became especially widespread during the Ming Dynasty when, for political, commercial, and religious reasons, the two cultures exchanged gifts of painted scrolls, sculpture, and musical instruments. The dragon was considered yin and the tiger, yang. Their complementary relationship held both in check because yin represented water, darkness, emptiness, and the female principle, and yang represented fire, light, movement in the heavens, and the male principle. The notion of harmonizing opposites permeates the entire spectrum of traditional Asian medicine.

Symbols for longevity that appear in Chinese painting include rocks and mountains, cranes, pine trees, and deer. The crane is a large gray bird with a long beak, very long legs, and a distinctive tuft of red feathers on its head. It elegantly strikes a pose. Animal icons in East Indian painting represent or accompany deities. I am reminded of beautiful Saraswati, the Hindu goddess of learning and culture, often portrayed as a woman riding a large, white swan. She, like an enlightened Dragon, is the essence of Water harmonized with Fire. Riding a waterfowl, she holds in her many hands an herb and a sword, shell, bow and arrows, trident, scepter, and other symbols of omnipotent power. The Hindu god Shiva—lord of dance and destruction that initiates positive change, half male and female—wears a tiger skin draped over one shoulder. Surrounded by a ring of sacred fire, he blends fury with gentleness. In the West, we love the mighty bear and give teddy bears to babies.

The dragon, bear, crane, and tiger are beautiful and beneficial to us in many ways. I chose them to represent our four energy types—instead of blood types or abstract humours such as wind, bile, and phlegm—because it is easier for us to identify with them. Following my diet advice for your type, presented in upcoming chapters, will help you improve your food karma. You may learn something useful and wonderful about yourself by discovering your animal energy. Animals can be bold, graceful, and loving in ways that we cannot. If you merely wish to lose 50 pounds or more, you can accomplish it easier and faster and keep it off better by eating according to your energy type.

The Five Animal Forms

The popular martial art and *qigong* exercises called the Five Animal Form was invented by Hua Tuo, a Han Dynasty physician who lived from AD 110 to 207. Born in a town now called Haoxian in Anhui Province, he is considered the Chinese father of surgery and has been compared, in this regard, with Jivaka of India (500 BC). Hua Tuo was a contemporary of ancient China's best-known herbalist, Zhang Zhongjing. In the *Chronicles of the Later Han Dynasty,* Hua Tuo was described as "still appearing in the prime of his life when he was almost 100, and so was regarded as immortal."

Hua Tuo's exercises imitated the free and easy movements of animals in nature. These movements have been compared to those of tigers, deer, bears, apes, and birds. One French source described them as tiger, dragon or serpent, bear, crane or eagle, and monkey. Hua Tuo believed that animals remained healthy by moving with graceful ease. These movements were later incorporated into various martial arts such as tai chi. You will learn simple movements adapted from Hua Tuo's animal form and other slimming exercises in Chapter 11. (For more information on Hua Tuo, see www.itmonline.org, a Web site devoted to Chinese herbal research.)

Our Four Energy Types

Five animals are too many to easily handle. Besides, most people reject being compared with a monkey or snake. In this book, I have narrowed them to four and described where and why each energy type gains extra weight.

- **Dragon:** The entire body is overweight from edema (water retention) and/or body fat. Overweight may be long-standing, due to illness, overwork, or hormonal imbalance.
- **Bear:** This type has a spare tire around the waist and hips—and a sweet tooth.
- **Crane:** Weights vary among this type. A Crane may be depressed or have problems with addictions or nutritional absorption.

- **Tiger:** This type has muscle weakness; joint discomfort; poor circulation; and cellulite at the waist, hips, and thighs.

The animal's shape, temperament, and dietary habits, including cravings and addictions, all go together to make up each energy type. You may identify with one or more of these.

The Dragon Energy Type

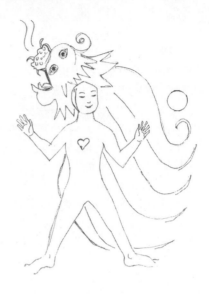

DRAGONS are miraculous creatures that spring from the imagination. The Dragon's heavy bottom half drags on the ground or lounges in swamps. The top half spouts fire. People who resemble Dragons may have round or oval facial features. Edema gives them puffiness under the eyes and swollen hands with soft nails. For an exhausted Dragon, the entire body feels bloated. The ankles may be thick if the heart becomes challenged. Illness or chronic fatigue increases the chances of thinning hair and chronic pain. Poor energy and low immunity lead to depression and sometimes a hypothyroid condition or hormonal imbalance. Hot flashes and night sweats indicate the Dragon's Fire and Water elements are out of balance. (We'll look at TCM elements and how they relate to the animal energy types in just a minute.)

People who resemble Dragons are go-getters until they collapse. Vivacious and commanding in the spotlight, they seem to fly through the air or hover in space. When fatigued, they can be reserved to the point of inertia. Long-term overweight often makes them emotional and self-protective. Dragons, who are psychic, enjoy magical thoughts of omnipotence or dramatic despair. Most often, Dragons ignore or reject their bodies, preferring to live in loftier thoughts, work, or art. They may hungrily consume books (along with junk food) or collect things. Dragons pile up work projects that time and chance often leave unfinished.

Dragons drive themselves with salt, sugar, chocolate, cola drinks, and foods with empty calories. Global overweight can accompany an irregular menstrual cycle because hormone balance, weight, and mood go hand in glove. Often highly motivated and multitalented, Dragons need to moderate their appetite and support adrenal vitality with herbs. Otherwise, they may develop insomnia, heart palpitations, or immune deficiency illnesses. Eventually, their vision, hearing, and memory suffer from lack of adequate rest.

The Bear Energy Type

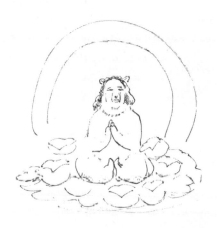

BEARS are happiest when they are entertaining family and friends or cooking up business deals. They are socializers who love to talk, eat, and kiss. When well fed, they revel at dinner parties, singing, telling jokes, and laughing. They may have square facial features and may or may not be stocky, but in either case, extra weight is carried in the middle. They have short, square hands and fingers. They like to digest (or obsess over) thoughts and feelings and communicate them freely. Bears with poor digestive *qi* lose energy mulling over ideas or projects that remain incomplete.

People who resemble Bears can be cuddly teddies or fierce grizzlies. They rapidly switch moods. Arguments give them stomach troubles.

Bears crave sweets and may binge on cookies, breads, or pastries. Overeating challenges their breathing and heart health. Bears require herbs for healthy digestive qi and blood sugar balance. High blood pressure and sleep apnea may come into the picture, especially for a large Ursa over age 60.

The Crane Energy Type

CRANES can be exquisite, slender artists, movie stars, models, and humanitarians—or lanky criminal offenders. They go to extremes.

They often have tall, slender frames with long facial features, hands, and fingers. They may fast for health or philosophical reasons or binge on one of their addictions without regard to their health or beauty. They may have to overcome bad habits like smoking or drug use. Poor food choices give them chronic sinus or breathing problems, energy deficiency, and skin blemishes. Their key issues are breathing, or getting enough oxygen; and communication, or distancing themselves from others in order to protect their vitality.

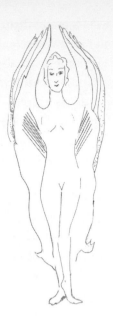

Cranes often prefer to work and be alone. Talking with others drains them. Cranes can be intensely tenacious in arguments or acquisitive with possessions. They need to rest and regroup after frenetic social activity. They can be dedicated, high-minded, and driven by their ideals or antisocial because they are naturally loners. Their addictions can make them feel persecuted or misunderstood. They need to support vitality and reduce the ill effects of poor food choices. Chinese herbs for withdrawal symptoms such as headache ease tension and improve sleep and digestion. In upcoming chapters, I recommend such herbs for all people going through major life changes, including important diet changes.

The Tiger Energy Type

TIGERS thrive or falter on the strength of their nervous energy and inner drive. They may have an athletic physique and angular facial features, along with cellulite from the waist down. Poorly fed Tigers suffer from swollen or achy joints, weak muscles or tremors, facial pallor or jaundice,

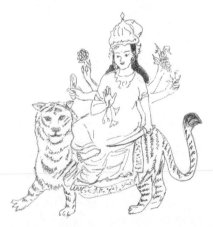

and poor circulation. Their hands are dry with many lines in the palms and brittle fingernails. Gregarious, charming, and moody, they become aggressive or develop flank or chest pain when frustrated. Their anger can flare or get stuck in a lump in their throat.

Tigers are used to prowling through the jungle. They love to glide gracefully and pounce with ease of movement. They can be highly ambitious and focused. One East Indian public relations executive retired early after creating the slogan "Put a tiger in your tank."

A ferocious appetite makes a Tiger combine fried and rich foods, sweets, alcohol, and hard-to-digest quarry, resulting in headaches, allergies, or skin rashes. Out-of-sorts Tigers can be crabby, hung-over, and jaundiced or attack other animals. Tigers need to reduce food allergies and indigestion with liver-cleansing foods and herbs. They do best with a varied diet that facilitates their natural bent for sexiness and adventure.

The Five Elements and Your Health

Western medicine describes bodily functions in terms of the circulatory, nervous, digestive, respiratory, and reproductive systems; the musculature; and the skeletal system. In TCM, these body functions as well as the internal organs and associated acupuncture meridians make up the anatomy and physiology of the five elements—Fire, Earth, Metal, Water, and Wood. Put another way, we humans and the earth are made of the same stuff. Our four energy types are also metaphorically made up of the five elements so that the types can be influenced by diet and other treatments. You will see that:

- The Dragon reflects the Fire and Water elements.
- The Bear reflects the Earth element.
- The Crane reflects the Metal element.
- The Tiger reflects the Wood element.

The Fire Element

In TCM, the Fire element—made up of the heart, pericardium, small intestine, and "triple heater" acupuncture meridians—regulates circulation, an aspect of absorption and elimination, and body temperature. Although any of the animal types can experience chronic feverish symptoms, including hot flashes or night sweats, the Dragon is defined by that imbalance: When vitality is low, the Dragon spouts fire.

A healthy, rosy facial hue and a natural capacity for joy and peace of mind are signs of health for the Fire element, whereas facial flushing, palpitations, mania, and insanity are signs of imbalance. Do you talk a lot, giggle, stutter, have nightmares or heart-pounding anxiety? These are signs of agitation in the Fire element. Do you know any Dragons who chatter and giggle?

The flavor most associated with the Fire element is bitter. Healthy cleansing and slimming bitter-tasting foods include salad greens such as endive, chicory, dandelion, tea, and Angostura digestive bitters. Overheated people addicted to a bitter/hot flavor often crave cigarettes, hot spices, and coffee with resulting acidity, nervous tension, and abdominal pain. The bitter flavor used as jet fuel results in an energy crash.

TCM doctors are trained to use subtle forms of diagnosis. They may notice a person's facial hue, posture, or mental attitude as being indicative of an imbalance. They may pay attention to vocal quality or odor. If a person has a predominantly bitter or burnt odor, the Fire element is overactive.

Sometimes during acupuncture treatment, an odor will arise that indicates an energy shift. Once I treated a European friend for high blood pressure. He was a brilliant professor known for his extroverted personality and bawdy jokes. He smoked and drank excessively. While the acupuncture needles reduced his hypertension, he suddenly broke into tears, complaining about his life. And the room was filled with his burnt and bitter perspiration odor. If you know someone whose odor tends to be burnt and bitter, that person may be challenging his heart with an overly stimulating diet or busy schedule.

People who have chronic inflammatory symptoms such as

menopausal hot flashes or night sweats need herbs to balance the Fire and Water elements.

Before we move on, here's a quick tip to rid the body of unpleasant odors while eliminating toxins and toning metabolism: Take alternating doses of homeopathic Kali mur 6X (potassium) and homeopathic Silicea 6X (silica), a mineral found naturally in rocks and grass. (Silica strengthens hair fiber, bones, and fingernails.) Put three pills of each remedy into separate glasses, each containing 4 ounces of water. Alternating, sip them every couple of hours throughout the day between meals. You will lose excess water weight and indigestion as your metabolism increases at the cellular level. Your tongue should look less coated, your digestive qi improved, and your odor reduced within 1 to 2 days of using this therapy.

The Water Element

The Water element is comprised of the kidney, urinary bladder, hormones, and vitality as they impact upon sexuality, fertility, and immunity to illness. The Water element regulates endurance, courage, and longevity. Water is the grounded half of Dragons. When kidney and adrenal energy are weakened from overwork, an unnourishing diet, or bad habits, Dragons, already weak from overweight, lose their bearings. It becomes hard to work, rest, and think.

Optimism, creativity, high vitality and endurance, strong immunity to illness, painless menstruation, and fertility are signs of health in the Water element. Chronic fatigue or infection; deep, relentless pain; incontinence; and sexual problems are among signs of imbalance. So are overweight and obesity. Since the adrenal glands and pituitary work together, as we age or develop chronic fatigue, hearing, vision, and memory are challenged.

Water is vital to every cell in the body. We do not drink enough of it. However, even when drinking eight glasses daily, we still need the right nutrients to ensure the vitality of fluids such as blood and semen. Among them are iron, B_{12}, and mixed trace minerals, including copper and gold. The herb nettle is a wonderful blood builder. Beets, green vegetables, black cherries, bee pollen, and chlorella are all good blood builders. Many overweight women cease menstruation or have an early or difficult menopause because their bodies become too weak to continue healthy blood production.

Stress, smoking, and illnesses cause a disconnect to occur: For Dragons, the Water element becomes deficient and Fire flares. They drag their legs when walking and may develop urinary incontinence or sexual problems accompanied by lumbar pain. At the same time, inflammatory problems in the upper body, such as hot flashes, chest pains, night sweats, insomnia, or anxiety, signal the Fire element.

Here is where the Asian idea of balance comes into play: Many chronic diseases and overweight resulting from exhaustion can be prevented and reversed with Asian foods and herbal treatments. Do you known anyone who has lower back pain from sitting at a computer? Does he or she munch salty snacks? That person is a Dragon. Addictions for the Water element include salty junk foods such as potato chips and (high-sodium) cola drinks. Chapter 6 recommends healthy foods for people who crave salty snacks.

The Water element gives us the basis of overall well-being. Without adrenal energy, life cannot exist. At times, our drive nearly kills us. I met a Dragon who raced through life catching trains, planes, and buses. She ate enormous health food meals because she thought they gave her energy. But her body was exhausted and her heart stressed by 80 extra pounds. Food cannot nourish when digestion is poor. Lacking adrenal energy, digestion falters. Exhausted people neither work effectively nor sleep at night.

When I inquired about diet, she looked at me intently and answered, "Food is my all." Food was her social life and support system, a closed circuit of consuming. It was as though her mad dash through life helped her avoid confronting her personal problems. It takes courage to stand still and say no to a harmful lifestyle.

The remedy I recommended cured her heart-pounding insomnia in 2 days. It was homeopathic Aconite 30C, often recommended for fear. She was not afraid of anything in particular, but her tired body was trapped in a fight-or-flight pattern that allowed her no rest. Her pulse revealed a fast, pounding heartbeat and low adrenal vitality—

that is, no energetic support for her high-wire act. The homeopathic remedy, three pills taken at bedtime, as needed, on an empty stomach, allowed her to rest and regroup. That gave food its proper place in her life. With proper rest and peace of mind, she could think about decreasing her food intake and increasing her exercise.

The Earth Element

The Earth element—made up of the stomach, spleen, and pancreas—regulates energy gained from digestion, blood sugar balance, and body shape. Bears live in their digestive center. They love food, family, and harmonious surroundings. They crave sweets and empty carbohydrates more often when tired or depressed. When in love, they call their favorite Ursa "honey," "sweetie," "cookie," and "cupcake."

Easy and adequate digestion and elimination are signs of health in the Earth element. Other tendencies are the capacity for mental clarity and concentration. Ancient Chinese texts stress the capacity for sympathy (caring for others) associated with the Earth element. Hypoglycemic spaciness, diabetes, obsessive thoughts, and worries are signs of imbalance.

If the Earth element is troubled by a difficult diet, daily worries, or medicines, Bears may crave especially sedating foods and empty calories—starches, carbohydrates, or sweets, which increase bloating and blood sugar problems. Rich, sweet, hard-to-digest sedating foods can neither cheer teddies nor clear their thinking. If you eat sweets for energy, why not take an herbal energy tonic instead and stay trim? I cover such tasty herbal tonics in Chapter 11.

Traditional Asian doctors pay a lot of attention to digestion because physical and emotional balance are central to the concept of health and longevity. They believe that if a person who is sick, even with a terrible illness, can maintain a healthy digestion, the chances of improvement are better. Chinese herbalists often recommend digestive remedies for people who are depressed and anxious, because these individuals feel better when they are "content in their center." Our digestive center is also our emotional center.

When Bears feel "off center," they whine and complain, ruminate, have stomach cramps, and eat sweets. The Earth element is speaking plainly, but we do not listen. When Bears' Earth element is troubled, their facial hue may be sallow or brownish, and water retention increases their waistlines. The Bear may have an unpleasant, sweet odor coming through the pores or from a vaginal discharge. Babies sometimes have a sour milk smell and colic if digestion is poor. Adult indigestion is just as painful.

Charcoal pills or homeopathic charcoal called Carbo vegetabilis 30C is useful for easing bloating and gas. Take the homeopathic remedy at least 15 minutes after eating. Zinc supplements are also recommended to generally reduce stress and aid the pancreas. Additional digestive remedies are described in the chapter devoted to Bears, which starts on page 172.

The Metal Element

The Metal element—comprised of the lungs, large intestine, and skin—regulates breathing, elimination, energy obtained from oxygen, and complexion. Traditional Chinese texts describe the Metal element as holding the body together. It may be a way of explaining that we absorb vital minerals such as calcium in the colon.

Oxygen absorbed in the lungs maintains life. The smoothness of our breathing creates a calming energy and mood. Yoga has long been practiced to establish a rhythmic breath as well as a limber body. The Crane's vital space is breath. Self-expression in creative work and comfortable space vis-à-vis other people is key to a Crane's character. If Cranes feel crowded by others, they withdraw into bad habits.

Adequate breath, smooth elimination, and a clear complexion are signs of health for the Metal element. Good mental focus and a so-called capacity to protect and preserve life are also signs of its health. It is interesting that ancient Chinese medicine practitioners believed that a healthy person strives to preserve health, whereas a sick person easily falls into destructive habits and addictions. In their view, improving general health, especially breathing, improves a desire for living. It speaks to people who would "die for a cigarette." Anxiety from lungs overheated by either illness or smoking creates feelings of isolation and persecution along with fast, breathy panting.

George Soulie de Morant went to China at the turn of the century and remained there for almost 2 decades. Returning to France in 1917, Soulie de Morant spent the next 40 years actively promoting acupuncture among medical professionals. In 1955, he wrote *l'Acupuncture Chinoise*, which led the first successful European acculturation of acupuncture. The 900-page book has recently become available in English. He may have been the first to use the French term *pervers* (perverse) when describing the Chinese concept of a death wish. The term, describing an aberration of the Metal element, stuck, and no wonder: Pleasure taken in something destructive of ourselves and others, such as smoking, is misguided. Reduced oxygen inevitably leads to mental fog and depression.

Do you know anyone who uses food to self-destruct? Addictions for the Metal element include those that impede energy, breathing, and elimination of impurities. Smoking and a diet of hot, spicy foods are overly drying and therefore increase anxiety. Overuse of dairy and rich, congesting foods is fattening and inhibits breathing. From a Chinese medical perspective, these foods are sedating.

In Chapter 8, I recommend antimucus foods that improve digestive qi and breathing. And, of course, homeopathic Pulsatilla 30C is helpful for people who easily weep, complain, or suffer from shortness of breath. It has also given remarkable weight loss results for people with water retention who eat to soothe depression. That sort of general weakness and vulnerability is often the result of deficient qi in both the Metal and Water elements. An overall deficiency of qi shows up as a large, puffy, or scalloped tongue.

The Wood Element

The Wood element, which encompasses the liver, gallbladder, muscles, and tendons, regulates digestion, movement, and vision. Good absorption of nutrients, a lack of spasm pain, ease of movement, and balanced emotions are signs of health for the Wood element. The pathways of the liver and gallbladder acupuncture meridians, because of their location, bathe the eyes with moisture and blood, ensuring sight. An old Chinese saying is, "The liver allows the eyes to show the soul." Very dry, staring, or squinting eyes are said to lack the milk of human kindness. It may also be an overdose of computer work.

Healthy Tigers move effortlessly through the forest, see clearly, and pounce upon their prey. When unimpeded by a river or a fence, they reach their goals. Illness occurs when a Tiger charges ahead too fast or is prevented from movement. Then his or her energy gets stuck. TCM doctors teach that the liver's energy chooses our actions, as an expression of our soul, and that the gallbladder's energy acts out those wishes. This is a hard concept to believe until you see the location of those acupuncture meridians. The liver meridian starts in the big toe and moves up the center of the body like a force in nature—the same dynamic force that renews plants in spring. The liver meridian continues up through the groin to the chest, the eyes, and the brain. All meridians are paired: Two work together to make an energy loop in the body. The liver meridian is paired with the gallbladder meridian, which starts on the outside of each eye and moves around the ears and down the shoulders, sides, hips, and legs to the fourth toe.

If energy gets stuck on the pathway of the liver, we suffer nausea, chest pain, dizziness, headache, cloudy vision, and possibly fainting. If energy gets stuck in the gallbladder meridian, spasm pains along its pathway lead to migraine headache, stiff neck, sore shoulders, chest pain, sciatica, hip and knee pain, and foot cramps. You can eventually get all of those symptoms from sitting at a computer for 7 hours a day. However, an overly rich diet, an injury, or emotional frustration can inhibit digestion and energy flow more acutely in those areas. If you know a Tiger who wants to pounce but is prevented, stay out of the way. Homeopathic Nux vomica 30C, a liver cleanser often recommended for hangover and crabbiness, could be helpful.

A healthy liver produces an enzyme that helps the body absorb calcium, which calms the nerves and gives strength to muscles and bones. An even temper, muscle strength and comfort, and comfortable menstruation and menopause are signs of health related to the Wood element.

Since drive, ambition, enthusiasm, and willpower define a Tiger, his or her addictions include hot, spicy foods and substances that overstimulate a charging Tiger. Alcohol can overstimulate or sedate nervous eating. Fried foods cause indigestion and liver congestion problems and stones. The opposite foods—cooling, cleansing, bitter-tasting laxative and diuretic herbs such as dandelion—reduce stones, fibroids, fat, and cellulite.

Do you begin to see how your energy type can create and maintain your cravings? You cannot change your energy type, but you can work within its dynamic to bring about new habits.

Weight Loss Questionnaire

The following questionnaire can help you to determine your energy type or at least to better understand your food cravings at present. A brief interpretation of this questionnaire follows. Please do not ponder your answers but mark quickly what most often applies to you.

____ I love hot spicy foods, sour pickles, fried foods, and alcoholic beverages.

____ I have lots of cellulite.

____ I have poor muscle tone.

____ I am a nervous eater. I keep snacks at work.

____ I eat when bored.

____ I have food allergies, especially to fat or fried foods and butter.

____ I easily become angry (especially with PMS).

____ I have arthritis.

____ I have lots of allergies.

___ I get nervous headaches or tics.

___ Sometimes I have a jaundiced complexion.

___ I have had hepatitis or other liver illness.

___ **Total = Tiger = Wood element**

___ I crave salty foods, fried foods, chips, peanuts, and bacon.

___ I have edema (water weight) in my entire body.

___ My ankles and legs are swollen with water weight.

___ I have been overweight since childhood.

___ I put on extra pounds during and after pregnancy.

___ I gained weight after an illness or emotional upset.

___ I gained weight after using medicine.

___ I eat when I am depressed.

___ I easily become weepy (especially with PMS).

___ My back and legs feel weak and painful from excess weight.

___ My immune function is low. I often get sick.

___ I am experiencing menopausal discomforts such as hot flashes.

___ **Total = Dragon = Fire and Water elements**

___ I am always hungry.

___ I crave sweet, rich foods.

___ I always keep cookies and sweets around as a snack.

___ I have an acid stomach or bad breath.

___ I frequently have a dessert after meals.

___ Sweets keep my energy up.

___ I need to slim my waist.

___ I binge on bread, pastry, candy, or chocolate.

___ I have sleep apnea and wake up choking.

___ I nap after meals.

___ I drink beer or wine with dinner.

___ I have diabetes.

___ **Total = Bear = Earth element**

___ I crave pizza, bread, and pasta.

___ I adore dairy products, especially cheese and ice cream.

___ I have some addictions I need to conquer.

___ I am often thirsty or have a dry mouth.

___ I have asthma, bronchitis, or chronic shortness of breath.

___ I have acne, eczema, or psoriasis now or I did as a child.

___ I have a sensitive stomach and easily develop diarrhea.

___ I have intestinal parasites.

___ I have cramps, indigestion, and constipation or diarrhea after eating.

___ I do not pay much attention to my foods or plan meals.

___ I would rather smoke than eat dessert.

___ My diet is part of my spiritual practice.

___ **Total = Crane = Metal element**

___ If I do not eat often, I get spacey.

___ I am often hungry and thirsty. I have frequent urination.

___ **Total = Blood sugar problems = More frequently Earth element**

Interpretation of the Weight Loss Questionnaire

The following review will help you interpret your answers. I divided the questionnaire into sections to address specific dietary and health issues that most frequently apply to the energy types. Where have you marked the most items? Those sections impact the most upon your energy type. You'll find detailed information about how to deal with weight loss for each energy type in Part 2. Here is the breakdown of types.

Tigers and Nervous Eaters

The first section applies to a large number of people who overeat to quiet nervous tension. Often they are Tigers. Tigers thrive on nervous energy, new projects, and excitement. They crave stimulation from work, relationships, and foods. As a result, they sometime get overstimulated and develop allergies, headaches, or emotional outbursts. Tigers, guided by the Wood element, have nervous or liver issues.

In my informal observational study, many participants indicated that they snacked as a response to nervous tension or boredom. One nutrition student wrote in the margin: "I overeat when I am stressed, overwhelmed, avoiding difficult tasks, socializing, bored, when tempted by ads or free samples. In other words, any excuse will do."

Whether or not you are a Tiger, your nervous habits should be addressed directly. If stress is from anxiety over work, future events, performance, or self-doubt, then homeopathic Gelsemium 30C might be in order. If you are an overdoer who always overeats and drinks too much, a workaholic who snacks constantly, then you might consider homeopathic Nux vomica 30C, a liver cleanser.

Dragons and Emotional Eaters

The next section of the questionnaire, which begins "I crave salty foods," is devoted to people who develop edema or excess water weight. They gain weight easily and cannot lose it until they gain vitality. They may have put on pounds following an illness because they never took the time necessary to recover. They may be emotionally vulnerable and binge on comfort foods. If they have been overweight since childhood, they are strongly invested in being heavy. It will take them longer than the other types to lose weight because their relationship to food—their food karma—runs so deep. As you will see, their health issues, which often originate from low energy and poor immunity, tend to be long term.

Edema, night sweats, an aching back and legs, and low immunity refer to the Dragon energy type. We will learn later that Dragons, men and women with low adrenal energy, can benefit from balancing Chinese herbal combinations that simultaneously quench the fire (hot flashes, palpitations, and night sweats) and strengthen water (kidney and adrenal vitality). In other words, we will use foods to balance and coordinate the Dragon's Fire and Water elements.

The statement "I eat when I am depressed" reveals the association of food addictions and mood that can affect any of the types. Some women binge and cry during PMS; others get angry and develop headaches and terrible cramps. Hypoglycemia (low blood sugar), resulting from fatigue, lethargy, or hormonal fluctuations, starts a cycle of bread, pastry, and chocolate bingeing that leads to blood sugar blues and sometimes candida yeast infection. Begin anywhere in the circle—blood sugar imbalances, sweet tooth addictions, depression, or chronic fatigue—and you stay in the same orbit.

The best success I have had with people who eat for comfort is a homeopathic remedy recommended for people who seek consolation from friends. Homeopathic Pulsatilla 30C is often recommended for sadness, yearning, complaining, and feelings of hopelessness. Interestingly, Pulsatilla also improves breathing. In that way, it may promote mental clarity and calmness, as does yoga deep breathing. Women with angry PMS, smokers, or people with chronic thirst may benefit more from homeopathic Nux vomica 30C, the liver cleanser, because it clears the senses and reduces headaches and irritability.

Bears and Sweet Eaters

The section in the questionnaire that begins "I am always hungry" describes Bears. Bears love sweets and may develop an acid stomach from stress or a high sugar intake. If they are prediabetic, they are likely to have frequent hunger and thirst.

People who rely on sweets to boost their energy accumulate fat in the middle. Many overweight people will be a combination of Dragon and Bear types. They will have global overweight with chronic fatigue and a sweet tooth. They need to treat both problems—edema and belly fat—with a balanced low-fat diet and additional energy tonics to support energy, immunity, and emotional balance. They can start with the Dragon diet and add foods and supplements from the Bear diet, depending on their addictions.

Cranes and Junk-Food or Cigarette Addicts

The section in the questionnaire that begins "I crave pizza, bread, and pasta" applies to soaring Cranes. However, those addictions might also apply to other types. What sets Cranes apart is their marginal association with food. Tigers eat for energy and adventure. They hunt for new restaurants and cuisines. Food may be part of their lifestyle. Dragons seek emotional comfort from foods. Bears live to eat. They plan vacations according to their favorite restaurants.

Cranes can either take or leave food. Food is a habit, often a bad one. Many Cranes are so wrapped up in work, travel, addictions, or spiritual pursuits that eating real food becomes secondary. They may be undernourished and overweight at the same time. Bread, pizza, pasta, and dairy products are simple and satisfying and turn quickly into sugar. Such foods take little preparation and can be consumed in flight. It may be difficult for Cranes to lose weight because, odd as it seems, they may not recognize the association of diet and overweight. They may believe they are overweight from some mysterious cause.

Additional Insights

If you are still confused, an overview of food addictions will help you to decide your energy type. After all, the energy type is only a working hypothesis. Use it as an operational model to treat addictions, improve vitality, and achieve emotional freedom from junk foods.

- **Dragons** crave salty or high-sodium foods, which encourage water retention.
- **Bears** crave sweets, which can lead to blood sugar problems.
- **Tigers** crave spice and alcohol, which can irritate the liver and nervous system.
- **Cranes** crave doughy foods such as pizza, bread, pasta, and dairy products, which increase mucus and cause breathing trouble, indigestion, and complexion problems.

Of course, there is usually some overlap between the energy types. Cheese and cake can be sweet and gooey to entice a Bear. One Bear wrote on her questionnaire: "I crave pizza, bread, pasta, cheese, and dairy products. I have sleep apnea: I wake up choking. I also have acne or eczema. I like creamy things: ice cream, pudding, melted cheese. A Chinese acupuncturist once told me to stop eating all dairy and sugar, which I did for 9 months. I had had a huge rash on my leg that diminished by about 75 percent. I still have the final 25 percent of the rash."

She was a Bear with Crane tendencies—complexion problems. Her Chinese doctor recognized that overuse of sugar and dairy foods tends to slow down healing. These foods underlie the chronic condition, including slow metabolism, that traditional Chinese herbalists describe as dampness. When she curbed her sweet tooth with an herb I recommend in Chapter 7, she lost weight and her complexion cleared.

Dietary habits point the way to the future; the questionnaire describes common illnesses associated with the energy types. For example, Bears develop spare tires from eating sweets and white bread because highly refined foods tax the pancreas and therefore deregulate blood sugar balance. If a spare tire is large and long term, it may lead to heart trouble. Bears may hover between hypoglycemia (low blood sugar) and diabetes (high blood sugar), never quite hitting the mark for either.

Cranes tend to have asthma, skin problems, or irritable bowels made worse by poor diet choices.

Tigers develop chronic joint pains, allergies, headaches, and bad tempers if they overindulge in foods that harm the liver and nervous system.

The association of food flavors, physical and emotional discomforts, and the five elements are an important part of TCM. They may not always be explained by modern dietary testing, but they are clearly proven in everyday observations.

Observe Your Animal Energy Type

Still not quite sure which energy type you are? It might be helpful to take a good look at yourself. Standing in front of a full-length mirror or mentally observing your body, ask yourself these questions.

- Where do I hold extra weight or cellulite?
- When and how do I expend the most energy daily?
- How many meals do I eat daily?
- What sort of exercise do I most enjoy?
- Do I sleep enough or too many hours?

You may have made some of these observations already for the questionnaire, but now is the time to look at and listen to your body. As a starting point:

- If you need to enhance vitality and lose total body weight, you are a Dragon.
- If you need to focus on slimming the middle, you are a Bear.
- If you are troubled by joint pain or allergies as well as fat and cellulite, you are a Tiger.
- If you can't pass up a pizza or you binge on ice cream when depressed, you are a Crane.

Each type has advantages as well as health challenges. For example, Dragons need to protect their hearts. Bears are more likely to have problems with insulin uptake, which puts them at risk for blood sugar imbalances resulting in hypoglycemia and diabetes. Tigers are usually up for a challenge, but their tireless enthusiasm and drive may also set them up for insomnia, allergies, and heightened autoimmune responses. Cranes may be sensitive, creative seekers of wisdom or people stuck in escapist addictions or self-blame.

How does knowing your energy type help you pass up a creamy dessert? Your craving has an energetic basis. Bears, people with weak digestion or blood sugar problems, often crave sweets. PMS can also increase a sweet tooth. Herbs recommended for improving digestion and menstruation can alter addictions. By knowing your energy type, you can check your progress according to your vitality and addictions. For example, if you are a Bear, watch your sweet tooth.

As another example, Dragons crave salt or high-sodium foods, colas, and junk foods that lead to water retention. Bloat is typical for Dragons. When Dragons feel stronger, sleep better, and experience less weakness and pain in their kidneys, lower backs, and legs, they start to live better. They feel confident trying new foods and improving their lifestyles. You can work within the bounds of your energy type to alter your cravings by improving your diet and digestive qi. You may not realize it yet, but addictions can be modified with diet.

A healthy person craves nourishing, slimming foods and has excellent vitality, strong digestion, and easy elimination. Someone chronically tired, sad, or anxious uses food to satisfy a physical and/or emotional need. Flavors that are bitter, sweet, pungent, salty, and sour—those associated with the five elements—affect both the body and mind. In TCM, the energy and flavors of foods as well as herbs are used in healing. The four animal types reflect the five elements, which influence your addictions.

There are times, especially with prolonged illness, menopause, or aging, when everything seems to go wrong at once. You may have

---

THREE WAYS TO WEIGHT LOSS

- Eat smaller portions.
- Increase fresh produce gradually to 60 percent raw foods and 40 percent cooked foods.
- Take a relaxing walk after meals.

symptoms associated with all four energy types. If you have symptoms associated with all four types, and you really can't figure out which type you are because aspects of all four seem to apply, start with the health and diet program recommended for the Dragon; it is the most supportive of overall vitality and immunity to illness. Then gradually add natural remedies from the energy type that most often applies to you.

Do not feel worried if you checked many of the items in every section. Anyone's energy and habits change over time, especially with a little help from the dietary practices appropriate for your animal totem. Getting to know your type means accepting the animal—or, if you prefer, Mother Nature—within. It hungers for food, adventure, and conquest. Each energy type offers great rewards.

In Part 2, I will describe the energy types along with their common weight loss and health issues, followed by menus to help fill in any remaining blanks. The following chapter will give you the tools to chart your success.

Chapter 4

Get Ready, Get Set

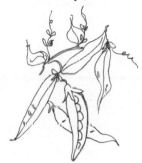

Lose weight now, live better and longer! This chapter offers practical guidelines to help you outline your dieting goals and observe your individual progress. Several studies by the Harvard University School of Public Health have shown that being overweight strongly increases your chances of having a heart attack, stroke, or other type of cardiovascular disease; developing diabetes; developing cancer of the colon, kidney, breast, or endometrium; having arthritis; developing gallstones; being infertile; developing adult asthma; snoring or suffering from sleep apnea; or developing cataracts.

In a 1999 study published in the *New England Journal of Medicine*, middle-aged people who gained 11 to 22 pounds after age 20 were three times more likely to develop heart disease, high blood pressure, type 2 diabetes, and gallstones than those who gained 5 pounds or fewer.

Waist size is another useful measurement because fat replaces abdominal muscle even when your weight remains the same. A larger waist size is a health warning. The National Institutes of Health has concluded that a waist larger than 40 inches for men and 35 inches for women increases the chances of developing heart disease, cancer, or other chronic diseases.

Few scientists consider how tough it actually is to lose weight

HOW'S YOUR RATIO?

Western health professionals use a ratio of weight to height called the body mass index, or BMI for short. It takes into account that taller people have more tissue than shorter people and tend to weigh more.

To calculate your BMI, multiply your weight by 703, divide that number by your height in inches, and then again by your height in inches.

Studies of more than a million adults have shown that a BMI above 25 is considered overweight and above 30 is obesity. However, nothing magic happens when you cross from a BMI of 24.9 to 25 or from 29.9 to 30. Muscle and bone are more dense than fat, so an athlete or muscular person may have a high BMI but not be fat. Since few adults add muscle and bone after their early twenties, nearly all the weight they've gained since age 20 is fat.

If your weight now is not more than 10 pounds over your weight at age 20, most medical professionals believe that you are on your way to achieving your ideal weight. But there is more to your healthy ideal weight than pounds! You might lose 30 pounds or more without reducing fatigue, cellulite, or poor muscle tone. In other words, you may lose weight while damaging vitality as a result of an unwise or extreme diet.

after age 40 or thereabouts, when metabolism slows to a crawl. Consider something as fundamental as exercising to lose weight. If you rode a stationary bike on a random course with little or no resistance—an aerobic workout—for nearly 20 minutes, reaching a total distance of 4 miles, you would burn only about 100 calories. That's the calories found in just one glass of wine or half a glass of beer!

Another factor to consider is enjoyment. You might continue with the Baseline Diet from now on to keep pounds and inches off. However, it is most important to maintain enthusiasm for dieting. That's where energy types come in. They individualize dieting. In addition, it is as important for your general health to incorporate foods and supplements that prevent extreme spikes in dietary fat intake or blood sugar fluctuations as it is to lose pounds. Those spikes put stress on

YOUR BODY MASS INDEX (BMI)

HEIGHT	WEIGHT (LB)													
4'10"	91	96	100	105	110	115	119	124	129	134	138	143	148	153
4'11"	94	99	104	109	114	119	124	128	133	138	143	148	153	158
5'0"	97	102	107	112	118	123	128	133	138	143	148	153	158	163
5'1"	100	106	111	116	122	127	132	137	143	148	153	158	164	169
5'2"	104	109	115	120	126	131	136	142	147	153	158	164	169	175
5'3"	107	113	118	124	130	135	141	146	152	158	163	169	175	180
5'4"	110	116	122	128	134	140	145	151	157	163	169	174	180	186
5'5"	114	120	126	132	138	144	150	156	162	168	174	180	186	192
5'6"	118	124	130	136	142	148	155	161	167	173	179	186	192	198
5'7"	121	127	134	140	146	153	159	166	172	178	185	191	198	204
5'8"	125	131	138	144	151	158	164	171	177	184	190	197	203	210
5'9"	128	135	142	149	155	162	169	176	182	189	196	203	209	216
5'10"	132	139	146	153	160	167	174	181	188	195	202	209	216	222
5'11"	136	143	150	157	165	172	179	186	193	200	208	215	222	229
6'0"	140	147	154	162	169	177	184	191	199	206	213	221	228	235
BMI	19	20	21	22	23	24	25	26	27	28	29	30	31	32

internal organs. Asian medical diagnosis provides a way to judge our actual success by observing our digestive *qi* (energy).

Traditional Asian Diagnosis

Traditional Asian medical diagnosis enables you to monitor your diet better than you can by watching a scale. By observing your facial and body shape and your tongue, an indicator of metabolism, you can observe your digestive qi—your body's capacity for digestion and absorption. In general, if you see puffiness or edema (water retention) in your face, tongue, or body, your digestive qi needs help. Do not expect to lose weight until your qi is strong enough to digest your food and eliminate excess water weight!

Observe Your Face

If you do not mark any of the points below, your digestive qi is in good order. However, there is always room for improvement.

___My complexion is lackluster or sallow.

___I have skin blemishes or a blotchy complexion.

___My face is puffy.

___I have bags or dark circles under my eyes.

A lackluster complexion indicates that digestion and/or breathing are troubled. Healthy skin breathes so that oxygen and nourishment fill the cells. It is not dull, thick, or rough from a lack of nutrients. A dull, grayish complexion indicates low vitality either from malnutrition or poor circulation. Blemishes may indicate that your diet is too sweet and spicy or that your body is not effectively eliminating acids and impurities. You may need to temporarily increase cleansing green foods that are laxative and diuretic and reduce acidic foods such as tomatoes, peppers, refined sugar, and hot spices.

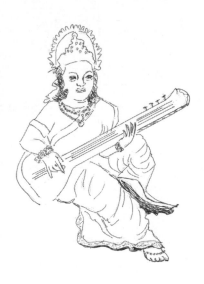

Low qi leads to a puffy face and water retention.

A puffy, waterlogged face and bags under the eyes are the best indication of facial edema resulting from inadequate digestive qi and vital energy. When you work long hours or travel long distances sitting in a car or airplane, your body backs up with excess water wastes. You may put on a pound or two, but excess weight usually leaves in a day. If you continually have a swollen face and eyelids, your digestive qi requires cleansing foods and herbs such as dandelion, alfalfa, or parsley to speed the elimination of water.

Observe your face and body regularly to monitor your energy as you add new foods.

Pay Attention to Vitality

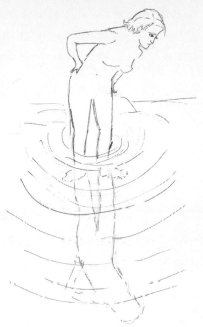

When your vitality is low, you have to be especially careful with diet. Here is an example of the importance of doing just that from my own health practice.

Sidney, age 70 and one of my clients, is sitting in the recovery room after cataract surgery. He is naturally pale and spacey after the procedure. His attention is excellent as he talks with his nurse. However, I can see that his vitality is low. His complexion is blotchy. His skin is thin and translucent with crusts of dry patches. He is tall and slender with long, bony fingers; thinning,

Dehydration of body fluids leads to chronic thirst, dry skin, and night sweats.

gray hair; and a long nose. Sidney is a Crane who teaches music. When we chat about his health, I learn that three of Sidney's brothers have died of prostate cancer, and his recent prostate test results were unfavorable. Sidney has heard about the importance of whole soy products to prevent prostate problems, so he eats soybeans daily. He makes a face, saying he is full of soybeans. Sidney has diabetes. The nurse gives him the usual apple juice fed to patients after surgery, although according to Chinese herbal experts, to maintain a healthy blood sugar balance, he should avoid all sweet foods, even beets and carrots. He drinks the juice passively. You don't have to be a genius to realize that Sidney is depressed and worried.

He asks my advice about foods for reducing prostate swelling. Because he is a Crane, Sidney will follow my advice to the letter and probably take it to extremes. Whole soy products; greens in the cabbage family; and anti-inflammatory, bitter, diuretic herbs such as dandelion, asparagus, and yucca are the best foods for Sidney's overall health and sensible weight loss. Fruit sugars are not useful for his diabetes, complexion issues, or latent prostate condition.

Observe Your Body

Put a check next to any observation that applies to you.

____I have water retention in my entire body.

____My legs and ankles are swollen.

____My muscles and flesh feel flabby.

____My muscle tone is poor.

____I drop things or bump into furniture when I am tired.

____I have lots of bruises that heal slowly.

____My excess weight is located at my abdomen and hips.

____I am overweight and out of shape from the chest to the groin.

In general, poor tone and excess water retention in the body indicate inadequate or troubled qi. Later in the book, we will determine its origin, which may be allergies or digestive and/or adrenal weakness. If you have poor coordination and drop things when you're tired, it may indicate poor muscle tone or fatigue, which requires rest.

Chronic slow healing, oozing wounds, bruises, and excess fat and cellulite indicate to a traditional Chinese doctor that the so-called spleen/pancreas needs attention. The Chinese medical concept of the spleen/pancreas is interesting. The organ system is supposed to keep the body in shape (prevent edema and cellulite) and prevent blood from escaping its vessels (excess bruising). The pancreas produces enzymes that facilitate the absorption of B vitamins. In other words, if digestive qi is weak, foods and supplements are washed through you without being absorbed. A diet that ignores your body's capacity for digestion, absorption, and elimination of wastes does only half its job.

The spleen/pancreas may be weakened from a diet of undernourishing or cold, raw foods or from chronic fatigue, illness, worry, or grief. If so, your body may not be able to absorb the nutrients necessary to reduce edema and cellulite and to strengthen blood vessels. I met a woman who had nursed her husband and lost him to cancer. She was overweight and had poor muscle tone and a large, puffy, pale tongue, indicating spleen/pancreas weakness and edema. She said that she was not depressed after the experience but that everything she ate turned into diarrhea and indigestion. A psychotherapist might say that she had "somatized" her loss—that is, experienced it as physical symptoms in place of emotional ones. A traditional Chinese medical specialist (a TCM doctor) would say that grief had weakened her spleen. Her reaction become part of her energy dynamic.

Overworking the spleen/pancreas by consuming overprocessed refined foods results in illness. Long before Western scientists discovered that the kitchen spice cinnamon increases insulin uptake and is, therefore, useful for diabetes, Chinese herbalists recommended pungent, drying herbs, including cinnamon, to heal and protect the spleen/pancreas. If you hold excess fat or water retention in the middle, your digestion needs attention. You may be spacey from hypoglycemia or always hungry from diabetes, but for now, we are concerned with your shape. (Special diets in Part 2 are recommended for both global edema and tummy fat.)

Observe Your Tongue

Asian tongue diagnosis is easy to use both for yourself and with your children. It lets you directly observe your present digestive energy. Put a checkmark next to any item that applies to you. Your tongue is:

___ Large, wet, and scalloped around the edges

___ Narrow, dry, red, or purplish

___ Very pale

___ Bright red with no coating

___ Coated with a watery film

___ Coated with a thick coating

___ Shaking

The appearance of your tongue may vary slightly from day to day, depending on your diet. However, we want to observe how it looks most often. Observe your tongue before brushing your teeth or eating so that no artificial color is added. Sit and look into a mirror, relax, and let it hang out. Observe daily how your tongue changes over a month.

How does a perfectly healthy tongue look? I probably have never seen one. Imagine a tongue that is neither too large nor too small, neither too wet nor too dry, neither too pale nor too red—a tongue that is right in the middle. The extremes are easier to notice because they indicate problems. First, we will observe the body of the tongue itself, not the coating.

SIZE: A large, pale tongue that is scalloped around the edges because it presses against the teeth indicates edema in the body from poor elimination of fluids. It would be wise to increase diuretic and strengthening foods such as ginger and mint tea; barley soup with parsley; cooked foods; and warming spices such as cardamom, clove, pepper, ginger, cinnamon, and asafoetida.

COLOR: A dry, red tongue indicates dehydration or inflammation and usually accompanies feverish illness or a chronic problem such as constant thirst, hot flashes, or night sweats. Often it is a smoker's tongue. People who exhaust natural fluids and vitality by working at night, have diabetes, or eat a very hot and spicy diet may have a dry, red tongue. You can begin to rehydrate your body with moistening foods such as American ginseng tea. You might also add cooling, cleansing foods (such as salads) and spices (such as cumin, coriander, and fennel) to your diet. A bright red or purple tongue with no coating shows even more inflammation and can indicate long-term illness or dehydration conditions.

COATING: The tongue coating indicates the acid/alkaline balance of the foods you are presently consuming. If your diet is alkaline or cold and raw, the coating will tend to be watery and pale. If your diet or stomach is too acidic, the coating will tend to be dry, thick, and yellow or dark.

SHAKING: A shaking tongue indicates nervous tension. Employ your nervous energy for weight loss by snacking with slimming foods, and use one of the homeopathic remedies recommended for emotional issues in Chapter 1.

Dealing with "Dampness"

Ancient Chinese and Ayurvedic medical texts addressed the individual causes of overweight, including slow digestion; a rich, sweet diet; emotional upset; and a humid climate that reduces vitality and increases edema. Like many of us, the Asian royal courts ate rich, complicated meals and suffered from body aches and indigestion. The herbal digestive treatments created to deal with these problems make up an essential part of your slimming program.

In Chinese medicine, overweight is treated as part of a larger category of imbalance called dampness (*shi*). Imagine a big, heavy cloud that fills your body with watery sludge. That is Chinese "dampness." The tongue looks thick, bloated, and coated. The person has a sluggish pulse and deep rheumatic pains that make the entire body feel leaden. People with edema drag their legs and feel short of breath when walking. People with dampness are weakened from slow digestion and a lack of oxygen. Their urine looks cloudy. They most likely sleep deeply and snore. Foods that are sweet and oily or rich and heavy destabilize blood sugar balance and increase these symptoms. A person with dampness can have either a pale or a red tongue, depending on his or her digestive qi.

In Ayurveda, a problem similar to dampness is called *kapha* imbalance. It involves excess *ama* (digestive wastes and poisons) resulting from poor digestion and a rich diet, which leads to excess phlegm, fat, body aches, tumors, and other conditions due to poor elimination of water and impurities from the body. The herbs, foods, and spices that treat both dampness and kapha conditions are digestive, cleansing, and stimulating.

You can use such TCM or Ayurvedic explanations as your guide. As your digestive qi improves, notice how your energy picks up, your tongue looks less coated and large, and your mental clarity and concentration return. They indicate that your digestion and metabolism have improved.

Doctors Frank Liu and Liu Yan Mau, in their 1980 book *Chinese Medical Terminology*, offer five commonsense warnings to avoid illness resulting from overeating.

- Avoid monotony in food choices and dietary habits.
- Avoid excess spicy foods—hot, sour, fried foods, salt, and sugar.
- Eat small meals and frequent snacks.
- Beware of exotic foods—snails, insects, etc.
- Do not let beverages take the place of food. Alcohol can cause serious damage to the liver.

Aside from the warning about eating snails, this resembles the current weight loss advice given by the Harvard University School of Public Health, which is:

- Eat less at meals, and eat slowly and at regular times of day.
- At restaurants, take home half your dish for a second meal.
- Exercise 1 hour a day.
- Drink lots of water and unsweetened juices.
- Choose healthy fats and eliminate trans fats.
- Avoid sugar and white flour products.
- Eat fruits, vegetables, whole grains, nuts, seeds, and healthy proteins.

Reading this long list of advice, you are likely to shrug and say, "That would be nice! Now give me the time and energy to do it." I do not blame you. Diets full of don'ts never last long. Stressing calories, portion sizes, and precise measures of harmful ingredients with a calculator in hand can make anyone give up. I personally do not count calories but sense when I feel out of shape or lethargic. That is enough for me to start my cleansing and slimming diet of bitter, pungent, and sour fresh fruits and vegetables and cleansing herbs. At the very least, I drink lots of strong green tea with and between meals to boost energy and metabolism.

Pay Attention to Portion Size

One thing that will help is to pay attention to the amount you eat, even when what's on your plate is slimming foods. First let's take a look at some new guidelines that *won't* be helpful. The government, as usual, has laid down rather complicated directions. *Bloomberg News* reported that the USDA recommends eating 3 ounces (85 grams) of whole grain foods, 2 cups of fruit, and 2½ cups of vegetables a day, as well as exercising daily for at least 30 minutes. The guidelines were recommended in January 2005 by a panel of scientists and doctors commissioned by the USDA and the US Department of Health and Human Services. For details, see the government Web site: www.mypyramid.gov.

The new food pyramid recommends calories that vary with age, sex, and physical activity. Here is their summary.

USDA Recommendations, Calories for Adults and Teens
- 1,600 for sedentary women and some older adults
- 2,200 for most children, teenage girls, active women, and sedentary men (more for pregnant or breastfeeding women)
- 2,800 for teenage boys, many active men, and very active women

According to the government's new food pyramid, if you are an active woman who needs about 2,200 calories a day, nine servings of breads, cereals, rice, or pasta are recommended, along with 6 ounces of meat or alternatives per day. If you follow these guidelines, the total fat (in the foods you choose, as well as fat used in cooking or added at the table) would be 73 grams per day. You won't lose weight that way, no matter how many times you take the stairs instead of the elevator!

Reading further into the pyramid, it gets even more complicated. You see that one serving of cooked cereal, rice, or pasta is equivalent to one slice of bread. For example: A slice of bread is one serving, so a sandwich equals two servings. A small bowl of cereal and one slice of toast for breakfast are two more servings. And if you have a cup of rice or pasta at dinner, that's two more servings. A snack of three or four small plain crackers adds yet another serving. One cup of milk or yogurt equals 1½ ounces of natural cheese or 2 ounces of processed cheese. But does a slice of pizza count as a serving of grain, dairy, or vegetable group?

For those of us who are mathematically challenged, weight loss comes as a result of sweating while figuring portion sizes when using the pyramid approach. It is enough to make you run screaming into an ice cream shop. Let's look at what the food pyramid recommends as lower, moderate, and higher portions.

Number of Daily Servings, According to the USDA

Lower Portions (about 1,600 calories)

Grains: 6 servings

Vegetables: 3 servings

Fruits: 2 servings

Milk products: 2 or 3 servings

Meats: 5 ounces

Total fat: 53 grams

Total added sugar: 6 teaspoons

Moderate Portions (about 2,200 calories)

Grains: 9 servings

Vegetables: 4 servings

Fruits: 4 servings

Milk products: 2 or 3 servings

Meats: 6 ounces

Total fat: 73 grams

Total added sugar: 12 teaspoons

Higher Portions (about 2,800 calories)

Grains: 11 servings

Vegetables: 5 servings

Fruits: 4 servings

Milk products: 2 or 3 servings

Meats: 7 ounces

Total fat: 93 grams

Total added sugar: 18 teaspoons

How could anyone of *any* size expect to lose weight eating 18 teaspoons of sugar a day? Get serious!

The government's answer is: "The best and simplest way to lose weight is to increase your physical activity and reduce the fat and sugars in your diet. But be sure to eat at least the lowest number of servings from the five major food groups in the Food Guide Pyramid." Using the MyPyramid.gov Web site, I entered information for several of my friends to check the results. To my surprise, two people with very different bodies were recommended a similar diet. The slender 5-foot-9 woman is 58 with strong digestion, and the overweight 5-foot-6 man is 68 with hypertension and poor digestion. But his number of recommended servings was higher than hers. Therefore, unfortunately, the food pyramid makes no allowance for individual differences such as body size, digestion, or illness. That's where this book comes in.

My Commonsense Guidelines

Simply telling people to eat less cannot work. The Baseline Diet prevents and treats illness, while promoting weight loss.

COMBINE YOUR FOODS WITH CARE. An important aspect of this diet that the government food pyramid fails to address is food combining. Reducing indigestion improves vitality and weight loss. When I have pasta, I avoid bread in the same meal because both increase dampness. (Cooking whole wheat pasta al dente reduces its stickiness.) I might have pasta with steamed vegetables and a light tomato sauce or a cheese-free pesto instead of a creamy sauce. When I have fish, I avoid milk, cheese, and eggs that day because they too are oily and fatty; the combination slows digestion (increases dampness.) That day becomes a fish day. Another day might be a dairy day.

PAY ATTENTION TO FLAVORS. Avoid combinations of rich, fat, oily, and sweet foods that hinder digestion. For example, don't have oysters, steak, creamed potatoes, and pie in the same meal or, better yet, the same day. If you consume a fatty food, add hot, spicy, pungent spices to speed digestion and bitter, sour tea to improve absorption and weight loss. Hot, sour, and bitter foods increase weight loss because they enhance cleansing.

CHOOSE VITALITY. It is important to consider the natural life force and flavor a food offers. This lifestyle considers the energy latent in foods and how it interacts with your qi. Every meal should enhance digestive qi. Savor the flavors and textures of wholesome foods. Reduce or eliminate animal fats and proteins, and you will soon see and feel the positive results.

TAKE YOUR TIME. Losing weight is easy when done carefully and gradually. You will improve your food karma as you feel stronger and less dependent on junk foods or stuck in negative emotions.

KEEP MOVING. Try to walk more often. Take the stairs. Rent an exercise bike to share with friends at the office. As you sit typing or watching the news, you might use an inexpensive electrical neuro-muscular stimulator to relax tense aching muscles and decrease your cellulite. (In Chapter 11, my chiropractor brother, Eric Hadady, and I offer slimming advice for people who do not like to exercise.)

BE KIND TO YOURSELF. High-powered, energizing herbs; relaxing hand and foot massages; herbal baths; and other treatments from this book are rejuvenating. Contact information for slimming products and home spa equipment are listed in the Natural Products and Information Resource Guide on page 348.

Observe Your Progress Daily

The better you observe and regulate your qi, the better you can improve weight loss. Take a few minutes daily to check these:

- **Tongue.** A pale tongue requires stimulating, digestive, warm cooked foods and pungent spices. A red, dry tongue requires more greens.
- **Facial tone and hue.** A puffy face may require more cleansing foods and diuretic teas. It may also indicate a need for rest and recuperation. A dull hue often indicates fatigue or the effects of addictions such as smoking.
- **Shape.** How do you feel in your body? Have you gained fat or water weight? Have fatigue, travel, or fatty or high-sodium

foods created water retention? Do you have achy legs or knees? We will learn targeted remedies that address these and other issues throughout this book.

Be Comfortable, Be Safe

Remember that it has required years for your body to take shape. Always be gentle with yourself when adding new foods and exercise. To avoid unpleasant side effects, never start the day with cold, raw foods, which weaken digestion. Also, use digestive remedies as needed for comfort.

Withdrawal symptoms may occur as the body fights against a dependency. By easing nervousness, irritability, or digestive discomforts with natural remedies, it becomes easier to reduce bad habits, lose weight, and gain lasting health. The table below indicates common withdrawal symptoms, ways to avoid them, and possible treatments.

SYMPTOM	PREVENTION	TREATMENT
Nausea	Reduce oily and fried foods.	Ginger tea
Headache	Avoid raw foods for breakfast.	Homeopathic Nux vomica 30C
Dizziness	Reduce dairy foods.	Ginger or mint tea
Acid reflux	Avoid hot spices.	¼ cup aloe vera juice in water 1–3 times daily, as needed
Diarrhea	Avoid excess salad.	Homeopathic Podophyllum 30C
Cramps/ indigestion	Simplify meals.	Licorice tea; homeopathic Lycopodium clavatum 30C
Irritability	Avoid hot spices and garlic.	Homeopathic Nux vomica 30C
Sinus congestion	Avoid dairy products.	Australian tea tree oil applied inside nose, using a cotton swab
Candida yeast	Avoid sugar and fruits.	1 drop Australian tea tree oil in water as tea 1–3 times daily
Depression	Reduce oily, sweet, and dairy foods.	Homeopathic Pulsatilla 30C

Pregnant women and new mothers are special cases. Childbirth dramatically pulls the energy meridians in the uterine area downward, which can cause a temporary prolapsed condition for internal organs and often results in diarrhea or incontinence. Women whose muscles are weakened by pregnancy may urinate a few drops when they sneeze. These women should avoid iced drinks and excess laxative foods and use tonic herbs such as astragalus (*huang qi*) to revive vital energy as quickly as possible. Simmer five to eight slices of astragalus root in 2 cups of water for 30 to 40 minutes, and drink the semisweet liquid throughout the day between meals.

Part 2

The Animal You

*The Baseline Diet in Part 1 fortifies digestion and absorption
for all persons. It detoxifies the body and prepares the mind
and spirit for a slenderizing lifestyle. Part 2 begins
the advanced level of this program. Use this section to
jump over a weight loss barrier and keep your slimming
program on track. In Part 2, you will address individual
weight and beauty issues according to your animal
energy type. You will talk to your totem.*

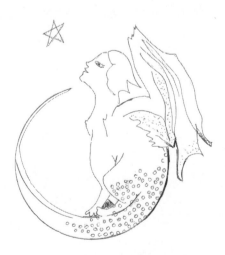

Chapter 5

Feed Your Tiger

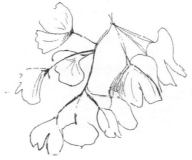

*D*ear Tiger,
I know you are too busy to eat properly. You would love to run, dance, swim, and work at all hours. This chapter suggests foods that nourish your nerves, muscles, and bones so that you may glide painlessly through your jungle. Asian herbs, including Siberian ginseng, gotu kola, and ginkgo, improve circulation and reduce cellulite. With them, you will create the endurance necessary to strive for your finest qualities, including patience. A wise cat learns to pace herself. To stand slender and strong, you need a solid foundation of good digestion, healthy blood production, and comfortable circulation.

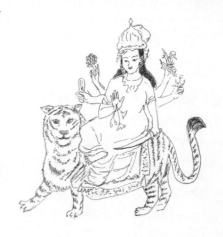

A Tiger has an oval face with regular features, engaging eyes, and a square chin. A healthy Tiger has an angular body with broad shoulders and no exceptional weight problems. Tigers troubled by poor circulation develop cellulite at the thighs and love handles at the hips. An excess acid condition resulting from poor digestion can aggravate swollen, painful joints; sharp nerve pains, such as facial neuralgia or sciatica; migraines; or allergies. Tigers tend to have poor calcium absorption and, thus, weak muscle tone and fragile bones. Calcium absorption affects muscles and circulation (because the heart is a muscle). Tense muscles lead to stiff shoulders, ringing in the ears, and vision problems.

You may spot a nearsighted Tiger with a dry, sallow complexion and liver spots squinting at a menu or wearing glasses. Deeply lined palms; dry, cracked skin on the hands and feet; and brittle fingernails with white spots indicate undernourished blood and inadequate calcium absorption. Tigers especially need vitamin D_3 daily from sunshine and from fatty fishes such as eel to discourage osteoporosis, autoimmune illnesses such as multiple sclerosis, prostate problems, and certain cancers.

Unlike group-oriented Bears, Tigers prowl alone or in small packs united by a competitive spirit. If something or someone gets in their way—watch out. They pounce upon new projects and personal relationships with zeal but become bored if unsuccessful. At their best, Tigers are ambitious, highly focused, and dedicated to a cause or relationship. Given the chance, they can be generous and understanding. A Tiger's natural enthusiasm makes him or her ready for any challenge. It shows up in a determined look and a tight jaw. Actress Katharine Hepburn's stunning performance on the screen or playing court demonstrates a Tiger's relentless climb to excellence. Tigers demand an open field.

When frustrated, a liverish Tiger develops headaches, liver pains, hives, rashes, cramps, and nervous tics. Timid Tigers simmer in a quiet rage for days or toss in bed during insomniac nights. Others explode in arguments and always feel better when they win. A Tiger's volcanic nature demands creative expression, or it may turn self-destructive. Chronic irritability or tunnel vision becomes possible when a Tiger remains isolated, bored, and frustrated too long.

Tigers make successful world travelers, athletes and sports pros, military personnel, police officers, firefighters, business executives, actors, designers, and dancers. Tigers work fast—if not constantly—and, of course, eat irregular meals. Overheated by stimulants or cold raw foods for breakfast, they usually develop an afternoon migraine. Digestive imbalance is indicated by a coated tongue and a wiry or bumpy, irregular pulse. Extreme diets, climate changes, and travel tie their digestion in knots. Tiger addictions tend to be spicy or fried foods, chips, nuts, chocolate, diet sodas, and alcohol. An addiction maintains homeostasis: Tigers are consummate nervous snackers who crave foods that overstimulate nervous habits.

Some Tigers are highly motivated dieters who follow weight loss directions to the letter. However, they change diets frequently. They need to realize that keeping fit requires a healthy lifestyle, not a battle. Tigers have problems with brick walls when they bump into one: If a diet does not meet their expectations, they blame the diet, not their poor digestive *qi*. Often their habits are not regular enough to maintain good digestion.

Tigers want a magic bullet: They are all about movement and transformation, not cooking and caring like Bears or exploration of personal feelings like Dragons. Restless Tigers thrive on challenges, real or imagined. Their drive and stamina seem to intensify from fatigue. Tigers embody the dynamic rebirth of spring. Among the Chinese five elements, the Tiger's is Wood, which engenders a yearning to procreate and roam free in the green, growing forest. Troubles occur when fire claims the trees.

This chapter helps Tigers—or anyone troubled by nervous eating habits, food allergies, and inflammatory nerve and joint pains—to safely reduce weight and cellulite. Stimulating, acidic foods that ordinarily slim a docile Bear or lethargic Dragon would severely irritate a Tiger, causing insomnia, a painful attack of sciatica, or a nasty bite for someone nearby.

One typical Tigress answered my weight loss questionnaire: "I hold all my weight in my thighs. I have given up sugar and dairy and all refined products. I am healthier since using your Baseline Diet. I now have energy to go to the gym and work out at home too. I have lost weight, from 152 down to 130, but I still have cellulite in really ugly thighs. I could jump out of my skin!"

Regulate Nervous Eating

Tigers are nervous snackers par excellence. Lack of exercise, prolonged mental activity, and excess caffeine equals poor muscle tone and cellulite. Tigers love the smell of fresh coffee and dark chocolate and the acidic bite of black tea. Some Tigers get so wrapped up in work that they forget to eat or to stop consuming caffeine stimulants. Then their muscles tense and shake. When famished, most people grab the wrong food. This chapter contains noncaffeinated slimming Tiger teas. There are a number of other things that can help.

HOMEOPATHIC NATRUM PHOSPHATE 6X. To ease nervous hunger, I recommend a natural acid neutralizer, homeopathic Natrum phosphate 6X (Sodium phosphate or Nat phos). Melt three pills under the tongue, or add three pills to 4 ounces of water and sip it between meals or 1 hour after eating. If you do not eat at all, sip the Nat phos water and breathe calmly for a moment every hour. That will help you to relax and think about something besides work.

Homeopathic Nat phos works as an antacid for the entire body. It facilitates the assimilation of fats and therefore melts the acid part of cellulite. A deficiency of natrum phosphate leads to a buildup of uric acid, causing joint stiffness and swelling, as well as water and fat trapped in the cells. When body fluids are alkaline, wastes, including cellulite, are discharged more effectively. Using Nat phos regularly also improves nervous tics, rashes, hives, and an acid stomach.

If your body requires Nat phos, you will notice dark urine, a yellow coating at the root of your tongue, nervous irritability, and insomnia. These symptoms go double for heavy drinkers of coffee and tea with caffeine. Bears, people who overeat sugary foods, also develop acidic blood and indigestion problems. If you get hungry at bedtime, become testy at PMS time, or suffer from rheumatism and lumbago, Nat phos may be all you need to reduce the acidic quality of your blood.

HOMEOPATHIC GELSEMIUM 30C. If you eat to soothe anxiety, find comfort, or relieve boredom, you may need something to directly address emotional balance. I recommend homeopathic Gelsemium 30C between meals. If you need both Gelsemium 30C for anxiety and Nat phos for acid burn, you might take Nat phos during the day and Gelsemium in the evening. When they start to work and acidity levels off, stop using the remedies until you need them again. You can expect to feel a difference within 1 to 3 days. During acute nervous attacks, you can alternate the remedies several times a day. In general, if nervous acidity feels emotional, with symptoms of anxiety, use Gelsemium. If it is physical, with burning indigestion, burping, constant hunger, gout, or an itchy rash, use Nat phos to put out the acid fire.

Diet and Withdrawal

Tigers—or anyone who tries to lose weight too quickly—are bound to develop withdrawal symptoms. I can't warn readers enough about dieting carefully and choosing healthy foods as a lifestyle instead of as a fast track on a crash course. Going to extremes in diet, adding new cleansing foods too quickly, or consuming raw foods first thing in the morning or when digestion is weak inevitably leads to headaches, dizziness, disorientation, and sometimes even hallucinations. The Tiger Diet offers protection while it helps cleanse the body.

We began with the Baseline Diet because it is slimming, cleansing, and balancing. Cleansing greens, fresh fruits, and raw vegetables are so rejuvenating, they unlock toxins and medical or street drugs that have been trapped in the body a long time. Sudden increased cleansing can temporarily throw you off balance.

Herbal digestive remedies can ease withdrawal symptoms for most people, especially those who have had a poor diet for many years or are recovering from illness or childbirth. As only one example, Ease Plus pills made by Health Concerns are based on a classic Chinese formula, Chai Hu Mu Li Long Gu Tang, recommended for nervousness, emotional distress, headache, withdrawal from tobacco, drugs, medicines, and addictions. It treats gastric acidity and ulcers, hiccupping, or belching.

I will describe how it works so that you can duplicate its actions with foods. The herbal pill combines calcium carbonate with herbs that condition the liver, such as bupleurum root (*chai hu*), skullcap, and rhubarb. Ginger and ginseng are stimulants that encourage digestion and absorption. Pinella and cinnamon are added to regulate the body's use of insulin and reduce phlegm and bloating. The manufacturer recommends the pills as a safe herbal Valium or Tagamet–type remedy.

Analyzing its components is useful when you're dealing with withdrawal. Liver-soothing, anti-inflammatory, and laxative herbs that enhance the flow of bile help calm nervous agitation. Rhubarb is laxative and helps eliminate uric acid. Ginger and warming spices enhance digestive qi. Calcium supports mental and emotional balance, as well as smooth circulation. This sure sounds like a remedy for PMS sufferers or anyone who goes overboard with angry or nervous emotions and food addictions. Knowing the energetic effects of herbs for withdrawal symptoms helps you to create a calming, balancing food substitute. (For example, see the Apple Rhubarb Pie recipe on page 129). To approximate the above herbal formula for withdrawal and transform it into a slimming meal, combine a slice of the pie with ginger tea and a slice of low-fat cheese.

Tiger Diet

To avoid problems associated with a Tiger's energy type, you can add the following specialized suggestions to the Baseline Diet as needed. I will make similar suggestions for the other energy types in later chapters. The Tiger Diet features mineral-rich, antacid, nonoily green foods, anti-inflammatory herbs, and balanced nutritional supplements that detoxify the liver and blood; tone metabolism; reduce fat and impurities; and support muscles, joints, and bones. Enhanced digestion and improved circulation reduce cellulite and facilitate free and easy movement. These dietary suggestions apply to athletes, people with arthritis or nerve diseases, women in perimenopause or menopause, and people with nervous eating habits, whether or not they are overweight.

Slimming Teas

Teas suitable for Tigers decrease stomach acidity, constipation, and water retention in the lower body. Enjoy at least 6 to 8 cups from among the following teas daily with and between meals.

- **Chinese bitter melon tea**, often sold as Cherry Grain Balsam Pear Tea, is made from dried, sliced bitter melon, a cooling, detoxifying vegetable. This tea also works well for Bears, especially when treating diabetes.
- **Tu Chung** is the name of a Chinese herbal tea that is made from *Eucommiae ulmoidis* bark. It is recommended for smooth joint action, backache, and hypertension. It can also help reduce arthritis pain. Tu Chung makes a pleasant tea you can sweeten with vanilla (sugar irritates nerve and joint pain).
- **Sorig Tripa Tea** is a Tibetan tea used for cooling and calming body and mind, restoring healthy blood pressure, and healing the liver. Order it from www.tibetan-medicine.org.
- **White and green teas** are more slimming than coffee. They contain no calories, and they improve metabolism. Unlike coffee, they neither overstimulate the kidneys nor cause digestive cramps. For jaundice or nausea, add sliced fresh ginger and mint leaves to stimulate liver function. White tea, which is low in caffeine, contains the most antioxidants and is the least processed tea. People with weak digestion, cancer, or chronic illness are advised to drink broccoli green tea.
- **Roasted chicory bark** works well for java drinkers. Caffeine from coffee and tea can increase nervous snacking and nerve pains. Simmer 1 teaspoon of dried roasted chicory powder per cup of hot water for 5 minutes. It tastes somewhat like espresso. Sweeten with a dash of cardamom powder, or add turmeric for an extrabitter taste. No sugar or honey, please.

- **Turmeric**, an anti-inflammatory root, resembles ginger and enhances circulation and digestion. It has proven anticancer effects and is recommended for arthritis pain and stiffness. Add ¼ teaspoon of turmeric powder, available from the supermarket, per cup of warm water or tea.
- **Several cooling, semibitter spices** reduce acidity. Add ¼ teaspoon each of coriander, fennel, and cumin powder to 1 cup of water as an antacid tea. Coriander is diuretic. Fennel reduces indigestion, and cumin reduces stomach acid burn. This is a good tea to use before and during allergy season to reduce irritating acid-related symptoms including irritability, rash, insomnia, dyspepsia, and ulcer pain.
- **Yin/Yang Sisters brand instant beverages** include eight beverages made by a Chinese hospital and sold online at www.eastearthherb.com and at some Chinese herb shops. Each foil packet contains finely powdered herbs that can be added to water or juice. The best ones for Tigers include Get Svelte, Clean Habits, and Happy Garden Tea. Get Svelte contains hawthorn berry, which strengthens the heart muscle and reduces harmful cholesterol. Drink one to three packs daily. Clean Habits, a bitter/sweet-tasting liver cleanser, reduces liver pain, jaundice, skin blemishes, and irritability. You might add it to your morning tea or to tomato juice. Happy Garden Tea is soothing for a calm night's sleep.

Coffee Substitutes

Caffeine found in coffee, tea, and chocolate irritates nerve pains and encourages insomnia. Overstimulating the body eventually leads to water retention and cellulite. Decaffeinated coffee is not your answer. In the decaffeination process, manufacturers use methylene chloride, which causes a carbon-to-chlorine bond in the body characteristic of toxic insecticides. *Earl Mindell's New Vitamin Bible* recommends using Chinese ginseng for an energy lift. Avoid it if you have insomnia, high blood pressure, or a fever condition, such as hot flashes and night sweats.

If avoiding coffee gives you a headache, consider using herbs for withdrawal, such as Ease Plus described on page 107. A homeopathic remedy called Coffea cruda 30C can be helpful for insomnia and anxiety. Another good remedy to take the edge off symptoms is Caffeine Withdrawal made by Natra-Bio. Its ingredients include homeopathic chamomile, Nux vomica, Spanish fly, and guarana. If you overuse caffeine today, tomorrow you may develop a backache, chronic fatigue, cellulite, and gum or tooth troubles.

Instead of using coffee to increase mental focus and memory, try gotu kola tea. Strong doses of 500 milligrams or more are recommended for preventing fatigue during athletic competitions. However, the tea is milder and more balancing. Gotu kola (*Brahmi*) is originally from India, where Ayurvedic herbal doctors sometimes called it the semen of Lord Shiva, because it improves mental powers and awakens universal understanding. You can enjoy gotu kola tea all day for promoting smooth, steady, and calm energy.

Cleansing, Balancing Foods

Since Tigers run on hype much of the time, their digestion and blood tend to be acidic, which causes all sorts of irritations and allergies, burping, indigestion, rashes, and insomnia. (If you get late-night phone calls, it is because Tigers believe that *everyone* gets to sleep at 3:00 a.m.) That's why foods that help deal with excess acid are perfect for Tigers.

Foods that neutralize acid include those that contain potassium—greens, vegetables, and some cereal grains. Also helpful are those that contain sodium—ripe fruit, whey, and okra. The silicon found in oatmeal is helpful, as is the magnesium found in apples, figs, ripe lemons, grapefruit, dark green vegetables, yellow corn, seeds, and nuts, especially almonds.

GREEN ALKALINE, CLEANSING FOODS stimulate the flow of laxative bile, helping to remove many impurities from the body.

Every day, have plenty of raw or steamed salad greens, especially parsley, celery, cucumber, watercress, asparagus, zucchini squash, okra, and cabbage (red, green, and Chinese). If foods in the cabbage family such as Brussels sprouts, cauliflower, and broccoli cause indigestion, steam them lightly in a little water with caraway and anise powder.

You can make a fat-free dressing to enjoy with your greens using mashed pumpkin, red pepper, lemon juice, and a little fresh garlic.

STIMULATING, SHARP, OR BITTER FLAVORS, such as watercress, are especially recommended for weight loss.

NATURAL HIGH-SODIUM FOODS include overripe plums, figs, apricots, and nearly rotten citrus. These help ensure comfortable joints and easy movement. I sun-ripen fruit in a metal basket hung in my window for more than a week after buying it green, hard, and tasteless from the supermarket. Natural sodium, which improves calcium absorption and reduces arthritis and bone spurs, tastes sweet, not salty. Soak all dried fruits overnight or bring them to a boil, soak for 15 minutes, and then discard the water, which contains most of the sugar.

FOODS HIGH IN MINERALS include fresh raw goat milk and Mt. Capra powdered goat whey, which can be added to teas, soups, or to raw goat cheese. Figs and goat dairy make a complete protein meal that supports joint comfort.

BARLEY is recommended by Ayurvedic doctors for the treatment of rheumatism because it is not "unctuous." Sticky foods such as yogurt, cream cheese, and rice congest circulation, whereas foods cooked with garlic and turmeric stir digestion and circulation.

SELECTED PROTEIN FOODS. A Tiger's best protein sources do not irritate the liver or impair circulation: for example, almonds and almond milk; small portions of fatty fishes such as tuna, salmon, and eel; goat or sheep dairy; or tofu served with vegetables. To avoid indigestion and cramps, never combine a dairy product with meat or fish. The Baseline Diet warns against mixing too many proteins, which taxes digestion and causes fat. A complete meal might be a handful of almonds with celery and an apple or figs and goat cheese.

To make almond milk, soak ¼ cup (2 ounces) of peeled almonds overnight in water, discard the liquid, then blend the nuts with 1 cup of water or low-fat milk. You may sweeten it with vanilla extract. One ounce of whole almonds yields 6 grams of protein, compared with 8 grams of protein for 1 ounce of lean roast beef.

Tiger Greens: Herbs and Supplements

Eating on the run and under stress increases acid stomach and cramps. Leafy greens make the body alkaline as they calm digestion and cleanse the blood of impurities, but Tigers are often challenged when it comes to getting their greens. Tigers who prefer restaurant hopping to cooking at home will appreciate the following green supplements. Dandelion reduces fat, fibroids, water retention, and stones. It is slightly laxative and diuretic. Alfalfa tablets and chlorophyll capsules make the digestive tract more alkaline and therefore enhance cleansing. All three greens help to soothe acidity. Here are several ways for Tiger's to get the benefits of greens. Which do you prefer?

- **DANDELION CAPSULES:** Take three or four with meals.
- **ALFALFA TABLETS:** Crack open three and swallow them with water with meals.
- **CHLOROPHYLL CONCENTRATE CAPSULES:** Take one to three with meals.
- **GARLIC/PARSLEY OIL CAPSULES:** Take one or two daily with meals. (One capsule can be used daily as a rectal suppository as an antiyeast and antiparasite treatment.)
- **POWER MUSHROOMS** by Health Concerns: Take six pills daily for energy and immunity. *Fu ling*, one of its diuretic ingredients, is helpful for cellulite and joint swelling. As a substitute, use 20 drops three times daily of reishi mushroom extract, an anti-inflammatory, anticancer mushroom that strongly supports energy in order to rid the body of wastes.
- **MIXED TRACE MINERAL SUPPLEMENT:** This contains manganese for liver health. Follow directions on the bottle.

Banishing Cellulite and Other Tiger Challenges

Think of cellulite as being made of fat, impurities, and water held in place by poor circulation and slow metabolism. Women most often develop cellulite at the abdomen, hips, and thighs after menopause because of reduced estrogen. This hormone makes the breasts and skin plump and youthful and delays menstruation until the correct time in the cycle. Especially with reduced estrogen, we need to help the body redistribute water in the cells and eliminate acid wastes that underlie cellulite.

The best order to follow when eliminating wastes from the body and enhancing circulation is to first reduce acidity and impurities with green foods and supplements and then increase circulation. To accomplish this, take the recommended green foods, such as chlorophyll and dandelion capsules, until some water retention is reduced from the legs and abdomen. Your bowel movements and urination will increase and will, of course, look green. You should use these supplements until signs of inflammation, such as fever, facial flushing, hot flashes, and night sweats, are reduced. Then you can add herbs to stimulate circulation and reduce cellulite. Otherwise, if unaddressed, excess acidity will continue to irritate, and you may develop complexion blemishes or other problems. Persons with fragile capillaries or varicose veins should proceed with caution.

Three basic herbs do the trick to enhance leg circulation and reduce cellulite anywhere in the body. They are Siberian ginseng, gotu kola, and ginkgo.

SIBERIAN GINSENG, like other adaptogenic herbs in the ginseng family, helps us adjust to fatigue, stress, and irregular and harsh climates. Because adaptogenic herbs help auto-regulate the body, they reduce many discomforts. Lower doses of Siberian ginseng, such as 500 milligrams per day, are enough to calm nervous energy and reduce nerve and muscle pain.

However, to reduce cellulite, you have to take enough to boost metabolism. That may be from 1,500 to 2,000 milligrams daily. Start by taking one capsule of 500 milligrams after one meal daily, and gradually increase the dose. If you are truly exhausted, you may need a nap after the first dose. Your body takes the stimulation it needs from adaptogenic herbs so that eventually you feel stronger. Cut back the dose if more than 1,000 milligrams daily makes you feel too hyper or gives you insomnia.

GOTU KOLA, already mentioned as a good substitute for coffee, is another adaptogenic herb that balances nervous energy and enhances circulation. It can also be taken in capsules. Smaller doses, such as 100 milligrams daily, are calming; larger doses, such as 500 to 1,000 milligrams, stimulate circulation in the legs. You might start with one 500-milligram capsule of Siberian ginseng along with two 500-milligram capsules of gotu kola daily between meals, then increase the dose as needed. You should feel a comfortable rush of circulation in the legs.

GINKGO, an herb often recommended for poor memory and sexual weakness, stimulates circulation in the small blood vessels of the brain and the entire body. It will bring nourishment from your green foods and supplements such as chlorophyll and dandelion to the surface of your skin, reducing cellulite. Use a dose that is equal to that of gotu kola.

You may need to use Siberian ginseng, gotu kola, and ginkgo for up to 6 months before you see marked improvements in your cellulite. Some people see and feel improvements in just 1 week. The rejuvenating treatment from these herbs has many lasting benefits, including improved elasticity of blood vessels.

During my clinical weight loss observations, I recommended a number of anticellulite products, including some Chinese diuretic herbs. The fastest results came from two Chinese herbal pills made by Health Concerns: Drain Dampness and Laminaria 4. It pays to analyze how they work energetically for problems of obesity, extreme widespread cellulite, or hypothyroid issues.

DRAIN DAMPNESS is traditionally recommended to reduce edema (water retention), joint swelling, a sensation of heaviness in the body, ascites (pockets of fluid in the abdomen) resulting from cirrhosis, urinary retention, and prostate swelling. It has also been used for gastroenteritis, hepatitis, and related low vitality. The pills combine diuretic herbs alisma (*ze xie*), poria (*fu ling*), and a medicinal fungus, *Polyporus clerotium* (*zhu ling*), known to prevent certain cancers. Also added are cinnamon, which tones spleen qi energy, and an aromatic middle-slimming herb called atractylodes (*bai zhu.*) The bottom line is that herbs that increase urination and sweating help reduce water retention. The traditional Chinese formula upon which Drain Dampness is based is called Wu Ling San.

Such an herbal formula might be used short term for leg swelling from jet travel or long term for swelling of the entire body or joint swelling in arthritis. You can combine some of these herbs on your own to make a daily tea to reduce water retention and cellulite. To use our recipe for Shiitake/Fu Ling Tea (page 45), add up to ¼ teaspoon of cinnamon per quart of tea. Drink as much as you like between meals, but stop at least 2 hours before bed.

LAMINARIA 4 pills contain laminaria and sargassum seaweeds and two seashells, all of which provide calcium, potassium, and iodine. I once asked a French endocrinologist, Yves Requena, MD, about the best herb for cellulite. His quick reply: laminaria seaweed, a form of kelp.

It looks light green and puffy in Chinese supermarkets, where it is sometimes labeled "*kun bu*" or simply "seaweed." Chinese products including seaweeds have been known to be mislabeled, however. A safe source is Laminaria 4 pills.

The Chinese remedy is often recommended for toning the thyroid and stimulating digestion and elimination. It can be used as an adjunct remedy for phlegmy fibroids. Hypothyroid (low thyroid) conditions commonly include listless energy and borderline depression.

A VARIETY OF SEAWEEDS might also prove helpful. If you feel heavy, sleepy, or phlegmy, or if your legs and belly are full of cellulite, you will benefit from ingesting stimulating seaweeds such as nori, hijiki, dulce, and laminaria. Nori provides protein; hijiki provides calcium; and dulce and laminaria are stimulating. Some Tigers should avoid kelp because it overworks the thyroid. Overstimulating the thyroid can drive a Tiger over the edge with emotional freak-outs and all-night insomnia. (Dragons with global edema need kelp more than Tigers do.)

Laminaria can be ordered online from Chinese herbal stores such as www.asiachi.com and cooked at home as a side dish with vegetables and fish. You have to soak and strain one handful of dried laminaria, changing the water many times until it is clear, because it comes full of soil and tiny shells from the China Sea.

For sources of seaweed from the coast of Maine, see the Natural Products and Information Resource Guide on page 348.

Varicose Veins

Heavy legs and varicose veins are common problems that arise along with cellulite.

HOMEOPATHIC CALCIUM FLUORIDE 6X can help with poor circulation resulting in cracked skin on hands and feet, bleeding gums, and varicose veins. Add three pills to 4 ounces of water, and sip it during your daily exercise or between meals.

Constipation

Constipation is not limited to Tigers, but it is a particular problem for this energy type. It results from stress, inactivity, or internal dryness. Tigers get tied in knots from nervous spasms and long car rides.

TRY A MASSAGE. Gently massage the abdomen downward from the navel toward the legs while breathing deeply and relaxing.

TAKE A LAXATIVE. My favorite stimulant laxative is a combination of one or two capsules of hawthorn berry, which tones circulation and reduces cholesterol, taken with one or two capsules of cascara sagrada, a bitter-tasting stimulant laxative that increases peristalsis. Take them once or twice daily as needed to promote effective fast-track elimination.

REACH FOR ALOE VERA GEL. You can add aloe vera gel to water, teas, or juice to soothe spasms and reverse dryness.

TRY A TRADITIONAL METHOD. Older Chinese people cook a handful of dried peach kernels in water and drink it as a moistening tea. Tamarind concentrate is a sour-tasting fruit paste that's used in Indian cooking. One-half teaspoon added to 1 cup of water works quickly and painlessly as a laxative.

STAY HYDRATED. Drinking lots of water does not always result in regularity, but it helps to flush impurities from the kidneys. For variety, simmer 1 to 2 cups of broccoli and other vegetables such as potato peelings, asparagus, artichoke, or carrot tops in 1 quart of water for 15 minutes. Drink the cooking water hot or cold.

Overweight, Arthritis, and Rheumatism

The connection between overweight and arthritis and rheumatism was made many years ago by Ayurvedic physicians. Think of joint pain and swelling as a result of impurities lodged in the body because of poor digestion, insufficient exercise, and a diet of sweet or oily, hard-to-digest foods and meat. A rich diet, napping after meals, and constipation can aggravate crippling pain. Impurities become trapped in the intestinal tract and eventually affect the joints and heart. The result is bloating, malaise, lethargy, feverish discomforts, and swollen and painful joints, bones, and cervical and thoracic vertebrae. Hip joint pain makes walking difficult. Scapula pain keeps the shoulders tense and reduces arm movements. There are a number of approaches to alleviating these conditions.

BE CAREFUL WHEN FASTING. Traditional Ayurvedic doctors Vaidya Bhagwan Dash and Acarya Manfred Junius in their book *A Hand Book of Ayurveda*, published in 1987, recommend avoiding excess fasting, which may result in aggravation of nervousness and pain.

SELECT THE RIGHT FLAVORS. Medicines and foods should be bitter, pungent, stimulating for digestion, and purgative (strongly laxative). By adding ginger, garlic, and turmeric to the diet, you can increase digestion and reduce impurities. You might add ¼ teaspoon of turmeric powder to your morning cup of tea or juice.

TRY INDIAN HERBS. One useful Indian herb is carminative (gas-relieving) haritaki churna (powdered *Terminalia chebula retz*), a rejuvenating fruit recommended for many digestive and nervous disorders, including vomiting, diarrhea or constipation, prolapsed uterus, malabsorption, bloating, intestinal parasites, tumors, jaundice, edema, nervousness, diseases affecting the spleen and heart, and skin rashes. Haritaki fruit is astringent: It makes your mouth pucker. Astringent herbs help eliminate impurities and check excessive discharges such as sweating, menstrual bleeding, vaginal discharge, and loss of sperm.

The best way to use haritaki is in a traditional formula made into a pill called triphala or a powder called triphala churna. The three dried fruits in triphala churna—haritaki, amla, and bibhitake—tone and recondition the digestive tract, eliminate poisons from the entire body, and regulate bowel movements, thus helping with either chronic constipation or diarrhea.

You can add ¼ teaspoon of either haritaki churna or triphala churna to tea, water, or juice once or twice daily with meals to speed weight loss, reduce digestive and other impurities, ease digestive discomforts, and tone abdominal muscles. Haritake is hotter—more pungent—than triphala. Both are safer than over-the-counter weight loss stimulants.

To normalize digestion and elimination and improve circulation for preventing and treating arthritis and rheumatism, use ginger, garlic, turmeric, triphala churna, or haritaki churna in tea. It's also helpful to take guggul capsules. You can read about guggul, a purifying and healing tree gum similar to myrrh, in the chapter for Bears. Bears overindulge in sweets and enjoy an afternoon nap, which sometimes turns into hibernation. They develop fat and aches from such habits. (After a lovely meal of leafy greens, fish, or tofu, it is better to take a stroll in the sun.)

Sunshine and Vitamin D

The sun lifts our spirits and for that reason enhances digestion, circulation, and well-being. The *Washington Post* (May 2004) reported another reason to bask in the sun. Most Americans, particularly African Americans, suffer from an unrecognized deficiency of vitamin D, which we get from sunshine. Ultraviolet rays act on the skin to produce the vitamin, which is absorbed into the body. The lack of vitamin D increases bone-thinning osteoporosis, life-threatening bone fractures, and severe tooth decay. A generation of sun avoiders is also beginning to see serious diseases related to vitamin D deficiency—many forms of cancer, high blood pressure, depression, and immune-system disorders, such as multiple sclerosis, rheumatoid arthritis, and diabetes.

Doctors have observed adults disabled by severe muscle weakness and pain until they were treated for a vitamin D deficiency. There is even a current rise in rickets cases, a bone disorder caused by vitamin D deficiency that leads to bowlegs and other bone malformations. Because the nutrient's apparently widespread functions in the body are just now being recognized, little research has been done to try to answer some of the most basic questions, such as how much is needed for optimal health.

One thing is clear: We need more vitamin D as we age and gain weight. Research has shown that vitamin D gets trapped in fat, so obese people have lower blood levels of D. They also have higher rates of cancer. People with diabetes are also prone to cancer, and their damaged kidneys have trouble converting vitamin D into a form the body can use.

The amount of vitamin D absorbed from the sun depends on where a person lives, skin pigment, age, and other factors. Dark-skinned people and anyone living in northern latitudes make far less than other groups. With people spending more time indoors and using sunscreen, and with smog obscuring the sun on many days, the amount of vitamin D people create naturally has become very low, many scientists say.

Milk is fortified with vitamin D, but most Americans get very little through their diets. That is not the case in Japan, where eel, a good source of vitamin D, is a favorite dish—and the number of people suffering from prostate and breast cancer is very low, compared with rates in America. Reinhold Vieth, PhD, a University of Toronto vitamin D researcher, has said, "There's been a lot of evidence emerging that indicates there's more to vitamin D than we thought. For me, it's a no-brainer: We're not getting enough."

A number of studies have found low levels of vitamin D in children, the elderly, and women. One federal study of women nationwide found that nearly half of African American women of childbearing age may be deficient.

Vitamin D interacts with every tissue in the body. The incidence of certain diseases seems to vary, depending on sun exposure and vitamin D levels. Breast, colon, and prostate cancer increase the farther you get from the equator, where exposure to ultraviolet light from the sun is greatest. "The highest rate of prostate cancer is among African Americans, followed by countries in northern Europe," said Gary G. Schwartz, PhD, MPH, a cancer researcher at Wake Forest University School of Medicine in Winston-Salem, North Carolina. "One way that they are alike is that both groups have very low levels of vitamin D."

Vitamin D appears to regulate the immune system, and researchers have found associations among sun exposure, vitamin D levels, and the incidence of autoimmune diseases such as multiple sclerosis, lupus, and diabetes—all diseases in which the immune system attacks the body. Some studies suggest vitamin D can reduce blood pressure, which would cut the risk for heart disease and strokes. Others suggest that low vitamin D levels may contribute to depression and other psychiatric conditions.

"It's a major health problem," said Michael F. Holick, PhD, MD, a Boston University scientist who is the most prominent proponent of the role of vitamin D in health. Dr. Holick argues that instead of the current recommended dose of 200 to 600 international units a day, most people should be getting at least 1,000 units a day. Dr. Holick agrees with nutritionist Bernard Jensen, PhD, who recommends exposing the face, hands, arms, legs, and back to the sun for 15 minutes a day, a few days a week.

Because ultraviolet light contained in sunlight may increase skin cancer and wrinkles, many experts say people can get enough safely by taking vitamin D supplements, sidestepping the contentious sunlight debate. Food sources of vitamin D include fish liver oils, sardines, herring, salmon, tuna, and fortified milk and dairy products. (Autoimmune illnesses are aggravated by cow dairy, not goat or sheep dairy.) If you have never eaten baked eel—*unagi*—from a Japanese restaurant, I strongly recommend its mildly sweet flavor. I enjoy baked eel along with hijiki seaweed salad, an excellent source of calcium. Grilled sardines are an excellent dish at fine Spanish and Portuguese tapas bars.

Vitamin D supplements work best when taken with vitamins A and C, choline, calcium, and phosphorus. Taken with vitamins A and C, it helps prevent colds and conjunctivitis (pinkeye). Vitamin D, being fat soluble, is absorbed with fats through the intestinal walls. A good time to take vitamins A and D, calcium, and other supplements for joint comfort is at breakfast with (naturally acidic) fruit and tea. The Vitamin Shoppe makes a dry, nonoily vitamin A and D capsule using cholecalciferol as vitamin D. For comfortable digestion, use non–fish oil vitamin D if your meal includes dairy or eggs.

If you live in an overcast or northern climate like New England or Seattle, increase your vitamin D intake, especially during the winter, when sunlight is reduced. Research done in Maine shows that we lose bone mass in the lower back and legs more during winter than at any other time of year. Vitamin D, calcium, and vitamin C improve circulation, muscle mass, and stamina, which helps reduce cellulite. Getting enough vitamin D certainly improves your form and endurance for running, walking, and swimming—a Tiger's favorite exercises.

Tiger Meals

The following dishes feature antacid ingredients that balance spicy or sharp flavors. In particular, cumin, coriander, fennel, mint, and dill reduce a Tiger's stomach acidity and help prevent reflux. Avoid butter, salt, and hot spices such as cayenne. In some cases, Chinese tree ear, also known as wood ear fungus (*Auricularia auricula*), is added as a blood-thinning ingredient helpful for hypertension and poor circulation. Turmeric powder lends a spicy flavor, stirs circulation, balances the pH of intestinal flora, and eases inflammatory nerve and joint pains. I would not be surprised if turmeric also reduced impurities that underlie cellulite. Tofu and tempeh are recommended throughout the book as substitutes for animal protein, known to aggravate calcium loss in the urine.

A Tiger Breakfast

A typical breakfast for feline friends includes one or two acidic fruits, a calcium source, and a low-fat protein. For example, fresh papaya, pineapple, apricots, berries, or black cherries can be enjoyed with a small container of low-fat yogurt and 1 teaspoon of milled flaxseeds. For convenience, black cherry concentrate can be added to water as a liver-cleansing juice. Flaxseeds provide protein and healthy omega-3 oils.

An apple and a handful of walnuts or no more than 2 ounces of sheep or goat cheese is also tasty. (Casein, the protein in cow dairy, aggravates the autoimmune responses that inflame arthritis and other discomforts.)

One block of tofu contains a day's quota of vitamins, calcium, and protein. I like tofu served cold and sliced, with a dash of soy sauce, vinegar, and dried seaweed, but it can be scrambled with onions, sesame salt, and grapeseed oil or steamed. The Chinese enjoy silken tofu warmed with a little sweet sauce such as maple syrup. People with diabetes can sweeten foods with stevia, an herbal powder that lowers blood sugar.

Hot green tea with lemon or a slimming herb tea such as Get Svelte rounds out the meal. Joint comfort supplements, including calcium, magnesium, and vitamins D, A, and C, would help to ensure bone and joint comfort.

Salads and Greens

Salads and steamed greens are mainstays of the Tiger diet because they are both nourishing and antacid. Bitter greens reduce a sweet tooth, energize digestion, and eliminate water retention, which maintains cellulite. Here are some helpful greens to add to salads: dandelion, endive, chicory, Chinese cabbage, red cabbage, beet greens, watercress, amaranth, raw asparagus, fresh herbs (such as mint, dill, parsley, and cilantro), and dried nori seaweed.

Steam kale, escarole, or endive, and serve with sesame seeds. They are high in vitamin A, iron, and potassium and make the body more alkaline.

For joint comfort, slice one or two raw okra spears into your salad. Okra, high in the natural sodium necessary for joints, is slimming for the body and moistening for the bowel.

Although carrots and beets contain a lot of sugar, their greens are high in potassium and iron. Simmer for 10 minutes in 1 cup of water a handful each of carrot tops, red radish tops, and white potato peelings. Strain well because radish tops contain spiny stickers that hurt the throat. Drink this brew as a natural mineral supplement, or add some to your salad dressing.

TIGER PAWS SALAD DRESSING

Tigers have problems with calcium absorption that often lead to joint, muscle, and bone pain. They usually respond well to diuretic herbs. Celery has been shown to reduce hypertension and ease movement. Lucky for us, it also reduces cellulite. I add celery extract to salad dressing because my hypertensive Bear complains that celery gets stuck in his teeth.

MAKES ENOUGH FOR ONE LARGE GREEN SALAD

> 4 tablespoons canola or extra-virgin olive oil
> Juice of ½ fresh lemon
> 1 clove minced garlic
> Dash of turmeric powder
> Chopped fresh parsley sprigs
> Fresh chervil, oregano, and dill (optional)
> 10–20 drops celery extract

Combine all the ingredients in a glass jar and shake until blended. This dressing keeps well for several days when refrigerated.

Potato Substitutes

Steamed parsnips, parsley root, and anise herb make delicious starch substitutes that are especially beneficial for the liver. Parsley root is blood purifying and stimulating for cleansing diets. It is high in iron, copper, and manganese, nutrients that are especially beneficial to the liver. You can add any of these substitutes to soups or enjoy them instead of potatoes. Cooked yucca, a Latin American favorite, provides nourishment and ease of movement for joints. Peel the hard skin from yucca found in the supermarket, and simmer it in water until it's tender enough to slice. Season with steamed garlic, onions, and a little grapeseed oil.

Bitter Melon

Momordica charantica is commonly known in America as bitter melon or balsam-pear bitter melon, in the Philippines as *ampalay*, in China as *ku gua* or *lai gua*, in India and the Caribbean as *karela*. Fresh green bitter melon can be found in Chinese and East Indian food shops in major American cities. Japanese bitter melon (*niga uri*) is among the foods eaten daily in Okinawa, an area where people commonly live to be over 100. Bitter melon is an annual climbing vine with hand-shaped leaves. The fruit is spindle shaped and light green. The form found most often in Indian markets has many small lumps and knobs. The one in Chinese markets has deep grooves that run lengthwise.

Since as early as the 1940s, scientific research in many countries has supported the traditional belief in bitter melon's health benefits. Several key compounds have been identified, including charantin, vicine, peptides, and polypeptide-p (a plant insulin). Eaten regularly, bitter melon is an important addition to a low-fat, high-fiber diet. It is often recommended in Asia for maintaining a healthy weight and blood sugar level.

Bitter melon contains protein, fat, calcium, phosphorus, iron, carotene, vitamins B_1, B_2, and C, proline, citrulline, and pectin, to name just a few nutrients. The flavor is bitter, but many people love it sautéed or added to soups.

A mild-tasting tea made from the dried sliced melon is sold online at www.asiachi.com as Cherry Grain Balsam Pear Tea. I add a handful of the tea to soups.

Dehydrating is a method of food preparation that retains 95 to 97 percent of the nutrients in fresh foods. To make dried bitter melon slices, blanch the melon in hot water, adding ½ teaspoon of salt. Let it soak for 5 minutes. Remove it from the water and slice the melon in half lengthwise to remove the core and seeds. Slice it crosswise into ⅛-inch pieces. Soak the slices in lemon juice for 5 minutes to protect the delicate green color, then drain on a paper towel to remove excess moisture. Place the slices in a single layer, so that they do not touch, in a dehydrator set at 120°F for 10 to 12 hours, until the slices are brittle. Store the dried bitter melon slices in a freezer zip-top bag for up to 1 year. If moisture appears on the inside of the bag, dry the slices again.

Bitter melon is famous throughout Asia and the Caribbean as a powerfully cleansing, slimming food. It has antiviral properties and is recommended for diabetes and hypertension. It cools heatstroke and strongly detoxifies the body, while it reduces fat and cellulite and helps treat diabetes. You can find more information about bitter melon, including testimonials from doctors and international sources for ordering it, at www.charanteausa.com.

Bitter Melon with Black Bean Sauce

This recipe makes a spicy side dish to accompany meats, vegetables, or brown rice.

MAKES 4 SERVINGS | PREPARATION TIME: 25 MINUTES

- *1 tablespoon dry sherry*
- *1 tablespoon light soy sauce*
- *1 tablespoon cornstarch*
- *1 pound bitter melon*
- *½ teaspoon salt*
- *2 tablespoons grapeseed oil, divided*
- *1 red bell pepper, thinly sliced*
- *2 cloves garlic, minced*
- *1 teaspoon grated fresh ginger*
- *2 tablespoons black bean sauce*
- *2 tablespoons chopped fresh coriander leaves*
- *Powdered green kelp to taste (optional)*

Combine the sherry, soy sauce, and cornstarch in a bowl. Cut the bitter melon lengthwise. Remove the inside pulp and seeds. Slice it thinly. Put the bitter melon into a bowl and sprinkle it with the salt. Let it sit for 20 minutes to remove some of the bitterness. Then, using cheesecloth or your hands, squeeze out the water from the bitter melon.

In a hot wok, heat 1 tablespoon of the oil. (I prefer grapeseed or peanut oil because they do not smoke at high cooking temperatures. Oils heated to the point of smoking become toxic, and their smoke is carcinogenic.) Add the bitter melon, red pepper, garlic, and ginger and stir-fry for up to 3 minutes. Add the sherry mixture, bean sauce, and 1 cup water. Cook for 1 minute longer, or until thick. After it has cooled slightly, you can add a few drops of the remaining grapeseed oil or sesame oil for richness if you wish. Garnish with the coriander. You also might add powdered green kelp to taste as a salt substitute.

HUNTER'S CHICKEN (OR TOFU)

This cacciatore dish is milder tasting and less acidic than those we have loved at small restaurants in the Triburtina section of Rome or outdoor garden cafés near the Corso Italia at Trieste. It combines tomato sauce with virgin coconut for a rich, sweet flavor. Schizandra berry (wu wei tse), a Chinese herb that has a hint of evergreen aroma and taste, is added to enhance endurance. Vegetarians can substitute extra firm tofu or tempeh for the chicken.

MAKES 4 SERVINGS | PREPARATION AND COOKING TIME: 1 HOUR

- 1 organic chicken, skinned
- 1 tablespoon grapeseed oil
- 1 medium yellow onion, sliced
- ¼ cup Chinese tree ear fungus
- 1 cup baby carrots or cut-up large
- 14 ounces spaghetti sauce
- ½ teaspoon each dried basil, rosemary, and oregano
- 1 bay leaf
- ¼ teaspoon cardamom powder
- ⅛ teaspoon turmeric powder
- ½ teaspoon each fennel, cumin, and coriander seeds
- 1 teaspoon dried schizandra berries
- 1–3 tablespoons unbleached all-purpose flour, if desired
- 1 tablespoon minced raw garlic
- Salt substitute and pepper to taste

Rinse, peel, and cut up the chicken. (I always mince the liver for my cats.) Coat the pieces with some flour and brown them in the oil in a large ceramic-coated pot. (If you prefer, virgin coconut oil gives tomatoes a mildly sweet flavor and does not burn at high temperatures.) In a different pan, brown the sliced onion in a little water over low heat. Soak the tree ears a few minutes in water until they are soft, then drain and add them to the onion, stirring to prevent sticking. Add the carrots, either baby carrots or large ones cut into 1" pieces.

Stir in the spaghetti sauce. I prefer Classico Tomato and Basil, which is nicely spiced with herbs and a little olive oil but low in fat and cholesterol. Add the basil, rosemary, and oregano.

Add the bay leaf and powdered spices and seeds. (If you cannot find fennel, cumin, and coriander seeds, the powdered versions will be fine.) Rinse and add the schizandra berries, which are available in Chinese herb shops and online.

Simmer the chicken in the sauce at low heat for about 40 minutes. Correct the seasonings. Add the flour to thicken the sauce, if necessary. Remove the chicken from the heat to allow the flavors to set for 10 minutes before serving. Most people overcook garlic by frying it in oil, which reduces its antibiotic effects and pungent flavors. If you mash your garlic and stir it into the sauce to steam at this point in the cooking, it will lose none of its curative effects. Remove the bay leaf before serving. This dish goes well with pasta or steamed potatoes garnished with parsley and cold cucumber salad.

APPLE RHUBARB PIE

MAKES 6 SERVINGS | PREPARATION TIME: 5 MINUTES | BAKING TIME: 1 HOUR
   3 red delicious apples
   2 stalks rhubarb, each 7" long
   1 tablespoon instant tapioca pudding
   1 tablespoon black cherry concentrate
   1 prepared graham cracker piecrust
   ½ teaspoon cardamom powder
   ½ teaspoon cinnamon powder

Preheat the oven to 425°F.

Wash the apples and rhubarb with the fruit and vegetable wash (page 31) to remove pesticides. Cut the apples into four pieces, then slice each piece into four or more pieces. Slice the rhubarb into 1" pieces. (Delicious apples are less acidic than other tart apples. Rhubarb eliminates uric acid and is laxative.)

Mix the tapioca and cherry concentrate (a liver cleanser) and place in the bottom of the piecrust to absorb excess moisture. If you want a really firm crust, apply a thin layer of egg white and bake for 10 minutes.

Arrange the sliced fruit on the piecrust and sprinkle with the cardamom and cinnamon. Cover with foil to seal in moisture as it bakes. Bake for 1 hour. Cool for 30 minutes before cutting.

Serve with ginger or mint tea. The pie makes a small meal when eaten with a calcium and protein source, such as a sliver of low-fat cheese.

Digestive Bitters

This homemade tonic reduces water retention as it speeds digestion and elimination. Be conservative: All liquor is fattening. Liquor is too stimulating and warming for people with chronic fevers, night sweats, and hot flashes.

The amount of herbs and spices used are according to your taste. I prefer a digestive tonic to remain bitter and somewhat sharp, which increases its digestive effects. Gentian root is used in most European after-dinner bitters. If you prefer a milder flavor, you can substitute dried dandelion root. Betel nut, an antiparasite herb, is sold plain or pleasantly flavored with rose essence in East Indian food shops and online.

MAKES 1 LITER | PREPARATION TIME: AT LEAST 3 WEEKS
2 tablespoons dried, sliced gentian root
2 tablespoons dried dandelion herb
½ teaspoon dried orange peel
½ teaspoon fennel seeds or powder
¼ teaspoon clove powder
¼ teaspoon cinnamon
1 teaspoon dried, sliced betel nut
1 tablespoon peeled, sliced raw ginger
1 handful chopped fresh mint or 1 teaspoon dried
1 liter gin or vodka, 80 proof or higher

Steep the herbs in an air-tight bottle of gin or vodka for 3 weeks. Allow a ½" space at the top of the bottle, so the herbs can expand. Store the bottle away from sunlight and heat.

To use, add 20 drops to a wine glass of seltzer before dinner, as needed. For most people, the brew resolves bloating and indigestion; for others, it may be a laxative.

Tiger Menus

Most nutritionists recommend dairy products daily as a source of calcium. Cornell University researcher T. Colin Campbell, PhD, author of *The China Study*, maintains that animal protein, especially milk, reduces the body's calcium content. Dr. Campbell does not differentiate between cow and goat or sheep milk. The latter two are considered easier to digest and cause fewer problems with the autoimmune system. Therefore, if you have dairy products at all, choose goat or sheep milk and cheese such as feta when ever possible.

If you have multiple sclerosis, lupus, or another autoimmune illness or food allergies, focus on fruits, vegetables, fish (other than shellfish), tofu, extra-virgin olive oil, and canola oil instead of meat and dairy products.

Tiger Menu 1

Before Breakfast
8 ounces half water, half pineapple juice

Breakfast
1 pot (up to 4 cups) hot green tea
1 cup fresh berries
1 slice whole grain toast sprinkled with a digestive spice
    powder such as star anise, caraway, fennel, or coriander
    powder

Snack
1 apple and tea
Optional: 2 ounces hard cheese

Lunch
Green salad with lots of different vegetables, dressed with
    canola oil and lemon juice
1 cup steamed asparagus or other green vegetable, with
    choice of:
- 3 whole grain crackers and tofu spread
- 1 cup whole grain pasta with pesto

Tea (people with weak digestion or chronic illness are
advised to drink broccoli green tea)

Snack (choose one)
- 2 rice cakes and 1 ounce of semisweet chocolate or other low-fat chocolate
- Raw carrots and celery
- 1 handful of nuts, seeds, dried dulse, or nori seaweed

Dinner
Green salad with oil and lemon juice or vinegar
4 ounces stewed tomatoes
1 baked sweet potato, with choice of:
- An egg white omelet
- 4 ounces baked low-fat fish

Tea

Before Bed (optional)
1 very ripe orange

Tiger Menu 2

Before Breakfast
4 prunes simmered for 1 minute

Breakfast
1 pot (up to 4 cups) hot green tea or broccoli green tea
1 cup cooked yellow cornmeal with raisins
1 handful of nuts, seeds, dried dulse, or nori seaweed
2 ounces goat or sheep feta cheese (optional)

Snack
2 or 3 figs
Tea or Get Svelte instant beverage

Lunch
Large green salad with vegetables such as cooked beets,
asparagus, potatoes, and black olives, dressed with
canola or grapeseed oil and lemon or vinegar
2 whole grain crackers with 1 tablespoon hummus

Snack

1 cup vegetable or bean soup

Dinner

Green salad with cucumbers and low-fat dressing, with one
    of the following:
- 2 chicken enchiladas
- 2 baked poblano peppers stuffed with canned nopales (cactus
  pads) or low-fat cheese

1 cooked green vegetable

Before Bed (optional)

Gelatin made with fruit juice and water

Tiger Menu 3

Before Breakfast

8 ounces half water, half juice (mango, grape, or cherry)

Breakfast

1 pot (up to 4 cups) hot green tea or 1 to 2 packs Get Svelte
    added to 8 ounces hot water
1 cup dried whole grain cereal with light soy milk
1 cup fresh berries or cherries

Snack

Tea or broccoli green tea
1 slice whole grain toast with 2 ounces cheese or
    1 tablespoon nut butter
Nori or dulse seaweed

Lunch

Salad with low-fat dressing
Miso soup
4 ounces steamed fish or sushi
Green tea or broccoli and vegetable cooking water (see the
    recipe for Broccoli Water on page 190)

Snack

Fresh fruit and tea

Dinner
Salad dressed with orange and tomato juices and raw garlic
2 servings cooked vegetables such as Brussels sprouts or
broccoli with lemon juice and grapeseed oil dressing,
with choice of:
- Tofu and vegetables
- Tofu pie made with 1 smashed block of tofu, 1 ripe banana,
1 beaten egg, and 1 teaspoon vanilla extract baked for 1 hour

Before Bed (optional)
Soy or low-fat yogurt

Tiger Menu 4

Before Breakfast
8 ounces half water, half grape juice

Breakfast
1½ cups cooked oatmeal, with flaxseeds, nuts, or raisins
Hot tea or coffee substitute

Snack
Oatstraw tea with black cherry concentrate added as sweetener

Lunch
Salad with low-fat dressing, with choice of:
- Vegetable lasagna
- Chinese bitter melon and garlic and black bean sauce and
brown rice

Tea

Snack
1 hard-cooked egg with raw celery and carrots
1 handful of nuts, seeds, dried dulse, or nori seaweed
Mixed vegetable juice or broccoli and vegetable cooking water

Dinner
Large salad with low-fat dressing, with choice of:
- 1 to 2 cups whole grain pasta and pesto
- 1 to 2 cups vegetable barley soup

Before Bed (optional)
1 very ripe grapefruit

Tiger Menu 5

Before Breakfast
Hot green tea and 1 pinch hingvastak (digestive) powder

Breakfast
1 cup fresh fruit
2 to 4 ounces sprout bread
2 ounces goat or sheep cheese
Hot tea

Snack
1 handful of nuts, seeds, dried dulse, or nori seaweed
Fresh fruit or 8 ounces half fruit juice, half water

Lunch
Salad with many vegetables and low-fat dressing
Vegetable wrap with tofu dressing
Tea or broccoli and vegetable cooking water

Snack
2 ounces nuts and celery

Dinner
Watercress and tomato salad with orange slices, oil and
    vinegar, or lemon juice
2 steamed green vegetables
4 ounces boiled white potato with nuts, celery, garlic,
    parsley, dill, oil, yogurt, hingvastak powder, and lemon
    juice
1 handful of nuts, seeds, dried dulse, or nori seaweed

Before Bed (optional)
Low-fat vanilla custard or low-fat milk

Tiger's Summary

- **Main problems:** weak muscles, nerve pains, food allergies, and
  cellulite

- **Traditional Chinese medicine (TCM) element and organs:** the Wood element affecting the liver, gallbladder, muscles, tendons, and eyes
- **TCM issues:** latter stages of digestion and elimination, calcium absorption, muscle and joint movement, circulation, vision, enthusiasm, and capacity to carry through with ideas and plans
- **Approach:** Reduce food allergies and excess acid conditions. Improve nervous snacking habits. Support endurance and ease of movement to facilitate muscle-toning exercise.

Recommended
- Homeopathic Natrum phosphate 6X and Gelsemium 30C as needed for nervous eating habits
- Bitter and pungent foods: celery, watercress, zucchini, garlic, okra, roasted chicory coffee substitute, and others
- Diuretic teas: Shiitake/Fu Ling Tea and pain-relief teas, such as Tu Chung
- Anti-inflammatory herbs that improve circulation: turmeric powder
- Anticellulite foods and herbs: laminaria seaweed, triphala churna to balance and tone digestion, and vitamins A, D, and C
- Herbs to ease withdrawal symptoms: Ease Plus or homeopathic Coffea cruda 30C or Nux vomica 30C

Chapter 6

Balance Your Dragon

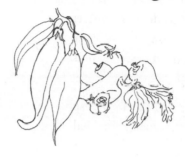

*D*ear Dragon,
You watch over everyone with care. You are a powerful presence that combines the water of compassion and the fire of imagination. When love arrives, you give your all. When exhausted, you retreat to a cozy cave and sleep. People rely on your patience and persistence. Tell those who would take advantage of your strength when it is time for you to rest. Are you trapped in a swamp of edema? Do you breathe fire from chronic fevers, palpitations, or hot flashes? Balancing foods and herbs will slenderize and refresh so that you can happily bask in the sun and feel a breeze in your hair.

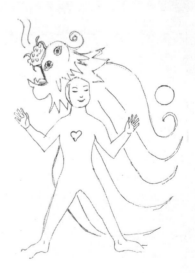

Dragons have round or square facial features and often a rosy or grayish complexion. Dragons tend to have edema (water retention)

resulting from poor digestive and kidney *qi*. They digest slowly, with difficulty, and cannot eliminate fluids effectively. Their entire bodies seem filled with water. Their puffy hands have small, fragile fingernails. A Dragon turns pink from hot flashes and looks flushed or blushes easily when the Fire element, especially the heart, cannot be moderated. A heart burdened by long-term overweight may give a Dragon chest pains or palpitations. Emotional agitation is revealed by a stutter, giggling, constant chatter, squeals of delight, or screaming.

Gray, somber Dragons suffer from adrenal weakness that harms the Water element. The results are weak, painful lower backs and legs that drag beneath them. Their eyes have dark circles or look puffy underneath, a result of many allergies. They may have thinning hair and tooth or gum problems. Dragons who develop a hypothyroid condition digest slowly and sleep many hours. Their low-pitched voices resemble groaning punctuated by nervous laughter. (For a good example, listen to actor Sydney Greenstreet.) Socializing and wearisome public appearances make them feel vulnerable, which usually makes them reach for comfort foods.

Dragons are more prone to "dampness" than the other energy types. Dampness (*she*), a Chinese medical term, is a chronic condition characterized by low vitality, poor metabolism, and water retention, which leads to excess phlegm and mucus congestion. Dampness may take the form of asthma, digestive bloating, or joint swelling discomforts. The tongue is usually overly large, puffy, and waterlogged. The pulse may be hard to find, deep and smooth, as though floating on water. Dampness—a heaviness in the body and cloudy thinking—is aggravated by rich, overly sweet and oily foods and by lack of exercise, at which overweight Dragons excel.

Because overweight Dragons have both energetic and emotional issues, their progress is often slow. One aspect of health may improve before the other. Typical comments from Dragons following the Baseline Diet are "I feel great, but the weight is not moving yet" or "I lost 5 pounds of water weight right away, then hit a plateau and stayed there for 9 months before losing 10 more pounds." Energy has to improve before a Dragon can lose weight and keep it off. Some Dragons have to alter lifelong emotional eating patterns, which takes time and patience. One Dragon reported that she felt great on the diet but found it hard to eat fewer carbohydrates. I recommended shirataki (konnyaku), a Japanese no-carb noodle featured in this and following chapters. Japanese high-fiber noodles and slimming teas are Dragon foods.

Physically fit Dragons are hard to find: They may be climbing mountains, crossing deserts, or building cities. Dragons like to think big and live big. When drawn to caring professions, they become nurses, healers, teachers, administrators, judges, and lawyers. You will find them among artists, writers, editors, religious mystics, and others who consider their work to be a calling.

Look into a Dragon's eyes, and you will see many lifetimes. That understanding comes from sharing kindness with others. At best, Dragons are guardians of culture that protect the treasures of the earth and its people. They feel, know, and understand. They are oceans of wisdom. At worst, they wallow in self-doubt or develop long-standing illnesses. The more exhausted Dragons become, the more empty calories they crave, and the less abundant their qi. Getting plenty of rest and nourishing foods is not enough for a cure. Herbs are needed to renew a healthful balance of the Dragon's Fire and Water elements.

This chapter helps Dragons—or anyone who gains weight easily; craves salt, sweets, bread, and oily foods; has weepy and angry PMS; is exhausted by work, illness, jet lag, postpartum depression, or grief; has been overweight since childhood; or became overweight after a serious illness or after taking an antidepressant drug or other medication—to overcome lethargy and edema.

Help from Homeopathy

Dragons are emotional eaters who crave foods that dampen their vitality. The trouble is, they rarely make a connection between their meals and their energy or emotions. Some diet experts recommend keeping a weight loss journal. However, those of us who write professionally know that everyone assumes an alter ego when writing. We at least want to sound interesting! A journal can become a way to kid yourself that you are getting better when you are not. Calling a friend or recording your meals may help track your progress but is not an end in itself. It is better to actually improve energy, digestion, and emotional discomforts with natural remedies.

Hunger is never for food alone. We too often eat to comfort emotions. Do you feel weepy or vulnerable when tired or worried, or during PMS? Do you call upon friends for support or eat snacks when you are upset? There are a number of things that can help with emotional eating.

HOMEOPATHIC PULSATILLA 30C is one answer to a deeply rooted problem of depression eating. It improves breathing, mental clarity, and absorption. Pulsatilla is an antimucus remedy useful for getting rid of parasites. This herb brings clarity and brightness. Homeopathic Pulsatilla is also recommended for people who rely on comfort food for emotional balance. They may enjoy eating sweets, gooey desserts, or cream dishes that impair breathing and digestion and cause bloating. For depression-related crying and bingeing, add three pills to a glass of water and sip it between meals all day.

OTHER HOMEOPATHIC REMEDIES to consider for down-in-the-dumps emotional eating are Hepar sulphuris calcareum (Calcium sulphide or Hepar sulph), Carbo vegetabilis (Carbo veg), and Ammonium muriaticum (Sal ammoniac). They work to dry or reduce excess moisture and gas in the body. In that way, they speed metabolism. Reducing unpleasant digestive complaints also improves vitality, absorption, and mood.

A classical homeopath would never mix remedies but work to find the one that best suits your individual needs. The following is a brief overview of these remedies to help you make your selection. (Remember, homeopathic remedies cannot be mixed with food, beverages, or toothpaste. And coffee or decaffeinated coffee is used to cancel a remedy. In other words, drinking a few sips of coffee will eliminate the remedy from your body and stop its actions.)

HEPAR SULPH is recommended for hypersensitive people troubled by weak, sluggish digestion and low energy, who tend to have glandular or lymphatic swelling and chapped skin. Sweating day and night, oozing wounds, and runny eyes and sinus congestion are characteristic problems. Chilly weather is very annoying for the person, for whom cold, dry wind can result in loss of voice, cough, and hoarseness.

The Hepar sulph person—someone suited to use the remedy—feels dejected and irritable, especially at night. She craves acidic foods, wine, and strong spices. There is bloating and burning in the stomach. There may be liver pain. Mouth and gums are painful and easily bleed. Stools are clay-colored, indicating a lack of bile, and contain undigested food. Urine is slow to void or greasy. Cold in any form—air, food, or weather—make the person feel worse. The remedy was once used to dry herpes, smallpox, or slow-healing wounds but, used correctly, can warm and energize weak, overweight people.

One dose (three pills or drops) of Hepar sulph 30C may be enough to stop runny, watery, hay-fever-like symptoms. (A low dilution such as 2X *increases* watery discharges.) Overuse of Hepar sulph may cause overheating, dryness, and burning symptoms. Postmenopausal women should use this remedy with care because frequent intake of dilutions can increase vaginal dryness. In 6X to 30C strengths, Hepar sulph is best for overweight people who feel chilly and have cold, wet, clammy hands and feet. Often one dose does the trick.

One homeopath even suggested using one dose of Hepar sulph 30C at the beginning of cold and flu season to ward off chills, weakness, and runny nose and prevent colds. It warms and energizes resistance and helps burn off phlegm, fat, and fatigue. Use it sparingly. Try one dose and see how it affects your energy and mood for the next 2 weeks. Hopefully, when your head clears after using Hepar sulph, you will be able to breathe deeper, feel energized and warmer, and crave fewer congesting foods.

In Chinese medicine terms, Hepar sulph works to correct problems associated with dampness and stuck liver qi, especially excess phlegm, abdominal bloating, and liver pain. It is suited to a person who is oversensitive. Everything irritates her—temperature changes, drafts, and noises. She craves acidic foods and has a yellowish (jaundiced) complexion because her liver energy, bile, and food are stuck. She feels heaviness and pressure in the stomach after eating a light meal. After using the remedy, these indigestion and breathing symptoms should disappear. The remedy may also be useful for yeast infections because it dries vaginal discharges that smell like old cheese.

You can decide whether or not to try a drying remedy such as Hepar sulph in the following way. Feel with your hand the area of your back closest to your kidneys—the same level as your navel. Imagine a string that goes from the navel to your back. That area has acupuncture points for the kidneys and a point called Life Gate, which controls energy, immunity, and metabolism. Is that area of your back cold and clammy? If so, you may benefit from a drying, energy remedy such as one dose of Hepar sulph. (One possible herbal equivalent of Hepar sulph—used to warm digestive and vital qi—is the spice cinnamon, which I have already mentioned using for diabetes and poor absorption.)

HOMEOPATHIC CARBO VEG can be used by anyone for intestinal gas. It is homeopathic charcoal that absorbs air from the intestine. Some people prefer to swallow charcoal pills to absorb gas. Remember that you may be making gas daily by combining fruits, sugar, and empty calories with protein, sodas, or other hard-to-digest foods. If you simplify your diet by following the food-combining suggestions for the Baseline Diet, you should be able to avoid gas and acid indigestion. If you use Carbo veg, wait at least 15 minutes after eating. Then melt three pills under your tongue.

AMMONIUM MURIATICUM (SAL AMMONIAC) is recommended for some of the same issues as Hepar sulph, but it works differently. Like Hepar sulph, it is often recommended for overweight people who feel sluggish and have breathing problems, but it treats grief and melancholy. An example will clarify its use.

Marjorie came to see me for weight loss, but her problems were emotional. She had lost her husband years before but was so troubled by grief, guilt, and loss that she could not take care of herself. Her apartment was a mess. She ate poorly. She cried every night and spoke about him as though he were still alive. Marjorie could not fall asleep at night until she drank wine, which helped her put on 40 pounds. Her grief made her grab for the wrong foods. She could not stop bingeing because she could not heal her emotions.

Ammonium muriaticum is recommended for people who desire to cry or change their lives but cannot; people who live under a cloud of melancholy, who feel vaguely apprehensive. They may crave lemonade or sour foods that weaken the liver. They feel nausea and regurgitate food and bitter-tasting liquid. They have gnawing stomach pain or abdominal pain after eating. They have pain around the navel, chronic liver congestion, excess fat in the abdomen, and gas pains. Mornings, they have a stuffy nose or cough; evenings, they have abdominal discomforts.

I recommended that Marjorie use the homeopathic remedy as part of a personal healing ritual. For example, honoring a departed loved one with an altar made of photos, flowers, and incense is a common practice in Buddhist temples. Some people do the same at home. Marjorie was pleased with the idea. She told me that after taking one dose of Ammonium muriaticum 30C during an afternoon of quiet meditation, within a few days she felt much better, stronger, and capable of taking better care of herself. She began her weight loss program and gradually was successful.

You may not be troubled by the same sort of grief as Marjorie, but you may feel unable to give up being overweight for your own reasons. When overweight is a such part of your life that you feel that you can never change, it brings melancholy—a dark cloud that obscures the light of reason. I believe that positive change is always possible because life—the vital energy we cannot dominate—demands renewal. An energizing natural remedy is a catalyst for your positive change because it engages that life force.

Describing these homeopathic remedies is not intended as a medical prescription. You know your symptoms best. A book cannot be your only health expert. However, Hepar sulph and Ammonium muriaticum illustrate how mood affects eating, digestion, and overweight. Grief, melancholy, loneliness, apathy, and a particular dissociation of mind and body are typical issues for Dragons. Sometimes they live as though they might endure any problem or digest anything. For a Dragon, the body is secondary to emotions.

Emotional Eating

Comparing Tigers and Dragons, you will find some overlap. To pinpoint the Energy Type and necessary remedies, you need to pay attention to the type and severity of the emotions and how they are expressed.

Tigers are nervous, agitated, jumpy, and aggressive. They cannot keep from fidgeting, tapping their fingers, or shaking their feet. They attack food as prey. They grab burgers, fries, or beer on the run, but their digestion is neither smooth nor predictable. They may feed a large appetite; however, they are really addicted to nervous stress. When Tigers start to relax, they become bored and immediately feel uncomfortable. Faced with a new situation where they are not in command, they become edgy. That is why for Tigers, I recommend homeopathic Natrum phosphate, an antacid remedy, as well as homeopathic Gelsemium, an anxiety remedy.

Dragons—many of them heavy over a lifetime—are more invested in their weight. For better or worse, fat is part of their self-image. They eat creamy, heavy, fattening, or salty foods to quench a need for emotional satisfaction that has no strings attached. Loving a cake is not like loving a person because compromise is unnecessary. Some Dragons, drained of energy from giving their all to work or family, need simple pleasures for themselves. Others may be committed to weight loss but not active enough to get out of their chairs. Exercise requires drive and breath.

Sadness, vulnerability, and mucus congestion are Dragon issues, which is why homeopathic Pulsatilla and Carbo veg work well for Dragons. Pulsatilla lifts sadness as it reduces phlegm and improves breathing and energy. Carbo veg reduces bloating and gas from unwise food combinations and slow digestion. These are the energy factors that affect Dragon overweight.

There is another more subtle cause for the Dragon's resistance to weight loss. In a nice Italian restaurant, my Bear and I had just finished a satisfying pasta, making sure to save half to take home. The family nearby was about to order, when the overweight mother and daughter, both giggling, left the table to peruse the pastries. There was no way that the little girl could keep her mother's approval and be slim. Fat was a female bond in that family. Meanwhile, the father admired slender women in the restaurant. I wondered if the scope of that couple's sensuality was limited to eating. The daughter would join that family tradition.

Remarkable changes take place when using natural remedies. All the body needs to start the healing process is a push in the right direction. One woman I know used a remedy to eliminate congestion and quickly felt energized. When I saw her a month later, she had changed her hair color, lost 15 pounds, and found a new friend. She told me that the remedy made her feel empowered. Her Dragon had claimed its brilliance.

Dragon Diet

Dragons will find our Baseline Diet to be a problem precisely because it is so simple. Most of them are used to eating everything at once—an appetizer, a main dish of protein and starch, a dessert, and coffee. That is most convenient to restaurateurs. To avoid indigestion and bloating, the Baseline Diet separates one starch meal from one protein meal daily. It recommends lots of greens and other bitter-tasting foods such as tea, which many people consider to be too healthy. Dragons, especially those living in their intellect or who are otherwise distracted, pay little attention to food combinations or what they eat. Anyone can change their diet completely by changing their eating rhythm. It sounds mysterious, but it is simple. Have your appetizer as a meal. Wait a few hours, then have a protein dish and a salad as a meal. Wait a few more hours, and then have a starch dish. Have your dessert with tea during midafternoon. Separate one restaurant-type meal into three, and you save money and lose weight.

Our Dragon diet features stimulating, nourishing foods that reduce water retention and excess hunger, along with herbs that speed metabolism.

Slimming Teas

Teas suitable for Dragons are simultaneously cleansing and energizing. They should protect the heart and adrenal energy, weak areas for those mighty beasts. Some Dragons are all heart, which is why their teas should support circulation. Others, courageous as lions, are prone to overwork or play until they have little energy left. A stimulating slimming tea is a good way to increase fluids and energy during the day. Enjoy mushroom beverages in the afternoon or evening (not with caffeine).

Daytime Teas

Slimming teas can be harsh especially when overused. Those containing senna increase cramps and may have cumulative effects that leave you gripping your stomach in surprise.

YIN/YANG SISTERS BRAND makes two healthy weight loss teas that can be used together: Get Svelte and Gorgeous You. They come individually foil wrapped as instant beverages made from powdered Chinese herbs. Get Svelte speeds digestion, reduces cholesterol, and regulates the heart with hawthorn. Added to hot water as a tea, Get Svelte seems to clear the senses and improve thinking. Gorgeous You boosts energy and immunity to illness. It takes energy to lose weight! Yin/Yang Sisters recommends one to three packets per day for each tea (a packet can also be added to juice). I prefer Get Svelte in the morning and Gorgeous You to boost energy at about 3:00 in the afternoon.

One participant in my weight loss observation, a nurse, wrote: "I have been totally enjoying the Get Svelte and Gorgeous You teas. I like them both and feel they have definitely shifted things, especially Get

Svelte, which I have every morning now in place of my usual herbal teas or juices. I try to also have another packet in the evening, since I work until 2:00 a.m.—keeps me energized without any speedy feelings. This, with your diet recommendations, has helped me feel a lot less bloated with water weight, and my digestion is working much better."

Yin/Yang Sisters brand is available from Lin Sister Herb Shop in New York or www.eastearthherb.com. (See the Natural Products and Information Resource Guide on page 348.)

SORIG BAD-KAN TEA is a Tibetan tea formulated to increase energy and metabolism and reduce excess weight. It can be enjoyed in the morning or anytime during cold weather to boost vitality. Order it from www.tibetan-medicine.org.

WHITE AND GREEN TEA (*Camellia sinensis*)—5 to 6 cups daily—reduces the risk of heart trouble by 40 percent, according to research done by Harvard cardiologist J. Michael Gaziano, MD. Andrew Weil, MD, recommends at least 10 to 12 cups of matcha Japanese green tea daily for prevention of cancer. Better yet, use a green tea extract.

The best teas for Dragons are white and green because they are the least processed and contain less caffeine than black tea or coffee. Chinese white teas, such as *shou mei*, contain the most antioxidants. Green tea, even with caffeine, has been proven useful for preventing breast cancer. Broccoli green tea or broccoli and vegetable cooking water work well as Dragon teas or in recipes.

If you need to sweeten teas, use pure vanilla extract, not sugar or lemon, which changes the character of teas and foods. Sugar is acidic, therefore irritating. Lemon is too astringent for Tigers with joint aches.

SHIITAKE/FU LING TEA WITH CINNAMON is recommended for Dragons who want to lose weight and boost energy and immunity. If your tongue is pale, use up to ¼ teaspoon of cinnamon per quart of mushroom tea. If your tongue is red and dry, cinnamon may be too stimulating for you. If you have candida, a yeast infection, avoid all mushrooms, including this tea.

ROOIBOS (AFRICAN RED BUSH TEA) is another useful tea for Dragons or anyone who wants to boost immunity.

Spiced Teas

You might flavor your tea with the most appropriate of the following stimulating spices—clove, cinnamon, cumin, and turmeric—or other helpful herbs.

CLOVE is a strongly warming and drying kidney and lung stimulant for shortness of breath, tuberculosis, wheezing asthma, frequent urination or incontinence, and low sex drive and vitality. It is a fast, hot energy boost for someone with a pale tongue and slow pulse. If you do not need heating, it will give you dry mouth, dizziness, or a headache.

CINNAMON warms the middle to speed reduction of belly fat. It tones the pancreas to treat blood sugar issues, including diabetes. (If you have diabetes, please refer to that section on page 182 in Chapter 7 for more tips.) Cinnamon frees stuck circulation and causes sweating to reduce joint and PMS abdominal pains. It is very warming. Don't use either clove or cinnamon if you have chronic fevers, hot flashes, or frequent headaches.

TURMERIC is recommended for poor circulation, joint inflammation pain, and low immunity to illness. It is mildly antibiotic and supports healthy intestinal flora. It can be added to tea, juice, yogurt, or cooked foods.

CUMIN reduces excess hunger and stomach burn, as do American ginseng tea and aloe vera gel added to water or tea. Cumin feels cooling but not especially moistening. It will not increase nausea the way some other antacids can.

AMERICAN GINSENG, also known as white ginseng, is cooling and moistening for dry mouth, chronic thirst, and excess hunger. It comes both as instant tea and as a root that can be sliced and simmered for at least 20 minutes.

ALOE VERA GEL OR JUICE, a health food remedy suitable for drinking, reduces stomach burn the same way that it reduces sunburn. It makes the digestive tract more alkaline. Either cumin or aloe is useful for settling the stomach, stopping cramps and spasm pains, and freshening bad breath. Up to ¼ cup of aloe vera gel added to tea, juice, or water, with a twist of lemon or lime, reduces excess hunger. It is cooling and soothing for a nervous stomach.

Stimulating Cooking Herbs

Kitchen herbs make satisfying teas. In most cases, use one pinch of herb per cup of tea.

SAGE LEAVES reduce excess perspiration and stimulate the body in a way similar to Chinese ginseng. The entire endocrine system is revved, which means that breathing, digestion, and elimination are stimulated. Sage, when overused, can increase fever. Avoid use with colds and flu, when you need to perspire.

ROSEMARY is strongly stimulating for the heart and adrenal energy. It must be used with caution—no more than a pinch of rosemary leaves per cup of tea. Avoid rosemary if you tend to be hot, feel dizzy, and have hot flashes.

CARDAMOM is a pleasant, semisweet spice that tones digestion and the heart. It lifts the spirits. However, it can increase hunger when overused. I like to add a dash instead of sugar to teas and pies.

Evening Teas

Nighttime hunger adds weight because when we are at rest, metabolism slows down. A harmful dietary practice is eating dinner, then watching television or going to sleep. Evening teas can be digestive and soothing for better sleep. Among delicious, soothing digestive favorites are mint, vervain, chamomile, jasmine green tea, and Happy Garden Tea, a Yin/Yang Sisters instant beverage.

The Java Jump

Coffee is tough on your kidneys and aggravates intestinal cramps. It takes vitamins, minerals, and electrolytes out of your body. It is a good temporary stimulant, and it stops a migraine for some because it narrows blood vessels in the brain to limit circulation. But coffee isn't helpful for either weight loss or energy. If you have been doing the java jump for years, you are bound to have acid indigestion, poor absorption, and a number of other nervous issues.

MATÉ TEA contains mateine, which is like caffeine but absorbed more gradually for a smoother energy source. It has few side effects. However, if you are not used to it, maté may keep you awake all night. Start with 1 cup during the day to judge the effects. Maté can be green and taste herby or toasted to taste like carob. It's a good source of antioxidants, chlorophyll, vitamins (A, C, E, and B vitamins), and minerals (magnesium, potassium, iron, pantothenic acid, and calcium), which makes it an immune booster against cancer and other chronic illnesses. Used for weight loss, maté is stimulating, reduces appetite, and speeds metabolism.

MATÉ LIQUID EXTRACT has a cumulative effect but acts like jet fuel. The recommended dose is one to two droppersful (each dropper is 30 drops) in juice, tea, or water or by mouth. But start with just 10 drops for increased energy, mental clarity, and alertness. My favorite source of maté products is the Maté Factor in Rutland, Vermont (www.matefactor.com).

Balancing Foods

Dragon foods reduce phlegm and water retention.

WATERCRESS is excellent Dragon food. It is semibitter, sharp, slightly sour—all the flavors that stimulate weight loss. Watercress makes a delicious salad or steamed vegetable dish.

BITTER FOODS such as dark leafy greens, cruciferous vegetables in the cabbage family, asparagus, and leeks are diuretic and stimulating. Sharp, bitter-tasting parsley and radish reduce phlegm.

SHARP AND SOUR FLAVORS such as lemon cleanse the liver and drain excess water from the body.

ALL SQUASHES AND PUMPKIN give you a satisfied feeling, similar to eating carbohydrates but without the fat and calories. Zucchini squash even reduces cholesterol. You might also enjoy a side dish of pumpkin pie filling—pureed pumpkin with pumpkin pie spice but no sugar.

PUNGENT HERBS AND SPICES that reduce phlegm and water

retention include cardamom, fresh sage, raw garlic, onions, ginger, and red pepper. Use them in salads.

CUMIN is diuretic and reduces excess hunger. Are you troubled by stomach acidity? Put ¼ teaspoon of cumin under your tongue to settle your stomach, or make a tea with cumin and coriander. Add cumin and coriander to sliced watermelon, mango, papaya, or grapefruit wedges for a refreshing meal.

AN OCCASIONAL LIQUID MEAL might work well for Dragons on the move. A juice made of beet greens, parsley, celery, and pineapple is slenderizing. If you want to add a protein, add 1 teaspoon of nut butter or protein powder. A good light lunch is ½ cup of cottage cheese flavored with apricot or peach nectar or apple juice. Blend a mixture of vegetables in a tomato, papaya, or pineapple juice base.

ONE PROTEIN SOURCE DAILY is allowed in our Baseline Diet. The best ones for Dragons are fish, egg whites, or extrafirm tofu with vegetables. Add some dulce seaweed to speed metabolism.

SHIRATAKI (also known as konnyaku) is a noncarbohydrate, no calorie, high-fiber noodle made from a Japanese yam called konjac. It is used as an anticholesterol fasting food in Japan. Made from a soluble fiber called glucomannan, the noodles have been used for diabetes, constipation, high blood pressure, cholesterol or glucose-reducing diets, triglyceride-reducing diets, heart trouble, obesity, and colon problems. The noodles are neither laxative nor diuretic, but the fiber reduces fat absorption.

Online at www.konjacfoods.com, you can find medical research or buy konjac sold as angel hair pasta, rigatoni, fettuccine, spaghetti, linguine, penne, lasagna, konjac flour, and tapioca pearls. Over 100 recipes are given on that Web site. This chapter has two of my favorites.

Shiratake or konnyaku noodles make perfectly satisfying, no-fuss Dragon dishes: Just rinse the noodles in cold water, blanch in boiling water for a moment, and use them in a variety of dishes—for cold sesame noodles, in soups, or with sauces. They are thin, translucent, and gelatinous, similar to Chinese glass noodles or bean threads, and have no taste but absorb the dominant flavors of the soup or dish to which they're added. They are the noodle used in Japanese sukiyaki. Shiratake noodles consist primarily of a glucomannan polysaccharide, plus calcium, and have a very low glycemic index; therefore, they are especially useful for people with diabetes. The noodles are sold in liquid-filled plastic bags in the refrigerator section of Chinese and Japanese food stores.

Dealing with Salt Cravings

You may not realize that you crave salt. But if you love peanuts, cashews, fried chicken, chips, soy sauce or miso, and popcorn, you probably crave their salt. If you pay attention to the energetic effects of salty foods, you may notice that they stimulate appetite, which is not useful for weight loss. They increase cellulite and can overstimulate the kidneys. If you frequently crave salty foods, it indicates that your kidneys are already stressed.

SEAWEED can help you deal with those cravings in a healthy way. Try dried nori seaweed, which is pure protein, or dried dulse seaweed, which is high in potassium. For additional information on seaweeds, visit www.seaweed.ie, a Web site maintained by the National University of Ireland in Galway.

HAJMOLA, an East Indian digestive pill recommended for bloating and gas, contains rock salt, cumin, and asafoetida and has a strong, spicy flavor that goes nicely with a cup of tea.

Herbs and Supplements for Water Retention

The first step for Dragons is always to strengthen vitality, which supports basic body functions such as digestion and elimination. That supports immunity to illness and chronic fatigue. Illnesses such as fibromyalgia, depression, arthritis, heart trouble, diabetes, high blood pressure, and most other problems are improved with weight loss. We all know that added weight stresses the body. Arriving at a happy medium that allows us to pursue our lifestyles and remain healthy is a balancing act. Years of "I don't care" catch up with us.

Therefore, supplements are necessary to ensure progress. The following herbal pills reduce chronic weakness and edema.

MEDICINAL MUSHROOM pills and extracts are not recommended for people with candida yeast infections or those allergic to mushrooms. Otherwise, Asian mushrooms, including shiitake, reishi, enoki, and oyster, can be used to enhance vitality and immunity. They have potent anticancer effects and reduce both cholesterol and arthritic pain because they contain 25 percent polysaccharides, a complex source of natural energy and immunity. An expert source of mushroom products, books, classes, and research information can be found at www.fungi.com.

If you use mushroom products, ingest them separately from caffeine, laxatives, and diuretic herbs to avoid losing the benefits. Coffee and tea other than maté are cleansers, but mushrooms are energy builders.

My favorite way to take medicinal mushrooms is to make a water extract by cooking mushrooms in a slow cooker for 6 to 8 hours. It saves money and is fun. Aside from use in Shiitake/Fu Ling Tea (page 45), reishi makes a fine extract. Cook one piece of dried reishi mushroom (*ling zhi*), along with one or two dried figs to sweeten the brew, for 8 hours. Drain the liquid into an empty wine bottle and drink it cold. Refrigerated, mushroom extracts stay fresh for up to 2 days. For smooth, steady energy, drink half a bottle during an afternoon and evening.

CHINESE HERBAL PILLS (already discussed) that improve edema include Drain Dampness and Laminaria 4 made by Health Concerns. For similar effects, you might cook one piece of dried reishi, a handful of fu ling, a handful of dried shiitake, 1 teaspoon cinnamon, and ½ teaspoon dulce seaweed powder. Take this brew cold—it tastes better—along with a large dose of vitamins A and D.

Achieve Balance

People who have survived health challenges, personal disappointments, and great success have all resembled Dragons at least temporarily. Under stress—even the positive stress of dieting—the body fights against starvation by storing fat. To make matters worse, our defensive energy gets stuck in a fight-or flight-anxiety pattern. When unchecked, this anxiety leads to hormone imbalances, thyroid problems, blood sugar issues, emotional upset, and more. There are a number of things that can help Dragons keep their balance in the face of stress.

IODINE: A Dragon, since she is mystical, fails to recognize her own capacities, which can seem limitless. One Dragon I know is a splendid opera singer with a huge voice. She skydives when on vacation, and at home, she sings Wagnerian roles. One winter, she developed pneumonia, then put on extra weight.

As an experiment, I asked her to put a drop of iodine on her wrist. The body absorbs the iodine it needs to feed the thyroid, the master gland that regulates energy, metabolism, and mood. If a drop of iodine disappears within 4 hours, it indicates the thyroid is under-active or exhausted. Hers was gone in 20 minutes. That one drop made her temporarily feel lighter, happier, and physically better.

If you wish to tone your thyroid with iodine, see how long it takes for one drop to disappear from the inside of your wrist. That indicates how quickly your body absorbs it. If it disappears within a few hours to a day, place another drop at the same time the following day. Repeat that until the iodine remains visible the next day at the same time or until you feel energized enough to quit for a few days. Learn to judge your energy capacity by watching the iodine disappear. Everyone's needs are different.

Some people do not enjoy stimulating the thyroid with iodine. They may feel nervous or irritable. In that case, use it when you feel comfortable and no more than once daily for a period of 1 month. Then consider the results.

LAMINARIA 4: Already mentioned as a cellulite treatment, it also tones the thyroid.

LIGHTER MEALS: My singer friend now enjoys a breakfast of apple and celery with hot green tea or Get Svelte instant beverage. She says it reduces mucus congestion, anathema to opera.

Tonics Help Maintain Balance

Many Dragon friends who answered my weight loss questionnaire were compulsive overeaters struggling with depression. They overate at night, an attempt to ground their flying Dragon energy in order to sleep. Their common complaints indicated what Chinese doctors call kidney weakness: poor circulation; lots of muscle pain and cramps; cellulite at the waist, hips, and thighs; an aching lower back; swollen knees; and painful legs. They needed a sane alternative to yo-yo dieting and a balancing energy tonic—one that would vary with personal needs.

A tonic is a food or herb that makes the body function better. It may stimulate energy or provide nourishment. A good tonic is much more than an upper. Dragons may have special needs brought about by menopause, chronic fatigue, or illness. For Dragons, the wisest tonic would support both the heart and adrenal energy—the Fire and Water elements.

THREE IMMORTALS made by Health Concerns is one such tonic, recommended for treating menopausal symptoms. It simultaneously reduces hot flashes with antifever herbs and builds adrenal strength with herbs that are precursors to testosterone.

KANG GU ZENG SHENG PIAN, a Chinese patent remedy, contains both moistening, nourishing *Rehmannia glutinosa* (*shu-di-huang*) and, among other warming, stimulating herbs, *Epimedium brevicornum* (*yin yang huo*), a precursor to testosterone. It is recommended to prevent and treat bone spurs and joint and bone problems. The label advises that the remedy promotes the health of the loins, kidneys, muscles, bones, blood, and nervous system.

A wide-reaching tonic made from nourishing, moistening foods and stimulating herbs suits the health issues of the Dragon. Here are two such tonics you can make at home.

USING FRUIT: Rinse 1 pound of berries such as blueberries, pitted black cherries, or blackberries. They provide iron and other nutrients. As a stimulating herb, you need one sliced Chinese ginseng root or 2 tablespoons of East Indian ashwagandha powder. Ashwagandha works better for chronic backache and sexual weakness. Add up to 1 cup of water and cook slowly over low heat for several hours, until the mixture turns into a thick paste. Let it cool. You may add a little raw honey if necessary. Eat 1 to 3 tablespoons or more daily.

USING CHINESE HERBS: Combine one handful each of lycium fruit (*gou qi zi*) and epimedium (*yin yang huo*). Simmer in 2 cups of water for 30 minutes, and drink the tea throughout the day. Gougi berries (also known as goji, gogi berries, wolfberries, and matrimony fruit) are similar in texture and size to raisins. They are known as a natural source of zeaxanthin, a carotenoid naturally found in healthy eyes, as well as many natural polysaccharides, antioxidants, and phytonutrients. The berries have been used as a tonic by herbalists to help bring a sense of well-being and harmony to the body and mind. They have become popular among herbal producers, who make many health claims for them and ask overly high prices. However, you can order these and other Asian herbs online at very reasonable prices. See the Natural Products and Information Resource Guide on page 348.

Finding Balance with Minerals

Trace minerals help improve your body's absorption ability. According to Yves Requena, MD, author of several books on traditional Chinese medicine and herbs, the trace mineral most important for adrenal vitality is gold. Traditional Ayurvedic physicians advise drinking water stored overnight in gold, silver, or copper containers. But where can I find a pure gold cup? For easy absorption, I prefer taking homeopathic minerals. My favorite source is a health food store product called Bioplasma, a combination of 12 essential minerals that are constituents of the body. The usual dose for adults is three to six tablets (two for children) dissolved under the tongue between meals three times daily.

Dragon Meals

For Dragons, I offer slenderizing variations on several classic dishes and a surprising beverage made with reishi mushroom extract. Dragons can moderate appetite, ease digestion, and calm nervousness daily by adding ⅛ cup of health food store aloe vera gel to a pot of tea, a glass of juice, or water. A twist of lemon adds tang. Aloe is soothing for acid reflux and improves irregularity, complexion problems, abdominal cramps, and Dragon breath.

A Dragon Breakfast

A large Scandinavian Dragon I once knew started the day with bacon, eggs, toast, and coffee mixed with bitter chocolate. A Bavarian friend served steamed veal sausage, sauerkraut, potato salad made with boiled eggs, and pastry. My Italian friend started the day with melon and prosciutto, toast and jam, fried eggs, and extrastrong coffee. In each case, breakfast had enough protein, fat, and starch to last the entire day. Sadly, those friends are gone now because of cancer, heart trouble, and stroke. I miss them but not their big breakfasts.

All you really need is fruit and either a little protein or a slice of whole grain toast. A cup of tasty dried dulse seaweed adds flavor and color to any meal. A small breakfast is no less romantic if served on pretty china along with a delicious tea, fresh flowers, and a smile. For example:

- Fresh fruit and a scoop of spiced cottage cheese
- Fruit-filled crepes and walnuts
- 1 baked or raw apple and Cheddar cheese
- ¼ cup fresh goat cheese, celery, and whole grain bread
- Stewed prunes or apricots and cooked yellow cornmeal
- One hard-cooked egg and melba toast with sugarless jam
- One chicken sausage with mustard and sauerkraut
- A small baked potato with 1 teaspoon canola oil, sauerkraut (optional), and a serving of low-fat cheese that is breakable, not soft and spreadable
- One small salmon steak and steamed asparagus
- ½ fresh papaya, a small bowl of high-fiber cereal, and fat-free milk
- Fresh fruit, a cup of plain low-fat yogurt, and 1 teaspoon ground flaxseeds

Dragon Recipes

Here are a number of tasty dishes that can be served for lunch or dinner.

LEEK PIE

This pie is rich enough to be served as a main course along with a green salad and steamed asparagus.

MAKES 6 SERVINGS | PREPARATION TIME: 1 HOUR

　2 *leeks, thinly sliced*
　1 *low-fat graham cracker piecrust (8")*
　½ *teaspoon instant tapioca pudding*
　1 *egg, slightly beaten*
　½ *cup low-fat milk*
　½ *teaspoon powdered green kelp seaweed (as a salt substitute)*
　¼ *teaspoon mace (optional)*
　　Pinch nutmeg

Preheat the oven to 425°F.

Soak the leeks in vegetable wash after slicing them, because they always contain sand.

Sprinkle the piecrust with the tapioca to absorb excess moisture. If you like a firmer pie, combine the tapioca with 1 egg white, spread onto the piecrust, and bake it for 8 minutes. Otherwise, use the entire egg in the filling. (People concerned about cholesterol can use eggs enhanced with omega-3 oils.)

After carefully rinsing the leeks, shake out the excess water. Place the sliced leeks in the piecrust. In a bowl, mix the egg, milk, powdered seaweed, and mace, if using. Pour onto the leeks. Using the back of a spoon, press the leeks into the egg mixture, so they are covered. Sprinkle a little nutmeg on top and bake for 50 minutes, or until golden brown. Cool the pie before cutting it.

Steamed Salmon in Pineapple Juice and Red Onion

This is one of my healthy favorites for any time of day. Use wild Atlantic salmon. Fish grown in crowded pens are likely to develop diseases. For that reason, manufacturers use chemical pesticides when raising them. High-quality fish tastes better when lightly steamed and fixed without creamy sauces that hide their natural flavor.

MAKES 4 SERVINGS | PREPARATION TIME: 15 MINUTES

   ½ medium red onion, sliced
   ½ cup unsweetened pineapple juice
   1 teaspoon powdered green kelp seaweed (as a salt substitute)
   1 pound salmon steak, cut into 4 pieces
   Fresh parsley

Steam the onion in a little water until soft. Mix the juice and the powdered seaweed, and pour them over the onion. Place the salmon on the onion. Cover and steam using low heat until the salmon is light pink inside. Garnish with parsley.

Al Dente Pasta and Tree Ears

Whole wheat pasta is underrated. Its taste is sweeter and richer than regular pasta. Fixed al dente, it resembles a whole grain dish because it adds fiber and a complex carbohydrate to the diet. Tree ears (Auricularia auricula) are a great addition to pasta dishes, soups, and steel-cut oatmeal. They thin the blood with a platelet-inhibitory effect. Aside from their obvious benefits in an anticholesterol, slimming diet, tree ears are fluffy, crunchy, and mild-tasting.

MAKES 4 SERVINGS | PREPARATION TIME: 20 MINUTES

   1 handful dried tree ear fungi
   1 clove fresh garlic, mashed (optional)
   2 cups whole wheat pasta
   ½ teaspoon dried chervil leaves
   ½ teaspoon dried marjoram leaves
   ¼ teaspoon chives, chopped
   ¼ teaspoon basil

½ *teaspoon parsley*
1 *tablespoon sesame seeds*
1 *tablespoon flaxseed oil*
Powdered dry seaweed to taste

Soak the tree ears in water for at least 5 minutes, or until they are soft. Squeeze them to find the hard, inedible parts, and discard those. Rinse the tree ears well. Simmer for 15 minutes in a small pot with water to cover. Drain, then add the garlic, if using. Very lightly steam in 1 tablespoon water and set the pot aside. Meanwhile, start the pasta. I usually add ¼ teaspoon turmeric to flavor and color the water.

When the pasta is al dente, rinse in cold water, so it is not sticky. Return it to the pot and add the tree ears and garlic, if using, with a little water to steam it until warmed. Toss with the herbs, seeds, oil, and seaweed. Serve hot.

Light Coq au Vin

This dish, easier to prepare and less fattening than the original recipe, omits bacon, butter, and the chicken's skin and dark meat.

MAKES 4 SERVINGS | PREPARATION TIME: 40 MINUTES
1 *egg white, slightly beaten*
1 *tablespoon cornstarch*
1 *large organic chicken breast, skinned and sliced into 2" pieces*
1 *teaspoon unbleached all-purpose flour*
1 *teaspoon grapeseed oil*
⅛ *cup scallions, cut into 1" pieces*
1 *cup dry red wine*
1 *teaspoon fresh parsley*
1 *tablespoon dried herbs de provençe or a bouquet garni*
Dash of nutmeg
Powdered green kelp seaweed to taste

Slightly beat the egg white. (I give the yolk to my cats.) Add the cornstarch. This is a secret borrowed from Chinese chefs: Marinate the chicken pieces in the cornstarch and egg for 10 minutes to make the meat tender and seal in the juices. Then sprinkle with the flour.

Heat the oil in a nonstick pan, but do not allow it to smoke. Brown the chicken, and add the scallions and wine. Add the parsley and dried herbs. (You may wish to make your own bouquet garni using fresh thyme, tarragon, chives, savory, marjoram, and basil or other provençal herbs tied together with a string.) Turn the heat down to simmer the chicken for about 20 minutes, or until it is tender but not overdone. (Remove the bouquet garni.) Thicken with a little flour as needed and add the nutmeg and powdered seaweed for richer flavor.

NOUVELLE RATATOUILLE

This colorful dish is especially pleasing for Bears and Dragons. Serve it with a crisp green salad, whole grain peasant bread, and a glass of chilled fruity rosé to complement its Provençal character.

MAKES 4 SERVINGS | PREPARATION TIME: 35 MINUTES

½ medium eggplant, cut into 1" pieces
1 large parsnip root, cut into 1" pieces
1 cup zucchini, sliced
¼ cup yellow onion, peeled and sliced
¼ cup celery, sliced
¼ cup cucumber, peeled and thickly sliced
½ teaspoon savory herb
1 large clove garlic, chopped
¼ teaspoon fennel seeds
1 teaspoon basil leaves
⅛ teaspoon rosemary leaves
1 bay leaf
   Dash of cardamom
1 can (14.5 ounces) organic stewed tomatoes
   Seaweed salt substitute and black pepper (optional)

Since this recipe calls for no oil, the ingredients are lightly steamed. Arrange the vegetables and herbs and spice in a ceramic-coated pot. Add the stewed tomatoes and bring to a boil. Cover, turn down the heat, and simmer for up to 20 minutes so that the vegetables remain slightly firm. Remove from the heat and allow the flavors to blend for 5 minutes before correcting the seasonings. Add salt substitute and pepper, if using. If you miss the taste of oil, add 1 teaspoon of extra-virgin olive oil after cooking.

INDONESIAN-STYLE NOODLES

Spicy noodles are a favorite in Amsterdam's cafes, along with sweet pancakes and a good cigar, or in New York with small sausages and strong lapsang souchong tea. At home, I serve them cold with salad.

MAKES 4 SERVINGS | PREPARATION TIME: 20 MINUTES

1½ cups chopped vegetables, including celery, carrots, red pepper, shiitake or oyster mushrooms, onion, garlic, and Chinese cabbage

2 packages (8 ounces each) shirataki noodles

2 teaspoons light soy sauce

¼ teaspoon (or less) chili paste

1 teaspoon raw ginger, peeled and thinly sliced

1 tablespoon Thai grated pickled turnip

1 tablespoon virgin coconut or flaxseed oil

¼ cup roasted peanut powder

Fresh cilantro and mint leaves

1 lime, sliced

1 carrot, peeled and finely grated in long strips

1 peeled daikon radish (about 2" long), finely grated in long strips

You can use your preference when selecting the vegetables. Slice mushrooms, onion, garlic, and cabbage into large pieces. The main thing is to have a nice variety of colors, tastes, and textures.

Wash off the sour-smelling packing liquid from the noodles and blanch them in boiling water for a few minutes, or until spongy and firm. Rinse in cold water and set aside.

In a covered wok or nonstick pan, cook the vegetables in a little water at medium heat for 5 minutes. Mix in the soy sauce and the chili paste and cook for another 2 minutes. Add the ginger with a little water, if necessary, and lightly steam for up to 15 minutes.

While the vegetables are still firm, toss with the noodles, turnip, and oil in a big bowl. For a lighter dish, use 2 teaspoons grapeseed or sesame oil in place of coconut oil. Sprinkle with peanut powder and garnish with the cilantro and mint, lime, carrot and radish. Asian chili paste gets hotter overnight, so finish this dish in one sitting.

SUKIYAKI

Japanese sukiyaki (pronounced "ski-yaki") is a party dish you can share with family and friends sitting around the table. Everyone does their own stir-frying. They help themselves from the pot, then replace the ingredients for the next person. If you use beef, buy it from a Japanese butcher who freezes it and slices it extra thin.

MAKES 4 TO 6 SERVINGS | PREPARATION TIME: 15 MINUTES

SAUCE

1 sachet instant dashi powder
1 cup hot water
½ cup Japanese light soy sauce
⅓ cup mirin vinegar
1 teaspoon stevia powder

SUKIYAKI

12 shiitake mushrooms
6 ounces eye fillet steak, sliced paper thin (optional)
4 tablespoons grapeseed oil
3 small onions, quartered
2 cups bean sprouts
½ Chinese cabbage, chopped
1 red pepper, sliced
6 green shallots, chopped
1 block firm tofu, cubed
1 packet shirataki (konnyaku) noodles, rinsed

To make the sauce: Combine all ingredients in a pan and bring to a boil.

To make the sukiyaki: Soak the mushrooms in hot water for 20 minutes, drain, and remove the stems. Heat 1 tablespoon of the oil in a nonstick wok, add about one-quarter of the steak, if using, and stir-fry quickly until well browned all over. Add one-quarter of the mushrooms, the rest of the vegetables, the tofu, and the noodles and stir-fry until tender. Pour one-quarter of the sauce over it and serve immediately. Repeat process until all ingredients are used.

COLD ARTICHOKE AND NOODLE SALAD

You can add Japanese no-calorie noodles to any salad or pasta dish for added fiber and fun.

MAKES 4 SERVINGS | PREPARATION TIME: 25 MINUTES

   6 fresh baby artichokes
   ¼ cup lemon juice + juice of 1 lemon
   ½ pound shirataki (konnyaku) noodles, rinsed
   ½ cup tomato juice
   2 tablespoons olive oil
   2 cloves garlic, minced
   3 tablespoons fresh parsley, minced
   3 tablespoons fresh basil or 1 teaspoon dried
   ½ teaspoon powdered green kelp seaweed (as a salt substitute)
   ¼ teaspoon black pepper
   ½ cup fresh tomato, chopped
   ½ cup Kalamata olives
   2 tablespoons capers
   ½ cup feta cheese (optional)

To steam the artichokes, cut the stems off and peel away the tough outer leaves to reveal the tender yellow-green hearts. Cut the artichokes into quarters. In a medium bowl, combine the ¼ cup lemon juice with 2 cups of water. Add the artichokes and toss to prevent discoloration.

Drain off the lemon juice and steam the artichokes in water until tender, about 20 minutes. Chill them.

In a large pot, rinse the noodles with cold water. Drain.

Place the tomato juice, oil, remaining lemon juice, garlic, parsley, basil, powdered seaweed, and pepper in a blender and blend for 30 seconds. In a large salad bowl, toss together the artichokes, noodles, tomato, olives, capers, and cheese, if using. Pour the dressing over and toss well.

Otherwise, if you are in a terrible hurry: Pour off the water from a small jar of pickled artichoke hearts and rinse them with water. Finely chop a tomato, some parsley, capers, and a piece of scallion. Rinse off the noodles and toss the ingredients together with a fresh vinaigrette made with a little prepared mustard, oil, and lemon juice.

CHOCOLATE BERRY PIE

This recipe makes a quick and delicious afternoon tea pie.

MAKES 8 SERVINGS | PREPARATION TIME: 15 MINUTES

- *2 teaspoons instant tapioca pudding*
- *2 tablespoons all-fruit jam (no sugar added) or black cherry concentrate*
- *1 low-fat graham cracker crust (8")*
- *2½ cups fresh berries (blackberries, blueberries, and strawberries)*
- *1 square bittersweet baker's chocolate, grated*

Preheat the oven to 450°F.

Mix the tapioca powder with the jam and a little water or cold Earl Grey tea. Spread the thick paste onto the bottom of the piecrust. Add the berries. Grate or melt the chocolate into a bowl and sprinkle on top of the berries.

Bake just long enough for the chocolate to melt and the fruit to become warm and soft, about 20 to 40 minutes, depending on the fruit used. Cool the pie before cutting into small slices.

Dragon Menus

Dragons require lots of energy to enhance vitality, immunity, and will-power for dieting. They often crave junk foods, salty and fried foods, and other snacks that may impede their weight loss progress. They may neglect regular meals and snack all day. They may develop hypo-thyroid conditions that lead to lethargy and extra pounds. To avoid indigestion, they should add slimming, stimulating spices such as star anise powder, rosemary, or sage to teas and use food supplements that are high in iodine, such as nori and kelp seaweeds. Reishi mushroom extract raises energy and immunity.

Dragon Menu 1

Before Breakfast
8 ounces half water, half grape juice

Breakfast
1 to 2 cups sliced apple, walnuts, canola oil, sesame seeds,
   and lemon juice
1 cup whole grain dried cereal and cranberry juice
1 pot or 4 cups hot green or white tea or red bush tea or 2
   cups of broccoli green tea or broccoli and vegetable
   cooking water (see Broccoli Water recipe on page 190)

Snack
Nori seaweed, 1 hard-cooked egg, 20 drops reishi
   mushroom extract

Lunch
Large salad with oil and vinegar or lemon juice
Unsweetened pumpkin pie filling
¼ cup nuts

Snack
8 ounces fresh lemonade and strawberries

Dinner
Large salad with steamed vegetables, greens, and canned
   sardines

2 whole grain crackers with tofu spread
20 drops reishi mushroom extract
1 cup vegetable soup with nori seaweed

Before Bed (optional)
Low-fat pudding and mint tea

Dragon Menu 2

Before Breakfast
8 ounces half water, half cranberry apple juice

Breakfast
Fresh fruit, with choice of:

- 2 ounces sheep feta cheese
- 1 slice whole grain toast with 1 tablespoon nut butter

Hot tea with lemon

Snack
Get Svelte instant beverage
Fresh pineapple or papaya slices

Lunch
Green salad with roasted, unsalted peanuts, cucumber, and
    avocado
4 ounces white meat chicken in lemon sauce
20 drops reishi mushroom extract
Noncaffeine tea

Snack
Mixed vegetable juice containing carrot, kale, and
    apple
1 handful of nuts, seeds, dried dulse or nori seaweed
2 cups of broccoli green tea or broccoli and vegetable
    cooking water

Dinner
Salad with low-fat dressing; add nori or sprinkle with kelp,
    with choice of:

- Shirataki cold sesame noodles and vegetables
- 1 block cold tofu with soy sauce, scallion, and balsamic vinegar

20 drops reishi mushroom extract
1 handful of nuts, seeds, dried dulse, or nori seaweed
Tomato aspic

Before Bed (optional)
Chamomile tea

Dragon Menu 3

Before Breakfast
8 ounces half water, half apple juice with 1 tablespoon
    lemon juice

Breakfast
Instant barley cooked with vegetables, including celery and
    carrot, onion, marjoram, and cumin; add powdered
    green kelp seaweed as a salt substitute
1 or 2 multigrain crackers with nut butter or Indian
    chyawanprash
Tea

Snack
Hummus and whole wheat pita with salad
2 cups of broccoli green tea or broccoli and vegetable
    cooking water

Lunch
Vegetable soup and salad
20 drops reishi mushroom extract in juice
1 handful of nuts, seeds, dried dulse or nori seaweed

Snack (choose one)
- 1 ounce semisweet baking chocolate
- 1 tube Chinese Extractum Astragali, a sweet, energizing
  tonic
Tea

Dinner
Salad with low-fat vinaigrette dressing
Salmon steamed in pineapple juice
½ cup whole grain pasta with tomato basil sauce

Before Bed (optional)
1 very ripe orange and warm mint tea

Dragon Menu 4

Before Breakfast
8 ounces half water, half apricot juice

Breakfast
1 cup Chinese Bojenmi slimming tea
2 or 3 rice cakes
1 hard-cooked egg with a dab of hot mustard
Nori or dulse seaweed
20 drops reishi mushroom extract in 1 cup V-8 or low-
    sodium tomato juice

Snack
1 to 2 tubes Chinese Extractum Astragali

Lunch
Large salad with low-fat dressing
Chicory coffee substitute or tea
2 cups of broccoli green tea or broccoli and vegetable
    cooking water

Snack
20 drops reishi mushroom extract in juice or 1 cup dried
    dulse seaweed

Dinner
Salad with greens and ripe grapefruit wedges
Baked potato with vegetable and tofu stuffing
3 ounces very thinly sliced beef with spicy ginger sauce
Tea

Before Bed (optional)
1 cup warm, unsweetened pure pumpkin pie filling with
    pumpkin pie spice

Dragon Menu 5

Before Breakfast
8 ounces half water, half Concord grape juice

Breakfast
1 pot hot green tea, with choice of:
- 1 cup multigrain cooked cereal
- 1 cup cooked yellow cornmeal with 3 stewed figs and ½ cup
  soy or low-fat milk

1 cup hot Bojenmi Tea or Get Svelte instant beverage

Snack
20 drops reishi mushroom extract in juice or vegetable soup
1 handful of nuts, seeds, dried dulse or nori seaweed

Lunch
Large salad
1½ cups chicken fricassee
1 cup cooked yucca with garlic
½ cup black beans
2 cups of broccoli green tea or broccoli and vegetable
    cooking water

Snack
3 chocolate-covered prunes and 1 rice cake

Dinner
Green salad with many vegetables
Split pea soup with 20 drops reishi mushroom extract
2 high-fiber crackers

Before Bed (optional)
1 very ripe orange

Dragon's Summary

- **Problems:** global overweight and edema, low energy, and immunity
- **Traditional Chinese medicine (TCM) element and organs:** the Water element affecting the kidney, bladder, hormone balance and sexuality, mental and emotional balance, memory, concentration, and hearing
- **Approach:** Reduce excess hunger, support adrenal vitality, calm anxiety, and support immunity to illness.

Recommended
- Homeopathic Pulsatilla and other remedies for emotional bingeing
- No-calorie shirataki (konnyaku noodles) and seaweeds
- Maté tea and extract and rooibos tea to boost metabolism and immunity
- Get Svelte instant beverage and Shiitake/Fu Ling Tea (page 45) and cinnamon tea for edema
- Mushrooms and other tonic herbs for long-term wellness and safe weight loss
- Tibetan Sorig Bad-Kan Tea for energy and weight loss

Chapter 7

Soothe Your Bear

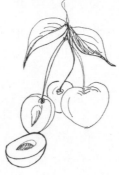

D*ear Bear,*
You crave comfort and fulfillment, not only from satisfying meals, but from happy work relations and congenial friends and family. Your enjoyment of food plays a part in feeling good about yourself. A pleasant meal creates a feeling of being at home with everything in its proper place. You may eat out often or be a chef. Comfort foods and sweet flavors ground you. Are you a cuddly teddy bear or a grizzly—i.e., Ursus horribilis? Do you digest your words, work, and relationships with ease or chew on ideas for hours and snap at sweet things?

Improve your digestion, and work, home life, and travel will become serene. Do not try to change your diet all at once. First add healthy sweet fresh fruits, whole grain breads and al dente pasta, and low-fat proteins, and then gradually reduce starches, refined foods, and cola drinks. Your energy and mood will brighten as you feel lighter.

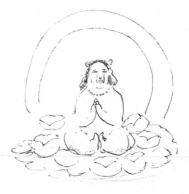

Bears have broad, round or square facial features. They may or may not be stocky, but their excess weight is carried in the middle. Bears can be identified by their squarish hands and short, plump fingers— just right for holding cookies. Gregarious, with rosy complexions, Bears are a joy to be with when they're happy. When depressed or anxious, they may withdraw to salve their wounds with a cake.

Ursa's energy and inspiration come from her breadbasket center. That's why she especially loves meals with friends and family gatherings. Her definition of family may encompass broad-ranging social issues such as world hunger or defending the rights of children. Cooperation among family members and peers and meaningful personal and professional relationships are Bears' ideals. Too frequently, they settle for a pastry.

Bears ruminate about words, thoughts, and feelings and freely communicate them. Bears can be found among writers, actors, attorneys, business executives, teachers, the clergy, and chefs. The Bear personifies the Earth element and represents all aspects of digestion, including blood sugar balance. For the Bear, language is an extension of the mouth and digestive center. A Bear's words and voice, though not always sweet, express a vital part of his or her personality. Highly attuned to music, a Bear's voice may be harmonious and sing-song or flat, depending upon mood.

Some Bears are naturally cuddly. You can tell at a glance that they are warm and accepting. Their handshakes are firm and generous. A teddy may turn into a hot-tempered grizzly if she misses a meal or her feelings are hurt. Sociable Bears give dinner parties at which they cook, sing, or tell jokes because they like to laugh. Arguments give Bears stomachaches. Divorce, changing jobs, and especially moving from one cave to another can bring on diarrhea or other uncomfortable digestive problems.

Halfway between hot-tempered, volatile Tigers and stoically entrenched Dragons, Bears go for the goods: In romance, they prefer liaisons that are short and sweet. They may accumulate several families and lots of children. Home for them is always the kitchen, no matter which one.

A lifetime of irregular or troubled digestion easily results in ulcers, acid dyspepsia, hiatal hernia, chest pains, or heart rhythm irregularities. Long-term overweight and crash dieting can lead to hypoglycemia and, eventually, diabetes—and any of the energy types may develop diabetes. People who live a sedentary life and regularly drink alcohol, eat junk foods containing refined sugars and starches, smoke, and live under stress are at high risk. The disease now affects children as much as adults. Bears have a particularly difficult time reducing their sweet-tooth habits. For that reason, I have included considerable information in this chapter about foods and herbs useful for diabetes, which in India is called the rich man's disease.

Traditional Chinese medicine (TCM) considers diabetes to be an inflammatory imbalance. Diabetes is translated as thirsting and wasting disease. In the United States, it seems that thirsting, hungering, and growing heavier most frequently apply to diabetes. The pancreas becomes overworked when fed a diet of simple sugars found in bread, white potatoes, pasta, cookies, bottled drinks, and other empty calories. Bears—or anyone who needs to lose weight and inches from the middle—do better with chewy whole grains and high-fiber foods. When we eat whole grains, which are filling, we consume fewer calories. High-fiber foods speed through the digestive tract, allowing less time for fatty acids and calories to be absorbed. If you are a Bear, think panda: They eat bamboo!

A large, puffy, coated tongue indicates water retention in the body and difficult digestion, accompanied by poor mental clarity and concentration. A dry, red tongue indicates possible internal inflammatory issues such as ulcers, chronic thirst, hunger, or diabetes. A Bear requires small, frequent, regular meals that do not challenge blood sugar balance. Otherwise, stress, emotional upset, and a diet of too many sweet and oily foods may lead to problems with cholesterol, triglycerides, high blood pressure, and diabetes.

Ultimately, Bears need to move beyond food to find strength within themselves. One typical Bear answered my questionnaire:

I have a spare tire around the waist and hips, cellulite, and an addictive personality (workaholic, foods, gave up smoking many years ago). I have an eating disorder. I have been a member of Overeaters Anonymous for years. Most of my history was compulsive dieting. I eat sugar foods—sometimes a whole cake. I want to feel good about my body and have confidence. OA did not work for me because all the foods I did not allow myself to eat I want now.

Comfort Foods

Foods cannot solve all our problems. This book may help you to recognize your relationship to food—your food karma. The roles you assign to foods can change as you develop. Former comfort foods may become less necessary, or you may find pleasing slimming substitutes.

The basics do not change: Meals require good digestion resulting from adequate energy (digestive *qi*) and peace of mind. One of the following homeopathic remedies may help you to achieve emotional balance in order to reduce addictive eating habits and improve your progress with weight loss. Melt three pills under your tongue as needed between meals once or twice daily for up to 1 week and see if there's a difference in your eating habits and energy. Stop taking the remedy as soon as you notice improvement.

Homeopathic remedies are not an end—the only answer—in themselves. However, if one seems appropriate, based on how you finish the following sentence, choose it.

I overeat the wrong foods when:
- I feel depressed—Pulsatilla 30C
- I feel anxious or nervous—Gelsemium 30C
- I feel exhausted and very weak—Arsenicum album 6X

We have already covered homeopathic Pulsatilla and Gelsemium. (Please refer to pages 140 and 107 for details on those remedies.)

People who participated in my weight loss clinical observation reported great results from both remedies.

HOMEOPATHIC ARSENICUM ALBUM, made from a trace of arsenic, is a strong energy booster sometimes given to tired racehorses. It picks you up off the floor when you have crashed. You may feel completely emptied or have exhaustion diarrhea. Do not abuse the remedy, but use one dose of homeopathic Arsenicum or another natural stimulant if you find yourself eating to maintain high energy. Why? It is better to address exhaustion directly: Digestion requires even more energy. Do not challenge your body when exhausted, but rest or take a tonic so that you are able to digest food.

One dose of homeopathic Arsenicum (for collapse) or Gelsemium (for weakness and anxiety) will probably be all you need to lift your spirits, focus your thoughts, and let you feel much stronger. Exhaustion makes everything, including food addictions, feel worse.

Daily Massage

Bears literally hold their stress in the middle. Eating under tension and on the run, in cars, or at your desk gives you cramps or chest pains. To ease the passage of food along the digestive tract, try this simple massage technique.

Lie flat on your back or sit comfortably, with your back leaning against the back of a chair and your feet flat on the floor. Relax and inhale quietly into the lower abdomen. With your thumbs together, gently push diagonally from the navel down and toward the right leg. Push until you feel relief. You may hear a gurgle of air as the ileosecal valve opens. The ileosecal valve is situated on the right side of the abdomen, halfway between the top of the pelvic bone and the groin. Pushing in that direction opens the valve so that food can pass from the small into the large intestine. Otherwise, you may feel uncomfortable as food and air back up.

SU JOK KOREAN HAND MASSAGE

Korean Su Jok hand massage offers a refreshing way to tone circulation for the entire body. It enhances energy, metabolism, and fitness without adding calories. It improves digestion and elimination of fat and toxins. This massage works well for children and older people who do not like full-body massage. The chart provided will help you to identify the parts of the body in the hands.

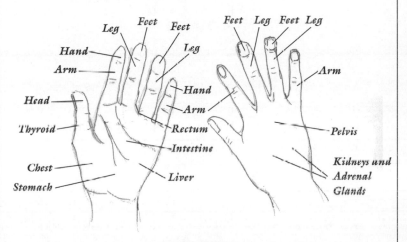

Su Jok Hand Massage

Massage the entire hand with a massage oil. If the hands are cold and stiff, life force is reduced or trapped by troubled circulation and emotions. To improve general circulation and mood, it is not important that you recognize every part of the body represented in the hands. However, it is important to know that painful points on the hands or feet indicate areas of the body where poor circulation or injury have caused problems. For weight loss, massage on the palmar side of each hand with slow, firm movements. Massage the entire palm from the wrist to the fingertips of the middle two fingers. That moves energy from the stomach, through the intestines, and to the extremities of the feet. The thumb on the palmar side corresponds to the thyroid and face. Massage all the fingers and the palms until they are warm.

Bear Diet

The Bear's special dishes are satisfying and slimming. Some of them are healthy sweets. Bears with diabetes can use herbal stevia powder as a sweetener. They should add ¼ teaspoon of cinnamon powder daily to water, tea, or cooked oatmeal. Cinnamon warms a Bear's tired digestion to reduce pain and bloating as it improves insulin uptake for the pancreas.

Slimming Teas

Slimming teas suitable for Bears also help to prevent and treat diabetes.

- **African red bush tea** is high in antioxidants. One tasty red bush tea, which combines cinnamon and other spices, is called Red Rooibos Moon Spice Tea. You can order it online from various Web sites, including www.myvitanet.com.
- **Cherry Grain Balsam Pear Tea** comes from China, but Chinese slimming teas at various price ranges can be ordered online. See www.asiachi.com. Other Chinese slimming teas that are laxative and diuretic include Bojenmi, broadleaf holly leaf (*Folium ilicis latifoliae*) tea, and Royal 1 & One black tea, once reserved only for the Chinese royal family. Get Svelte, a Yin/Yang Sisters instant beverage that contains hawthorn, a useful heart tonic, can be ordered from www.eastearthherb.com.
- **Digestive herbal teas** are soothing. They include mint, chamomile, and vervain.
- **Tibetan teas** are useful for emotional Bears. Sorig Loong Tea calms anxiety, Sorig Tripa Tea cools anger and frustration while it normalizes blood pressure, and Sorig Bad-Kan Tea boosts energy, warms the body, and lifts spirits to treat bingeing caused by depression.
- **Oatstraw tea**, which contains silica and iron, benefits Bears with thinning hair. Sweeten with health food store black cherry concentrate.

Food for Bears

Bears in the wild eat mostly fruit, berries, and seeds. Before hibernation, they purposely gain weight by eating lots of fish and fish eggs. The same diet applies for our Bears.

FRUIT: blackberries, blueberries, and other berries are good blood purifiers that provide necessary minerals. Figs, grapes, and grapefruit are cleansing and slimming. Ripe papaya is especially good for stomach and intestinal disorders. Papaya provides sodium, magnesium, and sulfur, and the seeds can be made into a cleansing tea. You should ripen citrus so that it tastes sweet. Overly ripe lemons, orange, and grapefruit improve calcium absorption and thus reduce joint pain and bone spurs. Ending the meal with a bite of orange is a traditional Chinese way to stimulate digestion and clear the palate.

THE CABBAGE FAMILY: Brussels sprouts, cauliflower, Chinese cabbage, and broccoli are good bodybuilders that also cleanse the body and protect immunity. The best middle-slimming Bear food in the cabbage family is sauerkraut. Sour is the opposite of sweet: It drains, cleanses, and purifies the digestive tract. Therefore, it slims and tones the middle. Buy organic, naturally processed sauerkraut without additives, and enjoy some for lunch with vegetables, goat cheese, or a baked potato. If digestion is weak, steam sauerkraut lightly or sauté it in grapeseed oil with caraway seeds and sliced onions.

THE BITTER FLAVOR: Chicory greens and chervil added to salads may be new foods to try for cleansing and enhancing Bear digestion, as well as for increasing minerals, especially potassium, iron, and sulfur. Additional slimming Bear foods are cooling and cleansing greens, including asparagus, watercress, and endive. They are all slightly bitter and sour and therefore cleansing.

VEGETABLE SOUPS: Some Bears enjoy making soups with a variety of vegetables. Some new ones to try may be potato substitutes such as parsnips. They are wonderfully light and sweet when steamed. Steamed or baked kohlrabi, a vitamin C–rich member of the cabbage family, is useful for the skeletal, digestive, and lymphatic systems. String beans are good sources of minerals. Pureed lima beans and lentils, both sources of potassium, phosphorus, and hormone-balancing isoflavones, are useful for stomach ulcers and are a good muscle-building food. In addition, baby limas provide calcium and iron.

FOODS CONTAINING OMEGA-3 OILS: Fish, such as organic or wild salmon, herring, sardines, and mackerel, is an excellent source of protein and omega-3 oils. If you are allergic to fish, you might use flaxseeds and flaxseed oil, hemp oil, or walnuts as a source of heart-protective omega-3s. Eggs can also be fortified with omega-3 fats by adjusting the chicken's feed.

RED YEAST RICE PILLS: Another way to protect the heart is a Chinese anticholesterol remedy that originates from rice. Red yeast rice pills, available from www.puritan.com and other Web sites, should be taken along with coenzyme Q_{10} daily. The dose recommended at the Columbia University Medical School conference on alternative medicine is two 600-milligram capsules of red yeast rice taken twice daily, along with one 50-milligram capsule of coenzyme Q_{10}. They reduce or normalize cholesterol within a few months, provided they are taken with a sensible diet and exercise routine. The only downside of red yeast rice is that it is best digested with a cup of coffee, not a big meal. Otherwise, it may cause bloating.

The Tree-Sap Cholesterol Cure

A Bear's love of sweet, rich, and congesting foods leads to chronic health problems beyond overweight. It is wise to prevent future discomforts and illness by using powerfully cleansing and slimming Asian herbs.

A treasure among East Indian rejuvenation tonics is the tree gum guggul (*Commiphora mukul*), a relative of myrrh. Guggul comes from India and is used for both incense and internal medicine. It is safer and more appropriate for weight loss than myrrh. Guggul disinfects secretions, including mucus, sweat, and urine. It clears the lungs, helps heal the skin, and enhances circulation, reducing fat, cellulite, and fibroids. A cleansing and slimming remedy par excellence, guggul is used for arthritis, rheumatism, gout, lumbago, diabetes, obesity, bronchitis, hemorrhoids, sores and ulcers, cystitis, and certain female disorders. Guggul should be avoided during acute kidney infections or acute rashes. (A better treatment for gout than guggul is homeopathic Formic acid 6X, taken several times daily between meals.)

The energetic effects of guggul are rejuvenating, stimulating, nervine (relaxes nervous irritability), antispasmodic, analgesic, expectorant, astringent, and antiseptic. It increases white blood cell count. Guggul steps up the action of other cleansing, healing herbs.

Guggul can be taken alone or with hawthorn to enhance circulation and reduce cholesterol. It can be added to digestive remedies to improve their middle-slimming, antifat properties. Guggul capsules can be combined with the herbs recommended for cellulite in Chapter 5, including gotu kola and ginkgo.

Guggul is also sold as powder (churna) and pills with various names such as Guggul Slim pills. Triphala guggul, a combination of three famous rejuvenating fruits and guggul, is a traditional Indian health tonic that balances the body and mind. Its ingredients include amla (*Emblica officinalis*), a cherry that provides a powerful food source of vitamin C and is used for acidity, edema, and hair loss; bibhitaki (*Terminalia belerica*), used for sore throat, catarrh, stones, and dysentery; and harıtakı (*Terminalia chebula*), used for bloating, hiccups, jaundice, heart disease, edema, and malabsorption. Triphala guggul tones digestion and circulation and improves energy and metabolism as it purifies the body.

You can find guggul in Vitamin Shoppe stores or other large chain stores, as well as in health food stores and online. If you plan to use guggul for slimming, take it between meals with a glass of water during the day because it may stir energy. Overuse may stimulate appetite or increase inflammatory conditions such as night sweats and hot flashes. As with all herbal products used for the first time, I recommend trying the lowest recommended dose once daily and watch for the effects.

People who will benefit the most from guggul have a large, puffy, pale, waterlogged tongue; a deep, sluggish pulse; low energy; and slow digestion. They may have a hypothyroid condition, chronic congestion, and edema like Dragons. They may have diabetes or kidney stones without having excess thirst or hunger. They may have slow-healing oozing wounds. Women with severe menstrual cramps and endometriosis, or anyone with burning stomach ulcers, should consult a natural health specialist. Guggul may be helpful but should be used with supervision. Otherwise, to balance guggul's drying effects, it can be combined with aloe vera gel.

Once, near a Delhi temple, I met a fellow who said that many Indian women fast on Monday, a day devoted to Lord Shiva, in order to stay slim and catch a husband. I can think of no more pleasant fast than fruits, tea with lemon or aloe vera, and guggul.

A Chinese Diet for Diabetes

China and Korea have a relatively low incidence of diabetes and obesity, compared with the United States, because their diet is generally less fatty and sweet than ours. In addition, many moistening foods and herbs are popular rejuvenation tonics in China. Visit a Chinese herb shop especially during the summer, and you will find people of all ages buying *Panax quinquefolium* (American ginseng) tea recommended for, among other things, excess dryness causing hunger and thirst, dry skin, and premature aging. American ginseng can be cooked as a tea or combined with other herbs to make a medicinal brew. In general, when cooking for diabetes, it is important to avoid sweet foods, including carrots and beets. However, beet greens can be added to salads, and carrot tops, cooked in soups, are a source of essential minerals.

TCM recognizes dryness and inflammation symptoms associated with diabetes in three problem areas—the lungs, stomach, and kidneys—called lung-fire syndrome, stomach-fire syndrome, and kidney yin-deficiency syndrome. Each area is treated with appropriate foods and herbs because inflammatory symptoms may vary. Following is an overview including recommended foods and Chinese patent remedies, which are herbal formulas made into pills, syrups, or capsules. Chinese herbal patent formulas, some of them dating from ancient times, are available today in Chinese food shops and online at numerous Web sites.

You may have the following symptoms without having diabetes. Chinese medicine quite often treats predisease discomforts. The recommended foods and herbs may help you to lose weight by reducing excess appetite and improving vitality.

Lung-Fire Syndrome

Smokers can easily develop this set of symptoms: chronic thirst, dry nose and mouth, dry cough, frequent urination, and vomiting blood. Lung-fire syndrome leads to dry skin, anxiety, and nervous snacking. In this case, foods should reduce lung tissue inflammation. They include asparagus, dried lily flowers added to soup or tea, and whole soy products such as cooked soy beans. Try duck eggs and green olives, too.

Stomach-Fire Syndrome

Stomach-fire syndrome, on the other hand, features a dry, bitter taste in the mouth; toothaches and bleeding gums; constipation from dryness; chronic excess hunger; fever; headache; hiccups; nausea; and vomiting blood. A diet of overly hot spices, excess alcohol, smoking, or stomach ulcers can aggravate these discomforts. Recommended cooling foods include carp, ripe banana, strawberry, bamboo shoots, steamed spinach, cucumber, beet greens, mung beans, peppermint tea, lily flowers, and a special edible fungus usually labeled as black fungus in Chinese groceries.

BLACK FUNGUS resembles crinkled paper that is black on one side and gray on the other. It is sometimes cooked with soybeans for up to 12 hours to reduce cholesterol and digestive inflammation. Soak one piece of black fungus the size of your palm in water until it becomes soft and doubles in size. Cut it into pieces and cook it with soups for up to 1 hour.

Kidney-Yin Deficiency

Finally, kidney-yin deficiency is one of the toughest problems faced by people with diabetes or anyone with chronic inflammatory and dehydration problems. Symptoms such as dry mouth and throat; hot palms and soles; fatigue; night sweats; pain in the heels; retention of urine or very thick, oily urine; insomnia; ringing in the ears; and sexual problems are worse at night. These discomforts are common for menopausal women who drink coffee and smoke; people with chronic infections; or people troubled by dehydration from illness, certain medicines, or other bad habits.

Some people literally wither their youth and sexuality with inflammatory habits. Eventually, vision, hearing, and memory suffer because reduced blood and body fluids fail to nourish the brain, nervous system, muscles, and internal organs. For kidney-yin deficiency, Chinese herbalists recommend cooling, nourishing foods such as abalone, asparagus, chicken and duck eggs, cuttlefish, white fungus, steamed oysters, royal jelly, water chestnuts, organic chicken liver, and a soup made with spinach and pork kidney. Broccoli green tea or broccoli and vegetable cooking water works well to hydrate the body and protect against cancer and diabetes.

WHITE FUNGUS (*Tremella fuciformis*; *bai mu er*), a puffy, beige fungus that resembles a dried sponge, is sold in Chinese grocery stores. It is recommended for reducing dry cough and chronic thirst, maintaining a youthful complexion, and reversing dryness and aging of the skin. It is thought to be rejuvenating for the lungs, stomach, and kidneys because it generates fluids. It contains B vitamins and trace minerals, including iron, sulfur, phosphate, magnesium, calcium, and potassium.

White fungus can be used as a rather tasteless, semisweet, and crunchy addition to soups, such as Chinese chicken and corn. Soak one piece in water for 1 to 3 hours, rinse, and remove specks of dirt. Using a kitchen scissors, cut off the hard yellow ridge from the bottom; it does not soften with cooking. Then rinse and simmer the white fungus in water for about ½ hour until it is soft.

REHMANNIA is an important rejuvenating herb made by cooking

Chinese foxglove herb in wine. It resembles sliced black tar and is said to recondition the tissue of the lungs, stomach, liver, and kidneys. Rehmannia tastes semisweet when cooked in herbal formulas for diabetes or other stress-related illnesses. Rehmannia contains extremely valuable components that reduce the common signs of aging and chronic inflammation. Among them are ß-sitosterol, a steroidal anti-inflammatory, and arginine. (People with herpes infections or other periodic rashes are warned to avoid excess arginine use because it can bring out a rash.) Used over time, rehmannia reduces high blood sugar.

MOISTENING AND NOURISHING HERBS can be useful for preventing premature aging and illnesses such as Alzheimer's. Many Chinese people use Liu Wei Di Huang Wan pills to improve vitality and reverse chronic thirst, menopausal complaints, and dry, aging skin. However, you have to watch as your symptoms change. Increasing moisture may not be the only answer to your problems. Moistening herbs may increase urination, diarrhea, abdominal pain, dizziness, or palpitations for some people. If those temporary discomforts develop, discontinue using rehmannia or formulas that include it.

The dose for Chinese patent remedies is always individualized. Most people prefer to use a smaller dose, such as six pills two or three times daily for a long period of time so that they can become accustomed to its effects.

It is advised to stop taking all tonics—either energy tonics or blood tonics (moistening herbs)—if you catch a cold. A cold is an acute problem that must be treated accordingly. Tonics are used long term to improve your general health.

Native American Miracle Herbs for Diabetes and Weight Loss

Our Native American herbal tradition encompasses desert plant medicines revered from New Mexico to India and the Middle East. America's most respected native herbalist, Tieraona Low Dog, MD, a Lakota who lives in New Mexico, is a beautiful, graceful, and vivacious woman with long, black hair, who's most often seen wearing a long skirt, turquoise jewelry, and a winning smile.

In 2001, *Time* magazine praised Dr. Low Dog as an outstanding innovator in complementary and alternative medicine. Currently, she is adjunct faculty at the University of Arizona in Tucson, where she works with Andrew Weil, MD, and his fellowship program in integrative medicine. In addition to her research, Dr. Low Dog is the author of *Gifts of the Earth: The Healing Way of Herbal Medicine.*

Dr. Low Dog's patient population in the Southwest is a proving ground for herbs. Overweight and diabetes are very common problems, and her women patients especially love herbs. And she has just the herb to treat these problems:

DEFATTED FENUGREEK SEEDS. When I asked Dr. Low Dog what she recommended most often for weight loss and diabetes, she did not hesitate a moment but answered, "I tell my patients to get defatted fenugreek seeds and whip up ¼ cup of them to make smoothies twice a day." I have enjoyed the spicy tea made from pungent yellow fenugreek seeds. Fenugreek, a stimulating aphrodisiac spice sometimes recommended for asthma, increases sweating; the tea makes your body aroma pleasantly spicy, like the seed.

Fenugreek (*Trigonella foenum-graecum*), native to North Africa and countries bordering the eastern Mediterranean, is widely cultivated in India, where the seeds are used to spice curries. Fenugreek seeds also have antidiabetic and anticholesterol properties. The fiber-rich, defatted portion of the seeds has nutritive and restorative properties that stimulate the digestive process. Fenugreek seeds are a rich source of fiber and protein. The protein fraction contains the amino acid 4-hydroxyisoleucine, which stimulates insulin production. Whole fenugreek seeds also contain 4.8 percent saponins, a plant nutrient that has steroidal properties.

A Google search for defatted fenugreek produced numerous medical and popular health Web sites. Some, like www.diabeticbar.com, offer scientific information and research; others, such as www.sedonalabs.com, sell products. For example, FenuMax is a pure, odorless fiber extract from fenugreek seed that helps regulate blood sugar spikes—jumps from relatively normal to high blood sugar. Other herb sites such as www.iherb.com sell blood sugar regulating products such as Blood Sugar Formula, which combines fenugreek seed, gymnema, and bitter melon. Such dietary supplements may prove to be a convenient way to suppress excess appetite and regulate weight. Finally, if you want to whip up your own smoothies, www.supplementwatch.com sells defatted fenugreek powder.

GYMNEMA. The other treatment Dr. Low Dog regularly recommends for overweight and diabetes is *Gymnema sylvestre*, a popular herb from India. It is sold in American health food stores and East Indian groceries as gymnema. The Web site www.himalayausa.com sells gymnema pills, and www.himalayanhealthcare.com fully describes the herb, including its pharmacology, actions, and important research findings.

Gymnema has antidiabetic properties because it has a regenerative effect on pancreatic beta cells and is insulinotropic. That means it rejuvenates the cells in the pancreas that secrete insulin. Gymnema leaf extract is a cardiovascular stimulant and digestive tonic. It reduces digestive discomforts and is mildly laxative and diuretic. Gymnema is a helpful herb for weight loss because it speeds and eases digestion.

Clinical tests on lab animals have shown the water-soluble extract to normalize blood pressure and glucose level after 60 days use. The alcohol extract of the leaves of gymnema was found to be effective in preventing liver damage.

Gymnema is definitely Bear food because it reduces an addictive craving for sugar, as well as high blood sugar. In India, the leaves are chewed because they neutralize the taste of sweet and slightly bitter foods for several hours. Whether or not you have diabetes, using gymnema to improve digestion or reduce appetite and a sweet tooth enhances weight loss. The recommended dose for diabetes is one 500-milligram capsule with a glass of water, twice daily before meals. When I tried it, being neither diabetic nor a Bear, the herb felt soothing and relaxing. It eased my nighttime hunger, which sometimes keeps me awake snacking. No side effects have been reported for gymnema. To be on the safe side, always separate by 2 hours taking an herb and a prescribed medication.

Since high blood sugar has been associated with overweight, heart trouble, and cancer, it is wise to keep it in check. When in doubt, you can observe your blood sugar with a simple over-the-counter test, and aim for a healthy range under 110 mg/dl.

An Ayurvedic Diet for Diabetes: Bitter, Cooling, and Rejuvenating

Ayurveda recognizes several forms of diabetes belonging to a group of 20 obstinate urinary diseases (*prameha*) brought on by a sedentary lifestyle; disturbed sleep patterns; and excess consumption of "unctuous" (sticky) foods such as yogurt, fish, crustaceans, and refined starches. Mental worries and stress also play important roles in diabetes, according to Ayurveda. The treatment reduces body fat, and the function of the pancreas is regulated to promote sugar metabolism.

Foods to avoid include sugary foods; starches such as rice, potato, bananas, and high carbohydrate cereals; and fats and oils. Ayurveda also has a number of recommendations concerning foods and herbs to add to the diet.

BITTER FOODS, such as bitter melon (in India called karela), are emphasized. The gourd and leaves are juiced raw, and 1 ounce is consumed twice daily on an empty stomach. I do not recommend it unless you love bitter flavors. It is easier to lightly steam sliced bitter melon using a few tablespoons of water or drink a strong tea made from Cherry Grain Balsam Pear Tea.

NEEM is another bitter herb very useful for detoxifying the entire body and reducing blood sugar. You can find capsules of neem in some health foods stores and online. Other useful foods include roasted chicory root as a beverage, chickpeas, turmeric, amla powder, guggul, and shilajit.

SHILAJIT CAPSULES are made from a refined form of bitumen, a coal product that contains many vitamins, minerals, and trace minerals.

It is cooling, moistening, and relaxing in nature. If you have a dry, red tongue; a fast or choppy pulse; chronic thirst; thinning hair; and dry skin, shilajit will feel rejuvenating.

I have recommended shilajit for a wide range of health and beauty issues, including premature aging, poor memory, insomnia, infertility, and reduced semen and sexual fluids. Imagine entering a dark, ancient cave and finding a fountain of youth. That is how shilajit smells, tastes, and feels when consumed. It is made from centuries of plant and animal life compressed under extreme pressure. In India, one form of shilajit is made by boiling rocks to make a foam, which is dried in the sun. In Russia, shilajit is used to set and heal broken bones in animals. It may be the closest thing we have to human bone marrow in the mineral world.

For general rejuvenation purposes and to de-stress internal organs, take one or two capsules of shilajit at bedtime. It is an aphrodisiac but not a stimulant. It works by gradually reconditioning tissue and fluids needed for youth and vigor. Can there by anything better for a Bear than to rest and rejuvenate during a long sleep in a cave?

AYURSLIM. An interesting herbal combination called AyurSlim, made by Himalaya Herbals, is sold in Indian food shops and at www.herbalsalon.com. It contains garcinia (*Garcinia cambogia*), guggul, gymnema, and a digestive and laxative fruit haritaki (*Terminalia chebula*). It is said to burn excess fat and reduce cholesterol and triglyceride levels. The recommended dose is two or three capsules 30 minutes before meals on an empty stomach.

Ginseng for Cholesterol and Chest Pains

Adaptogenic herbs help us survive stress by easing uncomfortable symptoms and supporting vitality. Adaptogens are substances that behave differently, depending upon what the body needs.

TIENCHI GINSENG is a great example. Raw tienchi powder can be added to water as a tea or to soups during cooking. It is cooling for the entire body. It reduces cholesterol and helps maintain blood vessel health and elasticity. It is useful for bruises, chest pains, and chronic inflammatory discomforts, including hot palms, heart palpitations, and high blood pressure.

Bears and others are not always overheated. Some people become weak and blood deficient because their vitality is low or after losing blood following an accident, childbirth, or an illness. They tend to feel chilled, wear heavy clothing, and use quilts on their beds during the entire year. More than likely, their tongues are pale and the pulse slow or deep and weak. They may have low blood pressure or hypo-adrenal (low adrenal gland) symptoms. They require a warming form of tienchi called steamed tienchi ginseng powder, which can be added to water as a tea. Tienchi, in other words, maintains healthy blood circulation but works differently depending on whether or not it is powdered, raw, or steamed.

Bears have to pay attention to unhealthy cholesterol because it can by aggravated by a Bear's favorite sweet, oily, and rich foods, as well as stress, indigestion, and family recipes (which are some of the causes of so-called genetic illnesses).

Reduce Your Sweet Tooth

Here is how you can become accustomed to enjoying foods that are less sweet.

- **Juice and water:** Start the day with a glass of half fruit juice and half water, and continue sipping throughout the day. Use apple, pineapple, pear, grape, or papaya, and avoid overly sweet orange or peach juices. Then, after a while, mix one-third juice and two-thirds water, so you become accustomed to less sweet flavors. Remember, the riper the fruits, the sweeter they taste. Allow citrus to shrivel and overripen in the window.
- **Broccoli water:** If you have diabetes, start the day with boiled broccoli water. It has tremendous healing effects, including preventing prostate trouble, cancer, and skin blemishes. This recipe is an adaptation of Dr. Ibrahim Saracoglu's "broccoli cure."

Simmer a handful of broccoli in 2 cups of water for 10 minutes. Drink the water and eat a piece or two of broccoli, then eat nothing else for 20 minutes. If you hate broccoli, pour the cooking water over green tea.

- **Bee pollen:** As a midmorning or midafternoon snack, have 1 teaspoon of health food store bee pollen, a source of B vitamins. It can be mixed with juices.
- **Green supplements:** To reduce acidity, end each meal with two capsules of chlorophyll concentrate or three capsules of dandelion, as needed. Cleansing the liver and blood and making the body more alkaline with these bitter foods will reduce acid and sweet cravings.
- **Aloe vera gel:** As a cooling, cleansing, alkaline, laxative drink, add ¼ cup of aloe vera gel to water, tea, or juice daily. If you have diabetes, add ¼ teaspoon of cinnamon powder per cup.
- **Minerals:** Add 60 to 100 milligrams daily of chromium picolinate and 30 milligrams zinc to your diet. Some doctors believe that we crave sweet foods because we lack chromium. Zinc reduces stress and supports the pancreas. Be sure to take a zinc supplement at night on an empty stomach because zinc can interfere with the absorption of other minerals such as copper and iron. Large intakes of zinc can cause nausea and diarrhea.

A Few Asian Sweets

Asians appreciate bitter foods, such as those in the cabbage family, teas (such as Shiitake/Fu Ling Tea on page 45), and bitter melon. That is one reason they live longer than many Americans. However, we cannot live on bitter foods alone.

Chyawanprash

When you want some chocolate, eat 1 teaspoon of chyawanprash, a semisweet health paste available in East Indian groceries or online at a number of Web sites, including www.bytheplanet.com. Chyawanprash, pronounced "cha-won-prosh," is a traditional Ayurvedic herbal jam made by Dabur and a few other major Indian manufacturers from a base of amalaki fruit. Amalaki or amla fruit, we have said, is the richest source of vitamin C known to man and is a powerful antioxidant and rejuvenator. While providing vitality to all the cells of the body, it both nourishes and strengthens the immune system.

Chyawanprash is formulated from more than 40 herbs, including ashwagandha, pippali (a rejuvenating pepper), digestive cardamom, nutmeg, and cinnamon in a base of clarified butter (ghee) and honey. This energizing formula is slightly warming and thus helps promote healthy digestion and stimulates the metabolism. It is suitable for adults and children. In fact, Indian mothers give a spoonful of the thick, sweet paste to their children as we would a multivitamin supplement. Enjoy chyawanaprash as a snack on crackers—1 teaspoon, two or three times per day.

Coconut Oil

Some people love coconut oil and add it while cooking to various dishes. It can also be used on pastas or taken by the spoonful as a slimming dessert. Others believe it is too heavy and avoid it. You have to decide for yourself. According to www.coconutdiet.com, "Researchers now know that weight loss associated with coconut oil is related to the length of the fatty acid chains contained in coconut oil."

Coconut oil has several practical advantages for healthy weight loss. One teaspoon of virgin coconut oil after a meal is rich, satisfying, and filling like a sweet treat. It is soothing for the digestive tract. Used internally and topically, it beautifies the skin and hair. It may be laxative for some people because it is moistening. Virgin coconut oil is available in health food stores and online. You may not lose more than a few pounds with it, but you will quickly feel and look better in your clothes—and you certainly will feel energized and less in need of dessert.

Bear Meals

Cooling, moistening foods and savory digestive spices satisfy a Bear's love of rich, sweet flavors. Among the Bear's preferred spices are anise, cumin, fennel, and cardamom. Black cherry concentrate is used to sweeten beverages and pies. Yeast-free breads and sugarless pies are fun ways to bring family and friends together.

A Bear Breakfast

Fresh fruit, one slice of whole grain bread, and ½ cup of low-fat vanilla yogurt make a natural Bear breakfast. A teaspoon of milled flaxseed sprinkled over yogurt or cereals provides healthy omega-3 oils. One block of tofu or a small filet of salmon along with a steamed vegetable provide adequate protein for the entire day.

If you eat fish, avoid eggs, red meat, and dairy foods during the same day. Those food combinations encourage digestive troubles and parasites. Most of the breakfast choices for Dragons apply equally for Bears, but Ursa prefers something sweet, like a sugar-free pie and a spiced tea. (To avoid added weight, think of desserts as a separate meal or snack with tea—not as part of a meal.)

Spices

Spiced teas are a practical way to incorporate digestive herbs into your daily diet. Add up to ¼ teaspoon of powdered spice per cup of tea. Read about and, if necessary, order spices online at www.botanical.com.

During Virgil's time, anise, cumin, and cardamom were used to make a digestive cake served after wedding feasts. Today, star anise is largely employed in France, Spain, Italy, and South America in the preparation of cordials. In China and India, anise oil is still added to water and used medicinally as an aromatic, carminative, and stimulant for bronchitis and asthma. It makes a healthy tea between meals for Bears and anyone who smokes.

To curb a sweet craving, pure fennel culinary oil—available in East Indian food shops or online—can be used as a relaxing perfume for the face and throat. Fennel seeds can be simmered in water as a tea.

WARMING SPICES: If you have a pale tongue, slow digestion, and wheezing from phlegmy congestion, you can benefit from warming, digestive spices anise, cardamom, ginger, pepper, clove, and caraway. Use only a dash of clove because it is strongly heating and best used for urinary incontinence or wheezing tuberculosis.

HINGVASHTAKA CHURNA: This spicy East Indian digestive powder reduces bloating, mucus congestion, and colic. It can be substituted for pepper in dishes or added to tea.

COOLING HERBS AND SPICES: If your tongue is red and you feel hungry or feverish much of the time, a cooling digestive spice is better. Cumin, coriander, fennel, mint, and dill are cooling, diuretic, and reduce acidity and excess hunger.

TURMERIC: This should be used by everyone daily. Turmeric grows as a tuber in India. In Indian food shops, it resembles a small gingerroot. The dried, bright yellow-orange spice powder is sold in your supermarket. Turmeric is anti-inflammatory for arthritis, has anticancer properties, and increases healthy intestinal flora. Try adding ½ teaspoon when cooking pasta, oatmeal, soups, or sauces. You can also sprinkle turmeric powder onto yogurt, juices and shakes, or starchy vegetables.

Here are several recipes that will help you incorporate healing spices into your daily diet.

SPICY CAULIFLOWER

To seal in natural flavors, lightly steam vegetables in a covered pot, using only a little water. Never throw away the cooking water but recycle it into soups or sauces. This dish uses cauliflower, but you can substitute Brussels sprouts, broccoli, or any root vegetable.

MAKES 4 SERVINGS | PREPARATION TIME: 15 MINUTES
- *1 head cauliflower*
- *1 tablespoon vinegar*
- *½ medium yellow onion, sliced*
- *Salt substitute or hingvashtaka powder (optional)*
- *¼ cup plain low-fat yogurt*
- *⅛ teaspoon turmeric powder*
- *⅛ teaspoon cumin powder*
- *½ teaspoon cinnamon powder*

Remove any dark spots from the cauliflower. Turn it upside down and cut out the center. Soak it in water and the vinegar for 10 minutes, or bring the vinegar water to a boil and blanch the cauliflower. Cut into florets.

Steam the onion in a little water until it is tender. Add the rinsed cauliflower and a little more water and steam for about 10 minutes. While the cauliflower is still slightly firm, turn off the heat and continue to steam for a few minutes. Remove from the heat and correct the seasonings with salt substitute or spicy hingvashtaka powder, if desired.

Gently mix the yogurt with the spices. Pour the mixture over the cauliflower. Serve warm or cold.

VEGETABLE SOUP WITH CORDYCEPS

This soup has a homey, sweet flavor and a few surprises. Tremella (white fungus) is crunchy and moistening for dry cough and dry skin. It is sometimes added to Chinese chicken soups. Cordyceps sinensis capsules, found in health food stores or Chinese herb shops, are made from a celebrated immune-enhancing herb shown to have antitumor activity. Cordyceps also eases chest circulation to counter stress. Japanese studies have shown the herb facilitates breathing and bloodflow to the heart, thus helping to prevent heart attack. It is also a traditional Chinese ingredient in duck soup.

MAKES 4 SERVINGS | PREPARATION TIME: 1 HOUR 15 MINUTES

> 1 piece Chinese white fungus
> 3 cups fresh vegetables cut into 1" pieces, such as yellow squash, parsnips, celery, broccoli or Chinese cabbage, yellow corn, peas, and spinach
> 1 clove garlic, minced
> 2 tablespoons tomato sauce
> ½ teaspoon coriander powder
> ¼ teaspoon caraway powder
> ½ teaspoon chervil
> Salt substitute
> 2 capsules Chinese cordyceps
> Dash of nutmeg
> 1 teaspoon virgin coconut oil or flaxseed oil (optional)

Soak the fungus for at least 1 hour or overnight. Remove the tough underside ridge with a sharp knife or scissors. Cut into 8 pieces and set aside.

Arrange the vegetables in your pot and add the garlic, tomato sauce, and all the seasonings. Add just enough water to cover the vegetables. Arrange the fungus on top. Cover the pot and simmer for 10 minutes. Turn off the heat and steam, covered, for 5 more minutes. If you want a richer, sweeter flavor, add the oil after cooking, if desired.

PARSNIP JAM

Quick and easy to make, you'll enjoy this inexpensive, healthy jam on breads. Parsnip jam was eaten during Lent, after the vegetable became sweet following a winter spent underground.

MAKES 1½ CUPS | PREPARATION TIME: ABOUT 1 HOUR

> 1 pound parsnip roots, grated
> ½ teaspoon stevia powder (optional)
> Anise powder to taste (optional)
> Juice of ½ lemon
> 1 teaspoon virgin coconut oil (optional)

I like parsnips' naturally sweet flavor, but you may wish to add some stevia or anise powder. Wash and grate the parsnips. Add 1 cup of water and boil until they are reduced to a thick pulp. Add the lemon juice and oil, if desired.

Pastries and Breads

Sweet breads and sugar-free pies can form the basis of a meal or snack and help a Bear satisfy that sweet tooth. Here are a number of sweet, healthy recipes that promote weight loss.

CRANBERRY APPLE BREAD

You may want to experiment with other spices. For example, cardamom tastes nice with apples.

MAKES 6 TO 8 SERVINGS | PREPARATION TIME: 10 MINUTES |
BAKING TIME: 40 MINUTES

> 2 tart apples
> 1 cup dried cranberries
> 2 cups whole wheat flour
> 2 teaspoons baking powder
> ½ teaspoon allspice powder

¼ teaspoon clove powder

½ teaspoon ginger powder

1 tablespoon cinnamon powder

1 tablespoon arrowroot or cornstarch

½ cup rice milk

¾ cup unsweetened applesauce

1 tablespoon vanilla extract

Preheat the oven to 400°F.

Wash the apples in the vegetable wash (page 31), then cut them into pieces. Place the cranberries in a pan, add water to cover, and bring to a boil, then drain off the liquid and excess sugar. Set aside.

In a large bowl, mix together the flour and other dry ingredients. In a separate bowl, mix the rice milk, applesauce, vanilla extract, reserved cranberries, and apples. Stir the wet ingredients into the dry ingredients. Using a spatula, scoop the mixture into a floured loaf pan and bake for about 40 minutes until firm and golden brown, or until an inserted toothpick comes out clean.

ESSENE BREAD

At home we call this mud loaf. You can really savor and chew the grains in this sweet, moist bread, a Bear favorite. Soft pastry wheat berries (sometimes called summer wheat berries) are available from natural food stores. Make sure the wheat berries are organic, or they will not sprout. Traditionally, Essene bread was baked on hot rocks under scorching sunlight, because preservation of the enzymes in sprouted bread requires baking at a low temperature for many hours. In this recipe, we steam the bread overnight in a slow cooker. This method is more convenient than baking it in a 200°F oven for 10 to 12 hours.

I have created several versions of this delicious recipe, combining organic wheat berries, rye or oat berries, and spelt berries along with spices such as cardamom, cinnamon, and star anise powder. Here is the simplest starter recipe, to which you may add up to ¼ cup of raisins, nuts, or seeds, and spices.

> *2 cups organic whole wheat berries (1 pound)*
> *2 cups cool water to cover*
> *1 tablespoon yellow cornmeal*
> *1 bag rooibos tea (optional)*

First you have to sprout the berries. Several days before you want to eat this bread, rinse the wheat berries in water, drain, and submerge in a jar or bowl with the cool water. Cover the bowl with a plate and allow the berries to stand at room temperature overnight. They will absorb most of the water.

The following day, rinse the berries in a colander and cover with a plate to prevent the berries from drying. You also can use a jar covered with cheesecloth. Set the colander in a dark cupboard or cold oven so the berries can sprout. Rinse the berries with cool water 5 times a day. In a day or two, the sprouts will reach their optimum length of about ¼". Their growth depends on moisture and temperature.

Grind the berry sprouts in a food processor for 5 minutes to make a thick paste. Pour the mashed sprouts into a large bowl. Squeeze and knead the grain for 5 to 10 minutes to develop its gluten. It will be sticky and heavy. Prepare your baking container: Use a medium soufflé dish with a high rim or a heavy Chinese soup bowl with a 7" diameter. Sprinkle the cornmeal into your container and scoop in the sprouted mash.

Pour water into a slow cooker to a depth of ½". Add the contents of the tea bag to season the water, if you wish. Without getting the dough wet, place the bowl of sprouted dough into the slow cooker. Replace the lid and cook at low heat for 12 hours, or until the bread is firm. Make sure that condensation appears on the lid. The bread is done when a silver knife stuck into the center of the loaf comes out clean.

Allow the bread to cool in the bowl for several hours. Store it in the refrigerator. You can scoop out large spoonfuls or, if the dough is firm enough, cut thin slices. You can drink the non-caffeine rooibos tea after cooking the bread; steeping or cooking it longer than 10 minutes increases its antioxidants.

REHMANNIA, CINNAMON, AND BLUEBERRY PIE

Rehmannia is a rejuvenating and moistening blood tonic. To moderate its laxative effects, I've added ginger and cinnamon. Blueberry, also cooling, moistening, and laxative, has been found to be useful for preventing chronic urinary infections. People with diarrhea, chronic digestive weakness, or herpes should avoid rehmannia and this pie.

MAKES 8 SERVINGS | PREPARATION TIME: 1 HOUR 10 MINUTES

½ *cup dried rehmannia (approximate; use enough to make ½ cup cooked rehmannia paste)*

1 *teaspoon apple cider vinegar*

1 *egg, slightly beaten*

1 *tablespoon pure vanilla extract*

1 *teaspoon cinnamon powder*

½ *teaspoon ginger powder*

½ *teaspoon stevia powder (optional)*

1 *pound fresh blueberries*

1 *low-fat graham cracker piecrust*

Rinse the rehmannia with boiling water and the vinegar to remove dust. Since the herb can be sliced in large or small pieces, you will not know the exact amount until it is cooked. Simmer in a little water for about 30 minutes, or until it is soft. Pour off the liquid and blend the rehmannia in your blender to make a smooth, thick paste. You need ½ cup of rehmannia paste.

Preheat the oven to 425°F.

Continue to blend the herb, adding the egg, vanilla extract, spices, and stevia powder (if using) until thoroughly mixed. Put the paste into a large bowl. Wash and drain the blueberries. Very gently fold the blueberries into the herb mixture. Then pour this into the piecrust.

Cover the pie with foil and bake for about 1 hour, or until firm. Let it cool completely on a rack before cutting. It can be baked the day before use and kept in the refrigerator.

SLIMMING APPLE PIE

Enjoy this refreshing meal with green tea. Its laxative action gets digestion moving. Hawthorn, a main ingredient in Get Svelte, reduces cholesterol. For additional protein and calcium, eat a serving of Slimming Apple Pie with 2 ounces of Cheddar cheese. Like all cleansing dishes, Slimming Apple Pie is best taken early in the day to allow for its slimming effects.

MAKES 4 SERVINGS | COOKING TIME: PREPARATION, 15 MINUTES; BAKE, 1 HOUR

> *3 organic red delicious apples*
> *1 packet Get Svelte*
> *¼ cup dried coconut flakes*
> *½ cup dried cranberries*
> *½ teaspoon caraway seed powder*
> *1 tablespoon Minute Tapioca*
> *¼ cup apple or cranberry juice*
> *1 tablespoon tamarind paste (optional)*
> *1 low-fat graham cracker piecrust*

Preheat the oven to 425°F.

Soak the apples in our fruit and vegetable wash for 10 minutes. Rinse and dry them. Cut into 4 pieces. Place in a food processor with the Get Svelte, coconut, cranberries, caraway, and tapioca. Add the juice. Process only briefly, to make large chunks. For a stronger laxative effect, you can add the tamarind paste.

Scrape the sides of the food processor with a spatula so everything is moistened. Allow the mixture to stand in the processor for 15 minutes, so the tapioca begins to thicken.

Pour into a piecrust and bake for about 1 hour or until done. Let cool at least 15 minutes before cutting.

Bear Menus

Bears require healthy, energizing nutrients that enhance digestion and emotional balance. Stevia herbal powder is the best sweetener for people with diabetes. Daily *Gymnema slyvestre* capsules may be necessary to lower blood sugar. Take the capsules ½ hour before meals. Gymnema reduces your sensation of sweet foods and thus reduces a fattening addiction, while it improves pancreas functioning. On cold days, add cinnamon powder to beverages—a recommendation for people with diabetes and hypothermia.

Digestive remedies such as Indian hingvashtaka, Chinese Xiao Yao Wan pills, Quiet Digestion, or other health food store digestive remedies will ease many Bear discomforts. Large doses of papaya enzyme pills—15 to 20 at a time, several times daily—will improve energy, speed digestion, reduce pain, and help satisfy a sweet tooth.

Bear Menu 1

Before Breakfast (choose one)
- 8 ounces half Concord grape juice, half water
- Water with 1 tablespoon liquid chlorophyll

Breakfast
1 hard-cooked egg and fresh vegetable salad with low-fat
    dressing
1 or 2 high-fiber crackers and spicy mustard
Tea with stevia, if desired

Snack
Hot tea or coffee substitute with stevia powder, with choice of:
- 4 prunes
- Sliced cucumber and celery sticks with 1 ounce low-fat cheese
- 2 cups broccoli green tea or broccoli and vegetable cooking
  water (see Broccoli Water recipe on page 190)

Lunch
Large salad with low-fat dressing
Mixed bean soup or bean burrito

Pico de gallo spicy chopped greens, tomato, and onion sauce
Tea or coffee substitute with stevia, if desired

Snack (choose one)
- ½ cup sliced cucumbers and buttermilk
- Pumpkin pie filling with pumpkin pie spice added
- A defatted fenugreek seed smoothie

Dinner
Salad
2 cooked vegetables
Egg white omelet with shiitake or oyster mushrooms
1 cup steamed or raw asparagus
Tea or vegetable juice

Before Bed (optional)
Low-calorie gelatin or low-fat custard

Bear Menu 2

Before Breakfast
8 ounces water with 1 tablespoon liquid chlorophyll

Breakfast
1 cup cooked oatmeal with up to ¼ teaspoon cinnamon
    powder
1 high-fiber cracker
1 handful of nuts or seeds
Get Svelte instant beverage or tea with stevia, if desired

Snack
1 or 2 tubes Chinese Extractum Astragali

Lunch
Large salad with cooked tomato and canned sardines
Tea or coffee substitute with stevia, if desired

Snack
8 ounces Chinese chrysanthemum flower tea, hot or cold

Dinner

Large salad

2 cups cooked squash, spinach, or kale dressed with oil, scallions, and lemon juice, with choice of:

- Tofu and vegetables
- Baked fish and brown rice

1 tablespoon dulse flakes or ⅛ teaspoon kelp powder

Cherry Grain Balsam Pear Tea

Before Bed (optional)

3 ounces Slimming Apple Pie (page 201) and mint tea

Bear Menu 3

Before Breakfast (choose one)

- 8 ounces water and 1 tablespoon liquid chlorophyll with a twist of lemon
- ¼ teaspoon Indian amla powder (a rich source of vitamin C)

Breakfast

2 ounces steamed salmon cooked with cranberries

2 rice cakes

Tea with a pinch of turmeric powder

Snack

Apple, papaya, or pineapple (for those with diabetes, avoid fruits and substitute 1 handful nuts or seeds)

Chrysanthemum flower tea or African red bush tea sweetened with vanilla

Lunch

Large mixed salad with low-fat dressing

1 cup kasha with mushroom gravy and horseradish

1 cup low-sodium borscht

Tea with lemon or broccoli green tea

Snack

8 ounces fresh vegetable juice or watermelon

Dinner

Large watercress and fresh orange salad
2 ounces steamed salmon cooked with cranberries
2 cups steamed broccoli with the cooking water
Tea or coffee substitute with stevia as needed

Before Bed (optional; choose one)

* Water with liquid chlorophyll
* 1 or 2 chlorophyll capsules

Bear Menu 4

Before Breakfast (choose one)

* 8 ounces water with 1 tablespoon liquid chlorophyll
* Half water, half orange juice

Breakfast

1 cup low-fat yogurt with protein powder added
1 or 2 high-fiber crackers
1 handful nuts or seeds
Tea or coffee substitute with stevia, if desired

Snack

1 cup cooked adzuki beans sweetened with stevia, if desired
Strong fresh-brewed oolong tea

Lunch

Large salad avocado, fenugreek, broccoli sprouts and
vinaigrette, with choice of:

* Chinese bitter melon and brown rice
* Mixed vegetables, including broccoli and eggplant

Snack

1 to 2 cups Bojenmi or oolong tea or Get Svelte instant
beverage

Dinner

½ to 1 cup braised sauerkraut with caraway and black
pepper or hingvashtaka powder

2 to 3 ounces soy sausage with spicy mustard

1 baked sweet potato

1 cup steamed green beans or asparagus

Before Bed *(optional; choose one)*

- Chamomile mint tea
- ½ cup low-fat yogurt with ¼ teaspoon turmeric powder

Bear Menu 5

Before Breakfast

8 ounces half water, half apple juice with ¼ teaspoon amla
   powder

Breakfast

1 cup vegetable barley soup

1 hard-cooked egg with a dab of spicy mustard

1 or 2 high-fiber crackers

Tea with stevia, if desired

Snack

8 ounces water with 1 tablespoon liquid chlorophyll

Raw vegetables

2 cups of broccoli green tea or broccoli and vegetable
   cooking water

Lunch

Large green salad

1 cup whole grain pasta with seafood diablo red sauce

Tea or coffee substitute

Snack

1 small wedge lemon pie

For those with diabetes: 1 or 2 rice cakes and 1 square of
   semisweet baking chocolate (optional)

Tea and stevia

Dinner

Large salad

1 cup grapefruit and orange wedges, scallions, nuts, and
   paprika

4 ounces baked fish
1 cup steamed zucchini with vinaigrette
Tea

Before Bed (optional)
8 ounces water with 1 tablespoon liquid chlorophyll

Bear's Summary

- **Problem:** Excess weight and cellulite at the waist and thighs
- **Traditional Chinese medicine (TCM) element and organs:** Earth element, affects the stomach and spleen/pancreas.
- **TCM issues:** the functions of digestion and assimilation and their impact on fat, cellulite, bruising, and mental clarity
- **Approach:** Enhance digestion and elimination. Improve sweet cravings.

Recommended
- Diet plan: More bitter, cleansing foods to reduce cholesterol, acidity, and sweet cravings; healthy sweets such as virgin coconut oil and chyawanprash; digestive remedies
- Get Svelte instant beverage, a digestive and heart tonic: 1 to 3 cups daily
- Green or black tea—5 or 6 cups daily—to protect the heart, reduce cholesterol and speed digestion; laxative slimming teas acceptable
- Mint tea or mint oil capsules or alfalfa tea or pills with meals
- Shiitake/Fu Ling Tea (page 45) for energy and balance
- Bitter, sour greens (dandelion, endive, arugula, celery, and artichoke): laxative and diuretic, reduce sweet cravings
- Pumpkin and squashes, radish, and parsnips to satisfy sweet tooth (instead of sugar, refined foods, turnips, rice, and fatty or oily foods)
- Kelp, dulce seaweeds, or Laminaria 4 pills to reduce phlegmy congestion, water retention, and tone slow thyroid; guggul to reduce fat, cellulite, and fibroids

- Quiet Digestion pills or Chinese Xiao Yao Wan pills for cramps, bloating, indigestion, and hypoglycemia; otherwise a digestive tea such as mint or ginger as needed
- A B-complex and C vitamin supplement (at least 1,000 milligrams of vitamin C), zinc (30 to 60 milligrams daily), and chromium picolinate (500 milligrams two or three times daily); one probiotic acidophilus capsule (at least 20 milligrams) twice daily to reduce discomfort and improve digestion
- Homeopathic Carbo veg 30C (charcoal) for gas and bloating

Useful for Diabetes and Weight Loss
- Cherry Grain Balsam Pear Tea, *Gymnema sylvestre*, AyurSlim
- Shilajit capsules for excess dryness and thirst

Chapter 8

Free Your Soaring Crane

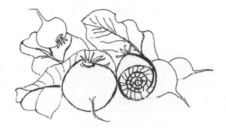

Dear Crane,
    You aspire to attain perfection. You may sparkle like a diamond, stand firm as a mountain, or burn out like a lightbulb: To achieve your aims, you must develop stamina and pursue your talents with care. You are a proud, sensitive, lovely bird who, with courage and dignity, aims high. Foods and herbs described in this chapter can help you—or anyone who has delved through jagged personal depths to rise above the abuse of alcohol, marijuana, cocaine, medical or street drugs, and yo-yo dieting. Detoxifying foods, nutritious sprouted whole grains, and pungent herbal teas help protect against colds, flu, and weak digestion. To prepare your flight from illness, addictions, and overweight, we will stroll through a forest of leaves, berries, and nuts. This chapter also features sea chlorella and rejuvenating Ayurvedic slimming aids that support vitality and beauty.

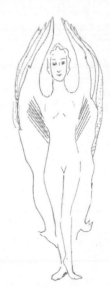

The Crane has narrow facial features and a striking appearance with features such as a high forehead, pointed chin, or prominent nose. Cranes can be further identified by their elongated palms and long, graceful hands or crooked fingers and bulblike fingernails. Wrinkled skin on the knuckles resembles knots in a tree. Cranes may be slender and willowy or massive. People always notice Cranes because they manage to look good wearing anything. Fashion models are always Cranes. Despite fragile health or harmful habits, Cranes remain attractive. Their commanding appearance gains attention.

The Crane personifies the Metal element, which encompasses *qi* energy affecting the lungs, large intestine, and skin. Typical Crane health issues include breathing, eliminating, and maintaining a clear complexion. Their illnesses may range from skin blemishes, shortness of breath, and constipation or diarrhea to chronic depression from low vitality. The Metal element's energy dynamic links consuming and eliminating, which makes Cranes natural subjects for bulimia, bingeing and purging, malnutrition accompanied by overweight, or the weakening effects of yo-yo dieting. Emotional upset can make a Crane reach for a food or addictive substance or run to the toilet.

Cranes protect their breathing space. They avoid people when speaking requires an effort. After public appearances, they withdraw to regroup. Preeminent French coloratura (and Crane) Mado Robin (1918–1960), beloved for her brilliant performances in *Lakmé*, *Mireille*, *Rigoletto*, *Hamlet*, *Barbiere*, and *Lucia* and listed in the *Guinness Book of World Records* for singing a B flat above high C, after performing an opera, added one drop of iodine to a glass of milk and retired for the evening. Several highly accomplished singers and actresses have told me that breath control used in singing has saved them from asthma attacks.

Cranes may be dedicated to their craft, highly spiritual, or politically active crusaders. Among accomplished artists and performers, religious leaders, gold-medal athletes, and world-class entrepreneurs are Cranes who have developed the self-discipline to become stars. Given the right flame, an otherwise cool and collected Crane will sizzle. Marilyn Monroe and Andy Warhol had both Dragon and

Crane energies. Despite personal insecurities, meager backgrounds, and poor health, they were celebrated worldwide.

Cranes and Addictions

Cranes' predominant energy issues influence addictions because vitality affects how we approach relationships. A Bear craves desserts and delights in a loved one's praise and sweet words. Sometimes cookies substitute for kindness. A Dragon, whose vitality stems from heart and kidney qi, may fear death if abandoned. A Dragon, when depressed, calls a friend for consolation or watches television and gulps salty chips or other stimulants. However, a Crane's long-term addictions are fences to keep people out of his or her personal breathing space. One woman told me she smoked to create privacy.

Because the Crane's energy dynamic, as defined by the Metal element, connects the most superficial organs (skin and lungs) to the deepest (the large intestine), Cranes are highly sensitive to their environment. A Crane who feels awkward or uncomfortable may be vulnerable to catching colds and flu. Cranes react strongly to opinions expressed about them. Harsh words penetrate deeply.

Timidity, anxiety, or illness may lead the Crane to seek protection from family, work environment, or external events with secretive, irregular dietary habits. Living under stressful conditions, Cranes are likely to develop constipation, diarrhea, intestinal cramps, or chronic prostate issues. A Crane may fade into the furniture or sink into a steely silence if insulted. Cranes have few natural defenses except escape. Unable to control their environments, many choose addictions to escape harsh surroundings, boredom, and loneliness.

There is more to any addiction than what meets the mouth. It says, "This is who I am." It may be a way of fitting in. When was the last time you shared a pastry, cigarette, coffee, or drug with a friend?

Cranes like to display their long hands. Smoking, eating, and drinking occupy their hands and quiet their nerves. As a tasty substitute for smoking, chew a long piece of cinnamon stick instead of a cigarette. Cinnamon's pungent, sweet aroma is stimulating and satisfying.

Its diaphoretic action (it facilitates sweating) and beneficial effects on the pancreas help free creative thought. Some experts recommend using licorice this way. Not a good idea! Licorice sticks are not useful for weight loss because they increase water retention and can raise blood pressure if overused.

I once met a lawyer, a confirmed cigar smoker, who had switched to chewing Chinese *dong quai* root. Now, this is a much better idea. The lawyer enjoyed the herb's toasty, semisweet flavor and rejuvenating effects. Dong quai's estrogenic action was not harmful for him. The herb improves circulation and increases T-cell count. However, I do not recommend it for anyone with an active cancer. Remedies for nervous habits mentioned in previous chapters, such as Gelsemium and Pulsatilla, and herbs for reducing withdrawal symptoms, such as Ease Plus pills, also apply to Cranes.

Vitality must be enhanced before anyone with addictive eating patterns can improve health and lose weight. No matter what your energy type, if you have menopausal discomforts or are recovering from an illness, chronic fatigue and low willpower will make your addictions difficult to handle. Barring a yeast infection, a reishi mushroom extract or Shiitake/Fu Ling Tea (page 45) can improve energy, immunity, and mood. Additional energy and immune system tonics will be covered in Chapter 11.

A Crane's dietary and energy needs are unique when compared with other types. Tigers require nourishment for pain-free movement, so they can exercise and reduce cellulite. Bears need to address their sweet tooth, regulate blood sugar balance, reduce cholesterol, and reduce a large waistline. Dragons must enhance energy and immunity before they can lose weight. Cranes need to recognize that they in fact have a body that responds to a diet. Some Cranes seem mentally and emotionally preoccupied to the point of free-floating through space. They try trendy diets with no regard for the consequences. One woman fasted on coffee and raw steak for a week, then broke the fast with a cake. Another fasted for weeks on water, then broke the fast with a pound of tomatoes! The acid from the tomatoes gave her hallucinations. The body cannot be abused without reacting: It is a law of nature unto itself.

How to Diet Successfully

If your life is crazy and superdemanding, you must create normalcy with balanced, nourishing foods and a regular eating schedule. Start with the Baseline Diet. That will help you eat more regularly and avoid irritating food combinations. Gradually add remedies for Cranes from this chapter that detoxify, fortify, and slenderize your body. A good general rule: Always address weakness and illness first, then add weight loss and addiction treatments. Here are a number of foods, supplements, and practices that should prove helpful.

REISHI MUSHROOM: Unless you have a candida yeast infection, add a balancing energy tonic made with *Ganoderma lucidum* (the reishi mushroom; in Chinese, *ling zhe*). Reishi+ liquid extract or Power Mushroom pills are both fine energy and immunity tonics.

DIGESTIVE SUPPLEMENTS: Consume something healthy every 3 to 4 hours during the day, until you feel emotionally settled, so that your digestion and metabolism can eventually function normally. Even if you do not eat a full meal, you should take a digestive supplement several times daily to even out the digestive process. If you have bloating, cramping, occasional constipation alternating with diarrhea, and poor absorption, add Quiet Digestion by Health Concerns or the Chinese herbal pill Xiao Yao Wan until you feel stronger. Both are useful for physical and emotional discomforts associated with blood sugar and digestive problems.

FOODS THAT SUPPORT QI: Cranes require pungent and rejuvenating foods that support breathing and, therefore, qi energy. They include green foods and salads with carrot, celery, broccoli sprouts, raw asparagus, radish, onions, ginger, and garlic; balancing whole grains, such as stone cut oatmeal, barley, and quinoa; whole soy foods that provide isoflavones (natural estrogen); nourishing, soothing almonds and almond milk; and antimucus fruits and vegetables, such as apple, papaya, and pineapple.

Important: Extreme diets and fasting lead Cranes to bipolar depression and boomerang eating habits. Lacking a sense of balance, a Crane may fast on water or health foods, while devouring cookies, cheese, and pizza.

The following natural remedies can help you achieve mental and physical balance.

Nux Vomica to Cleanse and Balance the Body

Homeopathic Nux vomica 30C, made from a bitter nut, is a good way to start a new health regimen. Its detoxifying action works very well if you feel stuffed with poorly digested foods and suffer from bad habits. It is recommended for hangovers, headaches with sinus congestion, crankiness, and overindulgence of any kind, especially of foods, drinks, drugs, medicines, work, or ongoing stress. It helps you to start fresh by cleansing the liver. This may be the break you have been waiting for. Nux vomica is useful for any of the energy types to regain balance after going overboard.

The typical Nux vomica patient is described as rather thin, spare, quick, active, nervous, and irritable. But don't believe it: An overweight person can overindulge. Mental work and a sedentary lifestyle are to blame. Someone with an addictive personality grabs for stimulants, coffee, and wine or sedative drugs. The real addiction is a stressful lifestyle. Exhaustion or long-term illness may make digestion, mental concentration, and sleep nearly impossible.

Nux vomica treats a sour taste in the mouth and morning nausea, nausea after eating, belching, colic, liver pain, constipation or diarrhea after eating spicy and rich foods, a feeling of weight and pain in the stomach, an irritated bladder, and the urge for frequent urination. Digestive discomforts such as bloating, flatulence, and ravenous hunger may feel worse a few hours after eating. If you experience such discomforts or crave fats, fried foods, pizza, hot spices, cheese, wine, beer, and strong coffee, you may need Nux vomica to improve weight loss.

One dose (three pills) of Nux vomica 30C taken on an empty stomach every evening for 1 month may solve many of your addiction problems. It should, at least, clear your head, calm your digestion, and help to keep your diet on track. Coffee cancels the remedy, so you need to take it 30 minutes after drinking coffee—regular or decaf. It's perfectly okay to take homeopathic Nux vomica 30C after breakfast and again before bed. If you must take natural remedies and medicines such as antidepressant drugs during the same day, separate them by at least 2 hours. Keep Nux vomica in your pocket for use anytime. Use it regularly, as needed, to prevent withdrawal symptoms.

Desert Herbs That Soothe and Rejuvenate

The following two herbal remedies are cooling, cleansing, and rejuvenating for all the energy types. I've included them here because they are typically recommended for problems ranging from indigestion and cramps to skin blemishes and hair loss. People who feel weakened by using bitter cleansing herbs can take them along with a cup of digestive ginger tea or a capsule of stimulating, astringent myrrh.

ALOE VERA juice soothes an irritated stomach and reduces acidity and appetite. You can drink ¼ cup or more of the health food store juice or gel daily to cleanse and soothe the digestive tract and rejuvenate internal organs. If you cut a branch from the aloe plant, shave off the bitter green exterior and wipe off the slimly liquid from inside. You can juice the pulp and add it to fruit juice. Reduce the dose if it gives you diarrhea.

ECLIPTA ALBA grows in the American desert Southwest, where it is considered a weed. In India, it is called bhringaraj and is used as a potent medicine to heal liver complaints, including chronic hepatitis, cirrhosis, enlargements of the liver and spleen, and anemia, as well as edema, skin diseases, loose teeth, and thinning hair. Chinese herbalists call the herb *han lian cao* and recommend it for premature graying and falling hair and to recondition the liver, blood, and bone marrow. If you take this herb, you'll normally feel an improvement in liver comfort within a week and see new hair growth within 1 month.

The herbal powder can be bought at Asian herb shops or online. Some people fill empty capsules to swallow the powder. Others add ¼ teaspoon to a little water and drink this bitter herb that tastes like mud. It is cooling and rejuvenating and should be avoided by people who have chronic chills. It can more easily be taken during hot weather or by people with chronic fever conditions. Eclipta is an ingredient in American-made herbal products that have liver-protective value, such as Ecliptex, made by Health Concerns.

Liver-Cleansing Home Brews

To balance the action of the liver (or another digestive organ), we stimulate, cleanse, and nourish at the same time. If liver-protective herbal combinations such as those mentioned above are not available, you can make your own home remedy by combining liver-cleansing herbs, liver-stimulating herbs, and balancing liver-protective herbs. You will have to adjust the amounts to suit your individual tastes and needs. But always combine all three sorts of herbs when making a liver tonic.

For liver and blood cleansing, use bitter plants such as skullcap leaf, dandelion leaf and root, or coptis (golden thread). They are laxative and diuretic herbs you might use for headache, complexion blemishes, hives, fever, or constipation. Liver-stimulating herbs include milk thistle. Liver-protective herbs and foods include reishi mushroom, cordyceps medicinal fungi, lycium fruit, schizandra berry, and eclipta. The overall taste of the combination is bitter, pungent, and muddy. If the taste is a problem for you, it may be best to have the herbs powdered by your local herb shop. You can use the powder to fill empty capsules that you get at the health food store.

You might prefer to mix these herbs with gin to make a liver-protective liquor. Add some dried figs to improve the taste. Use a total of about ½ cup of dried herbs per liter of alcohol. Wait 3 weeks before using.

The dose should be very small in the beginning. Try 1 teaspoon in 1 cup of water twice daily for 1 week. Then adjust the dose as needed. If you hate the taste, add it to apple or tomato juice. *Note:* People allergic to alcohol can use vinegar instead to make an extract that can be added to salad dressings.

A word of caution is necessary when using liver and blood-rehabilitating herbs such as eclipta, dandelion, or milk thistle. If you have used street drugs or medical chemotherapy in the past, a trace of the drug may still be in your body. You may experience a temporary mild flashback reaction as the drug leaves your liver, brain, or blood. Liver-cleansing herbs will also affect your menstrual flow and may increase clots as they reduce cramps. Adjust your diet to eliminate irritating spices or cold, raw foods for a while if your body is very sensitive.

Add cleansing herbs to your diet carefully. If your tongue is large, pale, and scalloped and your energy feels very low, you may be too weak to use bitter (laxative and diuretic) herbs unless you try them along with ginger and mint tea. To begin, take the lowest recommended dose of cleansing herbs—for example, one pill—and watch for the results. Gradually increase the dose so that your body becomes accustomed to the cleansing process. You may see great improvements very soon in your complexion, vision, digestion, and mood. Detoxifying the body eliminates fat, mucus, and impurities that would otherwise cause disharmony and disease. You will begin to find freedom from all sorts of poisons from the past.

You also have to realize that using detoxifying foods and herbs is a shock for your body. You will more than likely crave all your addictions twice as much while you destroy them. That is normal. The body tries to maintain any sort of imbalance. It has grown used to being out of shape and weak and functioning improperly. Give yourself time to heal, but stick to the cleansing foods and herbs for withdrawal. If you go back to your former habits, you will feel their ill effects stronger than before because your body has become healthier.

Everyday Drugs and Street Drugs

If you drink coffee, tea, and cola drinks and love chocolate, you should know caffeine's good and bad points. Caffeine acts directly on the central nervous system. A cup of coffee clears your head and lessens fatigue. Caffeine releases sugar stored in the liver, which accounts for its energy lift. However, according to *Earl Mindell's Vitamin Bible*, the release of stored sugar stresses the endocrine system and increases nervousness and withdrawal symptoms.

Research has shown that caffeine, which contains active chemicals called methylxanthines, can provoke fibrocystic breast disease and prostate problems. Caffeine robs the body of B vitamins, vitamin C, zinc, potassium, and other nutrients. It increases digestive acidity and may be implicated in bladder or lower urinary tract cancers. Decaffeinated coffees may be even more hazardous to health, depending on the chemicals used in the processing. Some are similar to pesticides. Either way, people who drink 5 cups of coffee daily are said to have a 50 percent greater chance of suffering heart attacks than non-coffee drinkers. Compare this with the recent research on tea, and you will throw away your coffeepot.

Robert McCaleb, president of the Herb Research Foundation in Boulder, Colorado, has suggested that if Americans drank tea (*Camellia sinensis*) instead of coffee, we could greatly reduce our fat intake. Tea reduces fat absorption in the digestive tract, and its acids speed digestion and elimination. Tea is McCaleb's favorite herb and weight-loss food. No matter if you drink white, green, red, oolong, or black tea; no matter if you add milk, lemon, or ice—tea has amazing health benefits. Depending on the type and how long it is brewed, 1 cup of tea contains about half as much caffeine as coffee.

Alcoholic Beverages

Alcohol, on the other hand, sedates the central nervous system. According to Dr. Mindell, long-term use can rupture veins, destroy brain cells, and deplete the body of a wide range of nutrients (vitamins B_1, B_2, B_6, B_{12}, C, and K; folic acid; and the minerals zinc, magnesium, and potassium).

Red wine is considered healthier than white wine or beer because of heart-protective acids found in red grape peels. However, four drinks a day are said to cause organ damage and severely hamper the liver's ability to process fat. Does knowing all this information stop us from drinking coffee or alcohol? No. We need to rebalance the scale in our favor with some remedies.

Dr. Mindell recommends vitamins to normalize the nervous system and help reduce an addictive craving. They include vitamins A, D, E, C, and all the B vitamins—especially B_{12}, B_6, and B_1—along with choline, inositol, and niacin and a high-protein diet. Other authorities recommend building up to five 200-milligram glutamine capsules (not glutamic acid) three times daily.

When reducing addictions, it pays to cleanse the body and keep the blood alkaline. Therefore, consume 2 to 4 cups of broccoli green tea or broccoli and vegetable cooking water daily.

Marijuana and Cocaine

Marijuana's use as a painkiller and appetite stimulant for cancer patients is under debate. It has positive and negative actions. According to Dr. Mindell, habitual use can raise blood pressure, increase heart rate, and lower body temperature and vitamin C levels in the blood. Like any substance for smoking, it is inflammatory and can cause lung damage. For protection from its harmful effects, Dr. Mindell recommends lots of citrus fruits and leafy greens, time-release vitamin C pills, and vitamin E to protect the lungs. I recommend lots of steamed and fresh greens, bee pollen, and medicinal mushroom extracts for chronic users of marijuana or cocaine.

Cocaine, a vasoconstrictor and stimulant to the central nervous system, blocks nerve impulses and produces a numbing effect. That may be one reason doctors such as Sigmund Freud, who did early research on its effects as a painkiller, quickly became addicted. He, certainly a Crane, smoked so many cigars that he died of mouth cancer. Short-lived effects of cocaine are usually euphoria and self-confidence. Because it requires ever bigger doses, dependence on cocaine is strong. Another danger is not knowing what the drug is cut with—lactose, cornstarch, talcum powder, or much worse.

Instead of antidepressants, many nutritionists recommend choline, calcium, magnesium, B vitamins, and L-phenylalanine. Considering the toxic substances some folks are currently using to fry their brains, these suggestions seem dated. For our purposes, it is better to address depression in relation to weight loss. A craving for empty calories is related to an imbalance of certain brain chemicals, as well as to poor digestion. Luckily, we have foods and natural supplements containing nutrients that benefit those brain chemicals.

Natural Antidepressants and Weight Loss

Lisa Licavoli, RD, CCN, a registered dietitian and board-certified clinical nutritionist who practices in Newport Beach, California, recommends reduced portions and special supplements for weight loss.

5-HTP. One natural supplement called Crave Arrest contains the serotonin precursor 5-HTP (hydroxytryptophan) along with tyrosine and nutrients to balance neurotransmitters. Serotonin is a neurotransmitter (brain chemical) needed for normal brain function. Serotonin deficiency is implicated in anxiety, panic disorders, bulimia, PMS, and hyperactivity. Clinical studies of 5-HTP in Europe and Japan have shown results equal to pharmaceutical antidepressants. Any such supplement should, of course, be combined with exercise, stress-reduction strategies, and counseling. Supplements that contain 5-HTP should not be combined with antidepressant drugs, especially MAO (monoamine oxidase) inhibitors, or selegiline, an anti-Parkinson's drug. They should not be taken while pregnant or given to young children. If nausea occurs, reduce the recommended dose or take the supplement with meals.

ENDOTRIM: Licavoli also recommends EndoTrim, which contains green tea to break down brown adipose tissue; *Coleus forskohli*, which helps thyroid hormones function properly; and other ingredients to support weight loss.

OMEGA 3 OILS: In conjunction with the two supplements mentioned, Licavoli recommends Nordic Natural omega-3 oils. She told me that a few of her clients have lost as much as 100 pounds by limiting portions and using her recommended remedies. For more information on Licavoli's integrative nutrition approach, see www. healthybodyimage.com.

Acupuncture Massage for Weight Loss

Acupuncturists have successfully treated all sorts of addictions by normalizing body functions and regenerating the scarred tissue of disturbed internal organs. Often treatments for addictions involve acupuncture points on the ear. During the 1980s and 1990s, public health clinics received financial support from the government so that acupuncture was supported in several New York hospitals and prisons for eliminating crack, cocaine, and methadone addictions.

Massaging the ears with organic lavender oil can be very soothing and relaxing for most people. If you find hard ridges and painful areas in the ear, massage them gently until they feel soft and supple. Your circulation and sense of well-being will improve.

Cranes especially benefit from acupuncture because many have a "try to help me" attitude: They won't believe anything works until it works for them. I usually tell them to ask their veterinary doctor about acupuncture. It's used for animals, which rarely are subject to placebo effects.

Crane Diet

The Crane's diet aims to improve irregular digestion and elimination, troubled breathing, low energy, sinus congestion, and chronic rashes. Antimucus foods improve digestive qi and breathing, which increases energy and reduces depression and addictive eating patterns. You might describe the Crane diet as cleansing, nourishing, grounding, and vitalizing.

Teas

Cleansing teas include white, green, red, and black varieties, adding ⅛ teaspoon of turmeric powder per cup. Other possible additions that improve digestion and breathing are tarragon, ginger, mint, cardamom, and orange peel. These spices can improve the taste of broccoli tea.

PU-ERH. James Leung, MD, a Chinese-born internist who practices in Vancouver, British Columbia, recommends pu-erh Chinese red tea for weight loss. It works well for some people who want to give up coffee. Pu-erh is made from an early picked tea leaf that is processed with a unique oxidization process. It is said to be fermented but is not. The process makes a rich-flavored tea that is more digestive than some other teas for people who overindulge in sweets, dairy foods, and red meat. Red tea (*hong cha*) is sometimes served with rich dim sum dishes. If you cannot find Chinese pu-erh locally, see www. inpursuitoftea.com or www.eastearthherb.com.

ROOIBOS AFRICAN RED BUSH TEA, or *Aspalathus linearis*, is indigenous to South Africa. It turns red in your cup and tastes mildly astringent, like Thai twig tea. Since it contains no caffeine or tannins, you can enjoy it anytime. Unlike black tea, rooibos does not reduce iron absorption. Rooibos contains iron, potassium, copper, calcium, manganese, fluoride, zinc, magnesium, and sodium and is considered particularly beneficial for healthy skin, hair, teeth, and bones. The Japanese use rooibos as an ingredient in bread, cosmetics, and sweets, as well as a favorite beverage.

Scientists in Japan have found rooibos to act as an antioxidant, slowing the process of aging and benefiting the immune system. It is also used medicinally to treat melancholy, insomnia, irritability, vascular disorders, allergies, respiratory conditions, blood sugar diseases, liver problems, cataracts, headache, indigestion, nausea, colic, stomach cramps, vomiting, heartburn, and constipation. Recent studies have reported rooibos tea as having antimutagenic (DNA protective) and anti-HIV activity. Other studies have reported strong antioxidant activity for the tea. Rooibos tea's active ingredients also include many healthful flavonoids, polyphenols, and many polysaccharides and oligosaccharides, which are useful for leukemia. The ascorbic acid content varies, depending on the method of preparation. Read more about the tea's ingredients and uses in the Herb and Supplement Encyclopedia found at www.florahealth.com.

YIN/YANG SISTERS INSTANT BEVERAGES include Happy Garden Tea—useful for digestion, poor circulation, a sour mood, nervousness, and emotional PMS. Clean Habits is a liver-cleansing beverage with a bitter aftertaste. I recommend adding one packet to juice once or twice daily. For Cranes who have breathing problems and chronic sinus congestion, Yin/Yang Sisters makes Breathe Free instant beverage, which is best used between meals.

TIBETAN TEAS can help to reduce addictions. Sorig Loong Tea reduces nervous snacking and emotional eating binges during PMS. Sorig Tripa Tea is useful for recovering food, alcohol, and substance abusers because it cleanses the liver and cools and refreshes the body. Sorig Bad-Kan Tea enhances courage and a positive attitude. It should be avoided during a cold, flu, or fever.

HERBS AND SPICES can provide stimulation for people like actors, dancers, and students who too often start the day with coffee, salted peanuts, and a candy bar. Consuming sugar, caffeine, and salt shift adrenal energy into high gear and raise anxiety levels but soon afterward result in fatigue and fat. Cranes can benefit from using stimulating spices added to soups and teas instead. Appropriate spices include ginger, mint, cardamom, a tiny pinch of asafoetida, clove, rosemary, cinnamon, sage, and thyme. Sage tea stops excess sweating. Clove is an adrenal stimulant for wheezing and low energy. Cardamom, a warming sweet and pungent spice, stimulates heart and digestion and is useful for depression.

Ayurvedic Slimming Remedies

As you read about the following Ayurvedic remedies, you may wonder how a digestive remedy treats so many discomforts at once. Ayurveda, a healing science that began some 4 to 5 thousand years ago, sees an individual's physical body, vital energy, and spirit as a unified whole. Ayurvedic physicians use herbs, foods, and other means to facilitate natural processes. Strong digestion is fundamental to supporting good health because it prevents poisons (*ama*) from creating harm. By increasing vitality and eliminating poor digestion and toxins, we prevent many discomforts and diseases.

Ayurvedic doctors today are wise enough to formulate herbal slimming remedies that treat discomforts stemming from our fast-paced eat-everything-at-once lifestyle. You will read more about their balanced formulas in chapters dealing with weight loss after age 40 and health problems related to travel. For long-term health and beauty, Indian herbalists combine rejuvenating herbs that gently detoxify the body as they enhance slimming. Anyone who has over-used stimulants or who smokes will have problems of premature aging, including dry skin, thinning hair, reduced sexual fluid, and chronic anxiety. Anyone who has combined dairy products with meat or fish or has traveled extensively is bound to have parasites. For these reasons, I recommend the following healthy slimming products from India. They are available in most Indian food shops and online.

GOOD CARE SLIMMING TEA has a spicy, invigorating flavor. Its major ingredients are nagarmotha (*Cyprus rotundus*) cypress bud, which increases circulation, relieves thirst, and expels intestinal worms; shatavari (*Asparagus racemosus*), wild asparagus that is used to treat water retention and acts as a moistening rejuvenator for sexual fluids, fertility, and mucus membranes; and vidang (*Embelia ribes*), which relieves constipation, expels worms, acts as a diuretic and laxative, and reduces body fat. The manufacturer, Goodcare Pharma in India, recommends adding 1 teaspoon of the dried herbs to a pot of regular tea. For a stronger brew, add ½ to 1 teaspoon of Slimming Tea per cup of boiling water. Enjoy 1 to 3 cups daily.

You can order Good Care Slimming Tea online at www. goodcarepharma.com. Butala Emporium sells this tea in their New York stores and online at www.indousplaza.com. Butala Emporium's *Ayurvedic Herbals and Beauty Care Products Catalog* sells it as Anti-Obesity Tea and lists the following ingredients: *Cyprus rotundus*, *Asparagus racemosus*, *Embelia ribes*, *Acorus calamus*, *Myrabolan*, and *Zingiber officinalis* (ginger).

I enjoy adding ½ teaspoon daily of Good Care Slimming Tea to my breakfast green tea. It is neither irritating nor enervating the way some antiparasite herbs are. Wild asparagus soothes and heals sexual dryness and constipation without causing bloating or diarrhea. One-quarter cup of Good Care Slimming Tea added to 1 liter of gin makes a tasty and bracing digestive bitter. You must wait 3 weeks to use it. After that time, add 1 teaspoon of the herbal tincture per cup of cold seltzer before meals.

MEDOHAR GUGULU is a popular slimming pill sold by many East Indian herbal shops and online at www.indousplaza.com. It contains stimulating and cleansing herbal combinations: triphala (made with three balancing fruits—amla, bibitaki, and haritaki), trikatu (made with black pepper; pippli, a rejuvenating long pepper; and ginger), and chtrakmul.

AYURVEDIC CHURNAS. If you prefer to spice teas with a pinch of digestive powder—Ayurvedic herbal powders are called churnas—try peppery tasting hingvashtaka churna, which sparks appetite and eliminates indigestion. Another Ayurvedic churna, avipattikar powder, is purgative (strongly laxative) and carminative (reduces bloating as it improves digestion and absorption of nutrients). Avipattikar powder is indicated in hyperacidity, indigestion, constipation, heartburn, vomiting, biliousness, melancholia, and rheumatic pains. The formula's main ingredients include trikatu, triphala, musta, ela, baibidang, tejpatra, clove, nishoth, and sugar.

From Your Kitchen

Oregano (*Origanum vulgare*) is a powerful germ and parasite killer likely found in your kitchen. We love its fragrant flavor in soups, Italian and Greek dishes, and salads. The best way to use oregano medicinally is the organic essential oil, in capsules. It is antiviral, antibacterial, antifungal, antiparasitic, analgesic, antiseptic, antispasmodic, diuretic, fungicidal, stimulating, and insecticidal. It supports overall health, especially the immune and respiratory systems. It has been used traditionally as a remedy for digestive problems, such as cramping and indigestion, and in China for fevers, headaches, rheumatism, and general aches and pains. Its warming herbal scent treats stomach upset and nausea.

Five to 10 drops of pure oregano oil can be diluted in equal parts of water and milk and applied topically to the stomach or added to your bath. Used as a tea, oregano oil must be diluted in hot water and a few drops of milk, which works as an emulsion, or else it may burn.

I enjoy using oregano in many ways. A cup of hot oregano tea made with 1 teaspoon of dried steeped leaves or a drop of the oil in green tea clears my senses. It can be used in ginger tea to divert an approaching cold or flu.

Used as a weight loss herb, oregano is an energizing and detoxifying remedy that burns fat and eliminates fungus and yeast. A capsule can be taken along with ¼ cup of aloe vera gel as an antiyeast treatment; as a bracing, deep-cleansing tea; and as energizing aromatherapy to lift your spirits.

Chlorella: A Green Superfood from Japan and China

Chlorophyll, made from air and light by green plants, resembles our blood chemistry. One potent green food that supports life on the planet is chlorella, a single-celled algae that's been on the earth since the Precambrian period—over 2.5 billion years.

Regular use of chlorella is said to strengthen the immune system, promote better digestion and elimination, and help in gentle detoxification, removing heavy metals and pesticides. That accounts for its success in treating acne, chronic fatigue, and anemia. The nutrients contained in chlorella include vegetable proteins, fiber, vitamins, minerals, and chlorophyll. Chlorophyll and its derivatives stimulate the formation of red blood cells, affect nutrition, and influence metabolism and respiration.

Laboratory tests have found chlorella beneficial for, among other things, preventing skin cancer and stress-induced stomach ulcer, reducing fibromyalgia pain, supporting the liver, and protecting against radiation poisons and cancer.

Chlorella and Weight Loss

Chlorella capsules can easily be incorporated into a well-balanced weight loss program. As the intestinal tract functions properly and toxins are eliminated, progress can be made toward permanent weight loss. Researchers found that chlorella stimulates the peristaltic action of the intestines, thus promoting a speedy, healthy digestive process. Chlorophyll feeds useful bacteria in the stomach and is a good neutralizer of stomach acids. It is a whole food that does not suppress a normal appetite but provides energy and well-being so people lose their cravings for junk foods.

Chlorella is popular in Europe as well as in Asia. See www.chlorella-europe.com for information on Japanese Yaeyama chlorella, which contains 67 percent protein. Meanwhile, in America, Puritan's Pride at www.puritan.com sells Chinese chlorella. The Web site reports that Chinese chlorella has over 10 times more chlorophyll than alfalfa. Chinese chlorella includes a rich supply of nutrients like organic germanium, nucleic acids, vitamins, minerals, and amino acids. I had hoped to find or create a recipe—something like chlorella noodles—but it requires a special process to break down chlorella's tough cell walls so it can be absorbed. For the present, we have to use supplements.

Chlorella contains calcium and a higher percentage of phenylalanine in its protein than does spirulina, another green superfood. An essential amino acid, phenylalanine reduces hunger, increases sexual interest, improves memory and mental alertness, and alleviates depression. (For appetite control, I recommend taking 250- to 500-milligram tablets of phenylalanine with juice or water 1 hour before meals.)

Tremella: Weight Loss Fungus

Mushrooms and other fungi are closer to humans in their DNA composition than they are to plants. They are ambassadors from the ancient world that bring good news for our survival. They detoxify the body and protect against industrial pollution, radiation, and chemical poisons. By consuming them, we harmonize our energy and essence with the enduring wealth of the natural world.

As discussed in Chapter 7, tremella (*bai mu er*) is a cooling, moistening food that makes a crunchy addition to soups. Tremella can be used as a low-calorie substitute for carbohydrates much the same way as shirataki or konnyaku noodles. If you crave pasta, white bread, or other empty carbohydrates, try tremella and enjoy its cooling moistening actions. Tremella specifically cools inflammation and moistens the lungs, nourishes stomach tissue, and produces fluids. Its healing action makes it beneficial for stomach ulcers, diabetes, excess hunger and thirst, parched skin, bad breath, and dry smoker's cough.

To cook tremella, see page 184. You might eat the cooked tremella seasoned with a little light soy sauce and seaweed flakes instead of rice or noodles.

A Quick Bedtime Beauty Treatment

Many people gain weight after eating a meal at bedtime, when digestive energy is low. Here is a satisfying facial beauty treatment that is best taken as a midnight snack. It enriches the body with protein and moistens the digestive tract, lungs, intestines, and skin.

TURMERIC AND PEARL POWDER: Add ¼ teaspoon of turmeric powder to 1 cup of low-fat yogurt. It makes a cooling, relaxing dish when taken on an empty stomach before bed. Turmeric is antibiotic and balances digestive flora for enhancing the complexion. To calm nervous tension while clearing a troubled complexion, mix one tiny tube of Chinese powdered pearl into the yogurt mixture. Pearl powder cools an irritated complexion, reduces acne and rosacea, soothes the nervous system, clears vision, and provides calcium carbonate.

The Crane can awaken refreshed and beautified. With moisturizing, relaxing, and rejuvenating foods, you can calmly take your place in the vast blue sky.

Crane Meals

Cranes who love spicy foods will relish our Asian-inspired dishes. Peppers, ginger, cumin, cilantro, clove, cardamom, garlic, curry leaves, and creamy coconut milk form the basis of all that is bright, hot, and delightful in Thai, Indian, and Szechuan dishes. A dash of chile peppers in appetizer dishes speeds digestion and reduces appetite. To quiet a flaming palate, I suggest yogurt and mango dishes and creative ways to use sprouts. Cranes love sweet fruits, nuts, and seeds. Soaking dried fruits overnight eliminates much of their sugar. Sprouting grains, nuts, and seeds improves their nutritional value and digestibility.

Crane Breakfast

Start the day with a juice that improves breathing and clears complexion blemishes. Also enjoy this juice between meals, when you need something stimulating and sweet: Mix half water and half pineapple, papaya, grape, or mango juice. If breakfast is your only meal until dinner, make sure you have a protein such as eggs, steamed fish, tofu, tempeh, yogurt with flaxseed meal, or a nut butter with sprout bread.

Have Good Care Slimming Tea, Get Svelte, or another slimming tea for breakfast and at midmorning. If you enjoy sour flavors and need a strong laxative, have up to 1 teaspoon of East Indian tamarind paste or add it to tea. It works fast without causing cramps.

Sprout Power

Sprouts are genuine Crane fare—perfect live foods filled with protein, vitamins, and minerals. Sprouts are clean, safe from pollution and pesticides, and easy to make in your kitchen, where you exercise omnipotence. The sprouts do all the work. All you have to do is rinse them. My steamed loaves made from sprouts cook overnight. Sprout dishes are powerful cleansing foods that build and tone the body. Only organic whole grains and seeds can sprout. However, some taste bitter and are harder to make. The best-tasting sprouts grow in 1 to 3 days from almonds, sunflower seeds, alfalfa seeds, lentils, mung beans, and soft pastry wheat berries. (See the recipe for Essene Bread on page 198.)

I bow to Ann Wigmore, the queen of sprouting. *The Sprouting Book*, like her other books, is informative, clearly written, and inspiring. I never met her, but her spirit shines through in her writings. Using her raw foods diet, she cured herself of colon cancer and arthritis in her fifties, founded the Ann Wigmore Institute in Boston and Puerto Rico, and remained the guiding light for several generations of health-minded people until 1993, when she died in a fire at age 83.

Chinese herbalists use dried barley sprouts in some herbal formulas and teas for treating poor digestion, weight loss, and baby's colic. A Chinese medical text from the late 16th century, *Pen Ts'ao Kang Mu* by Li Shih Chen, suggests using such sprouts for reducing inflammation, dropsy (a spare tire around the waist), and rheumatism. However, because of unsanitary growing practices, I never found raw sprouts or salads when I visited southern China during the 1980s to the 1990s. Sprouts would have been quite an improvement over the typical diet consisting of white rice, pork, doughy sugar buns, greasy soup, and boiled tea that I found in the impoverished Chinese countryside.

Sprouts can be grown in a glass jar or cotton sprouting bag. On the road, you can use a medium plastic zipper-lock bag into which you have made holes. That is placed into a larger bag without holes.

In a pinch, you might use a thin nylon sock. The simplest recipes call for soaking seeds or whole grains overnight in a jar of water. The next morning, pour off the soaking water, then cover the jar with cheesecloth fastened with a rubber band or foil in which you have punched a few holes. To make sprouts, keep the jar in a dark place, such as a cupboard. Rinse them three times daily with cool water. They grow at different rates, depending on the type of seed or grain used and their moisture and room temperature. Since making sprouts requires little space and no special talent, you can grow several varieties at once and use them for making salads, sprout cheese, and other appetizing dishes.

Sprouts are rich in protein; vitamins A, B, C, E, and K; and minerals, especially iron and trace elements. The table below shows you some of the varieties used to make sprouts, the hours of soaking time required, amount of dry seeds to use, optimal length of the sprout at harvest, usual number of days required for sprouting, and some suggested uses.

VARIETY	SOAKING TIME	DRY MEASURE OF SEEDS	LENGTH AT HARVEST	TIME REQUIRED	SUGGESTED USES
Adzuki	12 hr	1 c	½"–1"	3–5 days	Salad, loaf
Alfalfa	4–6 hr	3–4 Tbsp	1"–1½"	4–6 days	Salad
Almond	12 hr	1 c	0"	1 day	Milk, loaf, salad, bread
Clover	4–6 hr	3 Tbsp	1"–1½"	4–5 days	Salad
Fenugreek	8 hr	½ c	½"–1"	3–5 days	Smoothie
Lentils	12 hr	1 c	¼"–¾"	3–5 days	Salad, loaf
Mung beans	12 hr	½ c	½"–1½"	3–6 days	Salad, soup, loaf
Sesame seeds	4–6 hr	1 c	0"	1–2 days	Milk, bread, loaf, cheese
Sunflower seeds	8 hr	2 c	0"–½"	1–3 days	Salad, bread, pesto, cheese
Wheat berries	12 hr	1 c	¼"–½"	2–3 days	Bread, salad, loaf

REJUVELAC

Rejuvelac is a pleasant, mild-flavored, fermented wheatberry beverage that tones digestion, improves absorption, and reduces sluggish elimination. Consumed regularly, it slims the waistline and keeps digestion humming. Start with a cup or more at room temperature before meals and increase it to several glasses per day.

MAKES UP TO 1 GALLON | PREPARATION TIME: 2 DAYS
   ½ cup pastry whole wheat berries (soft wheat berries)
   6 cups spring or filtered water
      Sliced ginger and honey to taste (optional)

Soak the wheat berries in the water in a widemouthed half-gallon jar, covered with cheesecloth or nylon mesh screening, for 10 to 15 hours. Drain off the water. Let the wheat berries sprout as usual for 2 days. After this time, pour water over the sprouts using a 3:1 ratio of water to sprouts. Cover the jar and leave it at room temperature for 24 hours. Pour off the liquid Rejuvelac into another jar or plastic container, cover, and refrigerate. When refrigerated, it will keep for several days.

You can start making more Rejuvelac immediately by adding water to ferment the same wheat sprouts. If you consume eight or more glasses daily and use it in cooking, you might keep a jar of Rejuvelac unrefrigerated on your kitchen counter and add fresh water as you use it. Throw away any liquid and sprouts that turn sour or discolor. For variety, add peeled sliced fresh ginger and honey, if using, while fermenting the wheat berries.

Sprout Loaves

Sprout loaves and casseroles provide a rich source of quality protein, vitamins, and minerals. They can be made from many sorts of grains and seeds. Among them: adzuki, alfalfa, chickpeas, black-eyed peas, fenugreek seeds, whole dried green peas, lentils, millet, mung beans, oats, pumpkin seeds, and sunflower seeds. You will learn to recognize when the soaking time and sprouting are finished. Sprouts should smell lightly sweet or fragrant, never spoiled. Discard any bean hulls that float to the surface of the soaking water. In some cases, you can agitate the water to make the hulls rise, then scoop them out of the jar.

Adzuki, alfalfa, fenugreek, mung, and radish sprouts taste better with their hulls removed, and they store better and longer in the refrigerator without them. Lentils, peas, and grains need not be hulled.

VEGETARIAN MEAT LOAF

Raw-food mavens love serving raw sprout loaves. However, I find them cold and gripping, especially during winter months. I prefer to mash several kinds of sprouts mixed with raw vegetables, a little tomato sauce, and Italian herbs. I may coat the loaf with ground walnuts. I steam the loaf at low heat in my slow cooker until it has the consistency of a meat loaf.

MAKES 5 SERVINGS | PREPARATION TIME: 15 MINUTES;

STEAMING TIME: 6 TO 8 HOURS

Meat Loaf
1½ cups lentil sprouts
½ cup almond sprouts
1 cup sunflower sprouts
1 block tofu
1 egg, slightly beaten (optional)
1 carrot, thinly sliced
1 small yellow onion, chopped
½ cup celery, sliced
½ teaspoon caraway powder
½ teaspoon turmeric powder
    Salt substitute and black pepper to taste
½ cup fresh shiitake mushrooms, stems removed (optional)
    Fresh chopped parsley, thyme, rosemary, and savory to taste
½ teaspoon stevia powder
½ cup tomato sauce
1 bay leaf
1 tablespoon milled flaxseed or yellow cornmeal

Sauce
1 clove garlic
Pinch of salt substitute
Pinch of caraway powder

¼ cup orange juice
　Tomato sauce
2 tablespoons cornstarch

To make the meat loaf: Blend the sprouts, tofu, and egg, if using, until they are mixed but remain lumpy. (The egg makes a firmer loaf, but it can be left out.) Place in a large bowl and mix in the carrot, onion, celery, caraway, turmeric, and salt substitute and pepper. Rinse the mushrooms, if using, slice, and add to the mixture. Add the fresh herbs. Separately, mix the stevia into the tomato sauce. Moisten the sprout mixture with 3 to 4 tablespoons of the sweetened tomato sauce. Set aside the rest for the sauce.

Put ½" water and the bay leaf in the bottom of your slow cooker. Sprinkle the flaxseed or cornmeal in the bottom of a medium soufflé dish. Spoon the sprout mixture on top. Cover the sprout loaf with 2 tablespoons of sweetened tomato sauce. Put the loaf in the slow cooker and cook at low heat for up to 6 hours, or until firm. A knife inserted into the loaf should come out clean. Let cool before removing the soufflé dish from the slow cooker. Remove the bay leaf before serving.

Another method is to stuff hollowed green and red bell peppers with the sprout mixture and steam in your slow cooker or bake in a warm oven 125°F for 8 hours.

To make the sauce: Mash the garlic with the salt substitute and caraway in a bowl. Mix with the orange juice and the reserved tomato sauce.

Moisten 1 tablespoon of the cornstarch with 3 tablespoons of the tomato-orange mixture.

In a pan, bring the larger portion of the tomato-orange mixture to a simmer, and slowly add the cornstarch mixture until it thickens. Add enough of the remaining 1 tablespoon cornstarch to make a thick sauce. Pour it over the loaf at serving time. You might wish to serve the loaf with one of the following spicy Thai dipping sauces. They are normally used for meat and chicken dishes.

A word about Thai chile peppers, canned chili paste, and red and green curry paste: *Hot!!!* Most Thai recipes call for ½ to 1 teaspoon of chiles or canned red chili paste. Out of sympathy for our Western tongues, I have reduced the amount. Use your judgment and start with a pinch, not a spoon, for measure. Increase the dose as you like, but consider yourself warned.

Thai BBQ Sauce

This is a variation on the delicious hot barbecue sauce that goes with Thai barbecued chicken gai yang. I have added turmeric and cumin. It can be used over green vegetable salads that include grilled meat or fish. Try some with a sprout loaf to heat up the flavor. Use fresh mint as a garnish.

MAKES 6 TABLESPOONS | PREPARATION TIME: 5 MINUTES

    1 *teaspoon garlic, minced*
¼–½ *teaspoon minced chile or chili paste*
  ½ *teaspoon turmeric powder*
  ¼ *teaspoon cumin powder*
  4 *tablespoons water*
  4 *tablespoons sugar*
  ¼ *teaspoon salt*
  6 *tablespoons vinegar*

Bring all the ingredients to a boil and cook for 5 minutes, or until the liquid is reduced to 6 tablespoons. Let cool to form a thin juice.

Fresh Summer Rolls

Summer rolls, served as appetizers in Chinese, Vietnamese, and Thai restaurants, are a fresh, light, nonfried version of their cousins, spring rolls. They combine green herbs, sprouts, boiled shrimp, and "glass noodles" made from mung bean wrapped in a sheathe of white rice paper. Our version uses lettuce rolls instead of rice paper.

MAKES 6 SERVINGS | PREPARATION TIME: 20 MINUTES

Shrimp
  6 *large boiled deveined shrimp (optional)*
  ¼ *cup diced tempeh*

Dash of ground turmeric
Dash of ground cumin

Sauce

2 tablespoons fish sauce

2 tablespoons palm sugar or ¼ teaspoon stevia powder

3 tablespoons tamarind juice

1 clove garlic, minced

¼ teaspoon chili sauce

1 small onion, shredded

Crushed peanuts

Summer Rolls

Large lettuce leaves

1 large cucumber, peeled and shredded

1 carrot, finely shredded + additional for garnish

3 tablespoons chopped fresh cilantro leaves

1 cup alfalfa sprouts

Shredded radishes for garnish

To make the shrimp: If you are using shrimp, allow them to cool completely, and cut each in half lengthwise. Steam the tempeh in a little water. If you prefer, spice the tempeh with the turmeric and cumin.

To make the sauce: Bring the fish sauce, palm sugar or stevia, and tamarind juice to a boil and cook for 1 minute. Let cool to form a thick juice. Add the garlic, chili sauce, onion, and peanuts as desired.

To make the summer rolls: Take a large piece of curly leaf lettuce. Dip it into hot water just long enough for it to soften slightly. Take it in your left hand and fill it with your right. Add a pinch each of the shrimp, cucumber, carrot, cilantro, sprouts, and tempeh. Roll up the lettuce leaf, making a point on the bottom and sticking in the edges on top. Place the rolls onto a bed of lettuce along with the carrots and radish. Dip the lettuce rolls into the sauce.

Thai Shrimp (or Tofu) and Pineapple Curry

This looks nice served in half a pineapple. When buying fresh pineapple, sniff the bottom. It is ready to eat if the bottom has turned yellow and smells sweet. You can buy kaffir lime leaves at many Asian food markets and online at hundreds of Web sites, including www.importfood.com and www.fourwindsgrowers.com.

MAKES 4 SERVINGS | PREPARATION TIME: 30 MINUTES

1 large ripe pineapple with the outer skin and top leaves
½ pound shelled shrimp or 1½ cups sliced firm tofu
1 tablespoon red curry paste
1 tablespoon grapeseed oil
4 tablespoons + 1¼ cups coconut milk
2 tablespoons fish sauce
1 teaspoon sugar
1 teaspoon vinegar
¼ teaspoon ground paprika powder
4 kaffir lime leaves
1 cup fresh pineapple, chopped (from whole pineapple, above)

Wash the pineapple. Lay in it on a cutting board, and with a sharp, pointed knife, cut it lengthwise into two equal halves. Hollow out the center of one half with a serrated knife. That half will be your serving dish. Cut off the tough outer skin of the other half, remove the top leaves, and cut the pineapple into 1" square pieces.

Devein the shrimp and rinse and drain them. Stir-fry the curry paste, oil, and the 4 tablespoons coconut milk, using medium heat for a minute, until it turns fragrant. Add the fish sauce, sugar, vinegar, paprika, kaffir, pineapple, and the remaining 1¼ cups of coconut milk. Bring it to a boil. Add the shrimp and simmer until the color changes.

Pad Thai

These spicy noodles are enjoyed in outdoor markets all over Thailand. You can whip them up in a few minutes in front of your guests. I have substituted

stevia for sugar and no-calorie shirataki noodles for Thai sen lek rice noodles,
and added vegetables to the original recipe.

MAKES 4 SERVINGS | PREPARATION TIME: 15 MINUTES

¼ *pound shelled shrimp*
2 *packets shirataki noodles*
3 *tablespoons grapeseed oil*
2 *carrots, grated + extra for garnish*
1 *celery rib, sliced*
1 *small onion, chopped*
1 *teaspoon minced garlic*
¼ *teaspoon chili paste*
2 *eggs*
1½ *tablespoons fish sauce*
1½ *tablespoons tamarind juice or 1 tablespoon paste*
½ *teaspoon stevia powder*
¼ *teaspoon ground paprika*
¼ *cup fresh ginger, peeled and shredded*
⅓ *pound (1 cup) fresh sprouts*
2 *tablespoons crushed peanuts*
Juice of 1 lime
½ *cup thinly grated daikon radish*

Devein the shrimp, rinse, and drain. Rinse the noodles in cold water.

Heat 1 tablespoon of the oil and stir-fry the carrots, celery, and onion until the onion is transparent. Add the noodles and gently stir for a moment, until they are hot. Heat the remaining 2 tablespoons oil and stir-fry the garlic and chili paste until fragrant. Add the shrimp and stir-fry another minute. Add the eggs and stir-fry until slightly dry. Add the fish sauce, tamarind, stevia, paprika, ginger, sprouts, peanuts, and noodles and stir-fry briefly as you mix the ingredients. Sprinkle with the lime juice, garnish with the grated carrot and radish, and serve hot.

When I am in a hurry, I brown chopped vegetables with garlic and shirataki noodles, stir in an egg, add a spoon of unsweetened fruit jelly, and stir until it is thick. Then I sprinkle it with lime juice and peanuts. It takes no more than 5 minutes.

SEAWEED SALAD

To complement spicy foods and fish, and to ease digestion of protein meals, try a seaweed salad. It can be simple—a handful of dried seaweed flakes added to your regular salad—or it can be an exciting original creation.

This recipe uses Alaria seaweed (Alaria esculenta), which is high in calcium. It is similar to wakame, the sea vegetable used in miso soup.

MAKES 2 SERVINGS | PREPARATION TIME: 15 MINUTES

   ½–1 *cup dried alaria seaweed*
   1 *lemon in soaking water*
   ½ *lemon, juiced*
   ½ *orange, juiced*
   ¼ *teaspoon orange peel*
   1 *tablespoon grated ginger and its juice*
   1 *tablespoon grapeseed, canola, or sesame oil*
   ¼ *teaspoon mustard seeds*
   1 *tablespoon chopped red onion*
      Black or red pepper to taste
      Dash brown rice vinegar

Cut the dried alaria into strips with a pair of scissors. Do not blanch this delicate seaweed in boiling water. Rinse it once briefly in cold water, then soak it for 10 minutes in enough lemon water to soften it slightly. Keep the remaining soaking water.

Combine the lemon juice, orange juice, orange peel, ginger, oil, mustard, onion, pepper, and vinegar in a glass bowl. Add the alaria and marinate it in the bowl, adding just enough of the soaking water to keep it wet. The longer the seaweed soaks in the marinade, the softer it becomes.

Crane Menus

Strictly speaking, Cranes are people with long features and breathing problems, including asthma or itchy skin conditions, which are recognizable health issues associated with the Metal element in Chinese medicine. For our purposes, however, Cranes can be anyone with troubling addictions and very irregular eating habits. Too often Cranes fast and feast and need to create a healthy rhythm of meals and snacks to balance and tone digestion. Sometimes merely eating something the same time of day helps to develop better habits.

When regular meals are impossible, take a balancing supplement such as Chinese Xiao Yao Wan pills or Happy Garden Tea instant beverage every 4 hours until you crave regular meals. Instead of smoking a cigarette to calm your nerves, try doing the stretching, deep-breathing exercises for Cranes found on page 302. Take a daily dose (three pills) of Nux vomica 30C before bed on an empty stomach or 1 hour after eating until your addictions are better under control. If you have a yeast infection or intestinal parasites, avoid fruits and sugars, and use herbs to cure the problem. See the anti-yeast diet on page 273. For your convenience, the following menus involve minimal cooking.

Crane Menu 1

Before Breakfast (choose one)
- 8 ounces water with 1 tablespoon liquid chlorophyll and the juice of ½ lemon
- Half pineapple juice and half water with protein powder added

Breakfast
1 cup strawberries or other berries
1 cup low-fat yogurt with ¼ teaspoon turmeric powder
2 high-fiber crackers
Tea with ½ lemon and ¼ teaspoon molasses

Snack (choose one)
- 1 diet bar
- ¼ cup nuts or spicy seeds
- 10 to 20 drops of maté liquid extract for high energy
Tea

Lunch
High-protein drink and an apple or banana

Snack
Happy Garden Tea instant beverage in water or juice or
    2 cups of broccoli green tea or broccoli and vegetable
    cooking water (see Broccoli Water recipe on page 190)

Dinner
Large salad with low-fat or vinaigrette dressing
    or ½ cup hijiki seaweed or Seaweed Salad (page 238)
Veggie burger and pickles, tomato, and mustard
Tea

Before Bed (optional)
1 cup low-fat yogurt with ¼ teaspoon turmeric powder

Crane Menu 2

Before Breakfast
8 ounces half orange juice, half water

Breakfast
1 cup dry cereal, berries, and soy milk
Tea

Snack
1 handful nuts or seeds
2 cups of broccoli green tea or broccoli and vegetable
    cooking water

Lunch
Large salad with a hard-cooked egg or feta cheese added
Tea

Snack
Protein drink or 10 to 20 drops of maté extract for high energy

Dinner
Large salad with low-fat dressing, with choice of:
- 1 to 2 cups vegetarian chili
- A Greek spinach pie

Tea with lemon

Before Bed (optional)
1 cup berries with 2 ounces goat or sheep cheese

Crane Menu 3

Before Breakfast
8 ounces water with 1 teaspoon apple cider vinegar and
½ teaspoon molasses

Breakfast
1 raw apple
1 slice whole grain toast with applesauce
Whey protein drink
Tea

Snack (choose one)
- Happy Garden Tea instant beverage
- 1 cup Rejuvelac (page 231) only once daily

Lunch
Large mixed vegetable salad with sprouts and canned
sardines, salmon, or tuna
Tea or 2 cups of broccoli green tea or broccoli and vegetable
cooking water

Snack (choose one)
- 1 to 2 rice cakes and green tea
- 1 cup Rejuvelac (only once daily)
- 10 to 20 drops of maté extract for high energy

Dinner
Large salad with lemon juice
3 cooked vegetables
1 cup cooked whole grain—barley, kasha, or wheat
berries

Before Bed (optional)
1 cup pumpkin pie filling with pumpkin pie spice
Happy Garden Tea

Crane Menu 4

Before Breakfast
8 ounces half water, half apple juice

Breakfast
½ cup stewed prunes (laxative), as needed
Whey or egg protein drink
Tea

Snack
1 protein bar and tea or 10 to 20 drops of maté extract for
high energy

Lunch
Large salad with low-fat dressing
1½ cups steamed vegetables or vegetable soup
Tea or 2 cups of broccoli green tea or broccoli and vegetable
cooking water

Snack (choose one)
• Happy Garden Tea
• 1 cup Rejuvelac (only once daily)

Dinner
Caesar salad with extra-virgin olive oil vinaigrette
¼ cup egg salad on high-fiber crackers
Tea

Before Bed (optional)
Steamed green vegetables

Crane Menu 5

Before Breakfast
8 ounces water with 1 cup of apple juice and juice of ½ lemon

Breakfast
1 apple or banana
1 slice whole grain toast with 1 teaspoon chyawanprash
Tea with a dash of hingvashtaka, as needed

Snack
1 handful nuts or seeds
1 to 2 high-fiber crackers and soy spread
Tea

Lunch
Large salad with extra-virgin olive oil and vinegar
    dressing
1 slice whole grain toast with applesauce or low-fat spread
Tea or 2 cups of broccoli green tea or broccoli and vegetable
    cooking water

Snack
1 cup Rejuvelac

Dinner
Large salad with low-fat dressing or extra-virgin olive oil
    and lemon juice
1½ cups Pad Thai with vegetables, tofu, and optional
    chicken or shrimp (page 236)
1 to 2 cups fresh papaya
Tea

Before Bed (optional)
1 sliced apple with 1 tablespoon extra-virgin olive oil,
    walnuts, and raisins
Mint tea

Crane's Summary

- **Problem:** Poor dietary habits, addictions, and fixed ideas about
  eating
- **Traditional Chinese medicine (TCM) element and organs:**
  Metal element, which encompasses skin, lungs, and large intestine, breathing, absorption of oxygen and nutrients, and elimination of toxins and emotions held in the gut
- **Approach:** Support vitality; reduce ill effects of addictions.

Recommended

- Pungent cleansing fruits and vegetables such as apple, papaya, pineapple, radish, watercress
- Moistening rejuvenating foods: pumpkin, almonds
- Asian superfoods: chlorella, tremella fungi
- Homeopathic Nux vomica 30C for addictions
- Ease Plus for withdrawal nervousness, insomnia
- Aloe and eclipta for liver and blood cleansing and nourishing treatments
- Tremella and American ginseng pills for dry cough, chronic thirst, and serious viral infections
- Crave Arrest and other supplements that contain 5-HTP (hydroxytryptophan) for addictions
- Pu-erh and rooibos tea for antioxidants
- Good Care Slimming Tea for internal cleansing and balancing digestion
- Avipattikar powder (Ayurvedic medicine) for hyperacidity, indigestion, constipation, heartburn, vomiting, biliousness, melancholia, and rheumatic pains

Nearly any diet will stay interesting and functional for a week or so because slimming diet changes call our attention to the body in a positive way. However, to address real life issues that are complicated and long term, we need weight loss insurance—natural ways to stay slim and healthy in order to live longer and better.

Part 3

Get It Off, Keep It Off

This part begins the adventure of the rest of your life.
Live slim, live long.

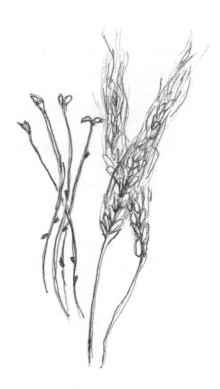

245

Chapter 9

Weight Loss Insurance

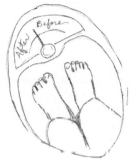

Weight loss fads promise fast results with no effort. The advertisements read something like this: Eat your favorite fattening foods and stay slim. With this book, we are as concerned with increasing health and longevity as we are with weight loss. In fact, you cannot have one without the other. What good is a diet that works fast but over time kills you faster? Part 3 addresses the weight loss needs of mature people and others with problems that we all face at one time or other. Longevity has become an important focus for research because we who strive to live fully desire to live longer and better.

We are entering an era when microbiology, genetic research, and nanotechnology—tiny robotic devices that destroy disease in the body—may well take the forefront in medicine. However, diet is not completely forgotten. While we wait—some say possibly as long as 50 or more years—for human genetic research to bear fruit, foods and herbs will continue to supply our needs for cell maintenance. In fact, there are already interesting crossovers in the latest research and our diet.

Cellular research for increasing human longevity is quietly being done by many private companies in the search for a cure for cancer, heart disease, and diabetes. However, university genetics laboratories carry the burden of proving the science behind new life-extension drugs. The scientists study enzymes, bacteria, and yeasts that can lengthen the life span of tiny animals. In an April 2006 report appearing in www.barrons.com, Michael Rose, MD, professor of evolutionary biology at the University of California at Irvine, said, "I am working on immortality." So far he has achieved breakthrough results extending the lives of fruit flies, as he notes, "Twenty years ago, the idea of postponing aging, let alone reversing it, was weird and off-the-wall. Today there are good reasons for thinking it is fundamentally possible." Although this is encouraging, we have a long way to go.

I wonder about the optimal fruit fly diet. Based on previous testing, it must be a low-protein, low-calorie diet. That is one way the Baseline Diet, which reduces food intake, especially animal protein, is similar to successful longevity experiments done in the laboratory. But to eat like fruit flies? No thanks.

Cell Cleansing

Eating less is only part of the solution to permanent weight loss and longevity. Another approach is to increase cleansing foods. That is how our diet, in principle, corresponds to groundbreaking genetic research done by geneticist Aubrey de Grey, PhD, Cambridge University researcher and de facto spokesman of the current antiaging crusade. He appears a slender, good-natured Crane with a foot-long red beard. Looking closer on his Web site, www.sens.org, you see he has an extraordinarily long list of scientific publications and his own journal, *Rejuvenation Research*. He is advisor for many scientific organizations dealing with aging—the British Society for Research on Ageing, American Aging Association, International Association of Biomedical Gerontology, Gerontological Society of America, International Coenzyme Q_{10} Association, and Mitochondrion Research Society, to name a few.

Dr. de Grey describes his research area as encompassing the role of all the accumulating and eventually pathogenic molecular and cellular side effects of metabolism that constitute mammalian aging and then designing interventions to reverse and/or obviate this accumulation. Part of that research is to seek out and destroy what he calls destructive junk inside and outside of cells. "Junk" refers to waste products such as plaque that lead to aging, impair cell function, and therefore hasten death. He is looking for specialized enzymes, bacteria, and fungi that destroy this junk.

Greatly simplified, Dr. de Grey's work strives to cleanse junk from cells. Cleansing and slimming are also the goals of the Feed Your Tiger diet. We stress digestive enzymes from foods such as papaya and the healing benefits of medicinal fungi. Our aim goes beyond temporary weight loss.

Dr. de Grey believes that barring accidents and suicide, most people now 40 years old or younger can expect to live for centuries. It sounds like science fiction, but it's pure science. Several mechanisms are known to extend life in flies; why not eventually in mammals? Dr. de Grey hopes to take a cohort of mice of a strain whose normal life expectancy is 3 years, do nothing to them until they are 2 years old, and get them to live an average of 3 more years, thereby tripling their remaining life expectancy. He calls it robust mouse rejuvenation, or RMR.

Dr. de Grey has said that, depending on funding and other factors, starting from the time the RMR mouse target is achieved, it could take at least 15 additional years to start human rejuvenation therapies. That's a long time to wait for practical ways to extend life, so I e-mailed the professor at his London laboratory, asking him to suggest foods and herbs that enhance longevity.

Quick as a wink he replied: "As you've gathered, my focus is on the molecular and cellular biology of aging other than on the dietary and pharmacological things we can already do to combat aging. However, some research has been published in my journal [*Rejuvenation Research*] on the antiaging potential of various phytochemicals that are Asian herbs."

A list of the articles concerning Asian herbs associated with longevity includes research on Asian tonic herbs used as stimulants. One of the articles covers yang-enhancing Chinese herbs. Such herbs are stimulating tonics used to treat chronic fatigue, asthma, backache, tired legs, and low libido for either sex. They are useful for memory and mental clarity and are frequently included in herbal rejuvenation treatments, hormone-balancing or menopausal remedies, and aphrodisiac pills. Many are precursors to testosterone, like cuscuta, epimedium, and others that enhance energy and sexuality besides affecting the mitochondria—the energy batteries inside our cells.

Withania (the Ayurvedic longevity herb ashwagandha) was also studied for its stimulating effects on the mitochondria. Ashwagandha is used for backache, low sexual energy, slow childbirth from weak muscles, and nerve illnesses with paralysis. Most people can use the herb to strengthen weak muscles and reverse physical and mental exhaustion by taking ¼ teaspoon of ashwagandha powder in hot water as a tea once or twice daily until energy returns. Avoid this and any energy tonic herbs during fever, cold, or flu, or severe dehydration.

I include this information on longevity research because it is important to keep our diet plan in perspective. To live long and well, weight loss must become a healthy lifestyle. On both the micro level of the cells and the macro level of diet, in order to promote longevity, it pays to consume smaller quantities and to emphasize deep-cleansing nutrients that rid the body of junk.

Weight Loss for Long Life

In Chapter 2, I established a Baseline Diet that anyone can follow to reach an ideal weight. In the same chapter, I added foods that jump-start weight loss when you hit a plateau. Part 2 concerns the special foods, supplements, and herbal treatments used to fine-tune weight loss for four energy types: Tiger, Dragon, Bear, and Crane.

Now we are ready to consider a weight loss lifestyle for health and longevity. This chapter combines elements of the Baseline Diet with a few suggestions useful for each energy type. It is your assurance of continued progress and protection from potential illness. The comprehensive diet plan presented here touches all bases because most people, at one time or other, develop complicated long-term health challenges resulting from poor digestion, illness, and, especially, aging.

To stay well and slender, you may continue using a version of this comprehensive diet from now on. You may vary it to accommodate seasonal foods, personal allergies, and your energy and time considerations. It protects against a broad range of discomforts. For example, many people who develop high blood pressure also eventually develop diabetes, overweight, gout, or skin rashes. They need a diet comprehensive enough to address all those issues in a practical way.

Using this chapter's comprehensive diet, Dragons will gain energy and immunity with an Asian mushroom. Bears will reduce their sweet tooth with gymnema. Cranes will enjoy spicy popcorn, a zesty, slimming grain. Tigers will reduce impurities and cellulite with chlorophyll capsules or alfalfa pills. Seaweed will protect all against radiation and excess weight resulting from sluggish digestion and elimination.

The overall weight you lose over time depends on your level of energy and your habits. We suggest small meals, including only one protein source daily. Limiting your diet and reducing impurities with herbs helps to fortify digestion and balance emotions, whereas digesting big meals of meat with rich sauces and starches, pizza with cheese, meat or fish, and greasy or fried junk foods taxes digestive *qi*, clogs the cells, and dulls the mind. Wastes build up in the body, and you gain weight and age prematurely.

If you fall off our cleansing diet, take a dose of homeopathic Nux vomica 30C to detoxify the body and lift your spirits. Start adding cleansing supplements such as three dandelion capsules, two chlorophyll concentrate capsules, or one raw carrot juice after meals to clean up your act. Then jump back on the diet again.

You may be a Bear who devours cake, bread, and wine; a Dragon who gobbles peanuts, chips, and diet drinks; or a Crane who starves and then binges. Some people are all of the energy types simultaneously. This comprehensive diet works for people who eat anything that adds weight. It smoothes out the wrinkles in any eating lifestyle. Its guiding principle is simple: Build qi to lose weight. Staying a little hungry and revved for adventure keeps you young and active as a cat. For that reason, we call this the Feed Your Tiger Diet. Sample menus are included.

The *Feed Your Tiger* Comprehensive Diet

Please use the following suggestions as a model for your experimentation, while respecting the acid/alkaline food ratio we established with the Baseline Diet. In other words, daily eat two or three fruits, six to nine vegetables, one protein, and one starch. That ratio keeps your daily food total 20 percent acid and 80 percent alkaline, which makes for healthy blood. Try to notice how you feel when you simplify meals. Are you lighter, livelier, and more cheerful? If you feel hungry, add juices, vegetables, and digestive remedies. They do not add weight.

Everyone who participated in my clinical weight loss observations reported that the Baseline Diet made them feel lighter, more confident, and calmer. Some felt more in control of their eating habits and their life. One woman said: "I have been totally enjoying the Get Svelte and Gorgeous You teas. I like them both and feel they have definitely shifted things. Get Svelte keeps me energized without any speedy feelings. I am also very excited to use the ganoderma products! They are great. I have added a bit more protein to my diet after a few years of not eating certain foods. I have also been eating more fruit . . . pineapple and apples, usually. Cooling for me. All of your recommendations have helped me feel a lot less bloated with water weight. My digestion is working much better too, since I have stepped away from eating too many heavy grains/pastas. I use them sparingly."

A shift in diet can be a wonderful way to reawaken your former healthier self. The body remembers when we urge our habits in the right direction.

To recondition your liver, blood, and digestion, gradually add the following supplements and practices.

CLEANSE WITH GREENS. At least three times per week, start the day with 2 cups of warm broccoli water and a few pieces of steamed broccoli. Simmer the broccoli in the water for 15 minutes, let cool, and drink the cooking liquid plain without any seasoning. Wait at least 20 minutes before eating breakfast. If you cannot tolerate broccoli water, pour it over organic green or white tea.

During or after meals, take three alfalfa tablets (chewed and washed down with water) or one capsule of chlorophyll concentrate (about 100 milligrams of chlorophyll copper complex). Eat at least 1 tablespoon of dried green kelp (laminaria) during the day. I enjoy kelp, alaria, nori, and dulse daily as a snack. Toast one handful of your favorite seaweed in a 200°F oven until crisp. You can crumble it over salads, dishes, or popcorn or eat it by the handful.

Larch Hanson, who has harvested seaweed in Steuben, Maine, for over 3 decades, recommends kelp, specifically *Laminaria longicuris* or *Laminaria saccharina,* as good daily food for maintaining adequate levels of iodine 127 in the body. He advises: "In the event of a nuclear catastrophe (like the one in Chernobyl, Russia), I recommend *Laminaria digitata.*"

DON'T HAVE DESSERT. After meals, to feel full and satisfy your sweet tooth, you may have 1 teaspoon of virgin coconut oil or no more than 2 tablespoons daily. If you still crave sweets or if coconut oil is too heavy for you, try 1 teaspoon of pure organic bee pollen to quench your craving for dessert. One slender Tiger I know eats a fresh lemon slice to clear her palate and eliminate her craving for dessert.

BE CAREFUL WITH FOOD COMBINATIONS. Fruit, a dairy food such as yogurt or cheese, and a slice of whole grain or sprout bread make a nice breakfast. Some people prefer 1 teaspoon of milled flaxseed mixed with yogurt or cereal. When possible, avoid consuming animal protein and starch in the same meal. Mixing fruits with protein or starch slows digestion (retards digestive qi) and therefore causes bloating or yeast problems. Our Baseline Diet protects against most food-combining errors.

DRINK PLENTY OF FLUIDS BETWEEN MEALS. If possible, drink six to eight glasses a day, choosing from green or white teas, Get Svelte instant beverage, homemade beverages of half water and half fruit or vegetable juice, broccoli water, and cleansing foods from Chapter 4. You may enjoy drinking Rejuvelac (page 231).

TAKE MUSHROOM SUPPLEMENTS. If possible, add these supplements to increase energy and balance immunity. At 10:00 a.m. and 3:00 p.m. daily, swallow 20 drops of reishi mushroom extract. If you do not like the taste of mushrooms, you can substitute four to six Power Mushroom pills made by Health Concerns or another mixed mushroom capsule available from www.fungi.com.

If you prefer to use foods, eat up to ½ pound of cooked shiitake or 4 ounces of cooked enoki mushrooms three times a week. My recipe for Shiitake/Fu Ling Tea is on page 45. You can drink up to 1 quart daily. Avoid all mushrooms if you are allergic to them or if you have a yeast infection.

PAY ATTENTION TO MINERALS. If you feel weak or are recovering from an illness, you may wish to add mixed trace minerals and chromium supplements. If you have a hypothyroid condition, you can add more seaweed such as kelp and dulse to your diet. That is my favorite way to supplement the diet with essential minerals. Some people prefer to use pills, such as Laminaria 4 pills. See the special instructions for ordering from Health Concerns in the Natural Products and Information Resource Guide on page 348.

It is less desirable to tone the thyroid daily by adding one drop of pure iodine to the inside of your palm or wrist, but it works in a pinch. If the iodine is absorbed by your skin and disappears within 4 hours, you are iodine deficient. Apply one drop twice daily, morning and afternoon, until the spot of iodine remains for the day. Continue to use it as needed or once a week. Reduce your use of iodine if it makes you feel too nervous or unable to sleep.

WATCH THOSE SWEETS. If you are diabetic, avoid all fruits and sweet vegetables, such as carrots and beets. Add two or three capsules daily of *Gymnema sylvestra* to lower blood sugar and reduce a sweet tooth.

VARY YOUR ROUTINE. People too often approach dietary suggestions as though they were laws written in stone. You should be flexible and vary your diet depending on your workday and energy level.

My Vermont summer diet of fruits, vegetables, raw goat dairy, dried seaweed mixed with nuts and seeds, whole grain pasta with mushroom sauce, and a bowl of spicy popcorn daily suits me fine because I see practically no one, hardly answer the phone, and get plenty of sunshine while gardening in the back field. My Florida winter diet contains lots of fresh fish and seaweed, but no dairy. In New York, whenever possible, I try to eat more as Japanese people do: a whole soy food daily or at least several times a week, the Baseline Diet, and sometimes a meal at a great restaurant.

ENJOY YOUR FOOD. The strength of your diet lies in how flexible it is and how it keeps you well. Your diet ought to allow you to enjoy life, the company of good friends, and the pleasures of health and happiness. It should give you the chance to break your diet rules and bounce back, using foods and supplements to regain the health, youth, and vigor you have lost.

Many depressed people punish themselves with food. They may feel guilty and apologize for eating poorly, which comes from a need to be scolded. I never scold my health clients. They already have an internal dialogue about food and overweight that keeps them feeling like children or sinners.

To me, food is fuel that supports health, growth, love, and wholeness of body, mind, and spirit. I use my diet to look and feel well and to create a healing home for my family and friends. Bernard Jensen, PhD, whose lifelong work with nutrition has helped a great many people, said it beautifully: "A man can eat the best foods, have the cleanest, strongest body, but if he lacks love in his heart, it is all for nothing."

LATE-NIGHT DINING

Most diet experts advise never eating a meal after 8:00 p.m. My response to that? Get real!

People who follow an active lifestyle often eat late and work at night. If that is the case with you, take a walk after your last meal of the day or have a digestive tea. Avoid napping or bathing immediately after eating. They slow digestion because digestive qi is not allowed to work properly.

Putting the Principles to Work

How do all of these principles play out in real life? Here are several menus that demonstrate how all of this can come together in a practical and enjoyable way.

Sample Menu 1

You'll find sample menus for all the energy types in each of the chapters in Part 2. In all the diet plans, I have left room for you to decide when you wish to consume your protein and starchy foods. Try to limit your daily portions to one 4-ounce serving of protein and one starch (a cup of cooked whole grains or pasta or two slices of whole grain bread, for example). That way you will consume more fruits and vegetables.

Currently, my favorite breakfast is hot green tea; sprout bread (made without yeast); fresh fruit; a handful of crisp, dried kelp or dulse; and sometimes a slice of goat cheese. The sprouted breads that I make with a combination of whole grains such as wheat berries, spelt, or rye kernels are dense enough to keep me satisfied until afternoon. You can substitute a slice of dense whole grain bread and a teaspoon of low-fat all-fruit jam or the Parsnip Jam on page 197. If you have your protein in the evening, combine it with cooked tomato or grapefruit sections to ease digestion.

Upon Rising
1 (8-ounce) glass half water, half fruit juice with the juice of
    ½ lemon, or Broccoli Water (page 190)
Exercise, walk around the yard, or stretch for 10 to 15 minutes.

Breakfast
3 cups hot tea or 1 to 3 cups Get Svelte instant beverage
1 cup raw fruit or ½ cup reconstituted dried fruit
¼ teaspoon cardamom or hingvashtaka powder added to
    fruit or tea to improve digestion as needed
Optional: 1 to 3 teaspoons virgin coconut oil (moistening)

Optional
If breakfast is a protein meal, choose one:

- 1 hard-cooked egg or an omelet made with 3 egg whites
- 4 ounces salmon steamed in pineapple juice, sliced red onion, and seaweed
- 2 ounces cheese you can break, not spread

If breakfast is your starch meal, choose one:
- ½ cup cooked yellow cornmeal with raisins (optional) and 1 teaspoon maple syrup (or stevia powder as needed if you have diabetes)
- ½ cup cooked rye, barley, brown rice, or millet with grated carrots, raisins, and vanilla extract; add powdered seaweed as a salt substitute
- 1 slice whole grain bread, sprout bread, or toast spread with ½ teaspoon coconut oil or 1 teaspoon chyawanprash, an East Indian paste made with ghee (clarified butter), sweet digestive spices, and rejuvenating herbs
- 3 alfalfa tablets cracked and swallowed with tea or 2 chlorophyll concentrate capsules

Note: People allergic or otherwise unable to eat fruit can have raw and steamed vegetables and a protein source. Have 2 cups of broccoli green tea or broccoli and vegetable cooking water daily.

Midmorning Snack
20 drops reishi mushroom extract or 8 ounces shiitake tea, with choice of:
- 1 apple, 4 or 5 prunes, or 1 cup raw vegetables
- 2 whole grain crackers and 1 tablespoon tofu spread or hummus
- 1 to 2 glasses of half water, half fruit or vegetable juice
- Get Svelte instant beverage
- 10 to 20 drops of maté extract for high energy
- ¼ cup dried whole dulse seaweed and a rice cake

Lunch
A big salad with many different kinds of raw vegetables, sprouts, and seeds with a dressing made with grapeseed, canola, or olive oil and lemon; with (optional) choice of:

- An omelet
- 4 ounces steamed fish with seaweed
- Sushi or sashimi; cooked vegetables and seaweed
- Vegetable barley soup
- Tofu and vegetables sprinkled with dried seaweed
- 2 to 4 ounces naturally fermented sauerkraut and a baked potato with a dab of low-fat sour cream

Tea or Get Svelte instant beverage

1 to 3 teaspoons coconut oil or up to 2 tablespoons grated unsweetened raw coconut (optional)

Alfalfa tablets or chlorophyll concentrate capsules

3:00 p.m. Snack

20 drops reishi mushroom extract or 8 ounces shiitake tea, with choice of:

- 1 cup raw vegetables
- 1 to 2 glasses half water, half juice
- 1 to 3 cups tea or 1 Get Svelte and 1 Gorgeous You instant beverage
- 1 square semisweet baking chocolate and an unsalted rice cake
- 1 to 2 cups spicy popcorn (1 cup counts as 2 servings of a whole grain) made with air-popped corn, 1 tablespoon canola oil, salt substitute, turmeric powder, and a pinch of asafoetida powder
- 10 to 20 drops of maté extract for high energy

Dinner

Salad, cooked vegetables (sweet, steamed parsnips instead of potato)

2 to 4 ounces protein (fish, eggs, chicken white meat, nuts, or tofu) served with stewed tomato or ripe, raw grapefruit wedges

2 to 3 cups tea

Optional: 1 glass of red wine with 20 drops of reishi mushroom extract

Alfalfa tablets or chlorophyll concentrate capsules

Before Bed (choose one as needed)
- 1 cup yogurt with ½ teaspoon turmeric (to discourage intestinal parasites, do not eat dairy the same day as fish or red meat)
- Happy Garden Tea or mint, chamomile, or vervain tea
- 20 drops of reishi mushroom extract in water
- 2 to 4 ounces baked pumpkin or orange squash with a dash of nutmeg
- 1 very ripe sweet grapefruit (not commercial grapefruit juice)

Sample Menu 2

This menu, simpler than number one, fits into a leisurely fasting or cleansing schedule. You might want to follow it one afternoon a week. Take care to rest and eat lightly during the day. Take acidophilus capsules or chlorella with meals, or eat ½ cup of yogurt, adding ¼ teaspoon turmeric powder for one meal. Give yourself an enema followed after several hours by a hot bath at night, and sleep enough to feel refreshed.

Daily
Have 2 cups of broccoli green tea or 1 cup of broccoli and its cooking water. Choose a time either first thing in the morning on an empty stomach or when you will not eat anything afterwards for several hours. Use no spices with the broccoli.

Upon Rising (choose one)
- 1 to 2 glasses half water, half fruit juice
- 1 glass water with the juice of ½ lemon
- 3 cups hot tea or Get Svelte instant beverage
- 1 cup raw fruit or ½ cup reconstituted dried fruit, with cardamom or hingvashtaka powder
- 3 alfalfa tablets or 2 chlorophyll concentrate capsules
- 1 to 3 teaspoons virgin coconut oil

Midmorning Snack
20 drops reishi mushroom extract in water or 8 ounces shiitake tea, with one of the following:

- 1 to 2 glasses half water, half fruit or vegetable juice
- Get Svelte instant beverage
- 10 to 20 drops of maté extract for energy
- ½ cup dried whole dulse seaweed

Lunch

A big raw vegetable salad (optional salad dressing) with fenugreek sprouts (if you have diabetes), with choice of:
- Vegetable barley soup with miso and alaria seaweed
- Tofu and vegetables
- Up to 1 cup Onion–Tree Ear Soup (page 47)
- Mixed vegetable smoothie made with 1 tablespoon coconut meat or 1 teaspoon coconut oil (add soaked defatted fenugreek if you have diabetes)

Tea or Get Svelte instant beverage
Alfalfa tablets or chlorophyll concentrate capsules
1 to 3 teaspoons coconut oil or 2 tablespoons raw coconut

3:00 p.m. Snack

20 drops reishi mushroom extract in water, with choice of:
- 1 to 2 glasses half water, half vegetable juice
- Up to 1 cup Onion–Tree Ear Soup
- 3 alfalfa tablets or 2 chlorophyll concentrate capsules

Dinner

Juice of one orange, lemon, or lime added to 1 glass of water, with choice of:
- 2 steamed green vegetables such as kale or watercress
- 1 to 2 cups tomato cabbage soup
- 2 cups soup made with potato, corn, red pepper, peas, kelp seaweed, and soy milk

Optional: Raw vegetable salad

Before Bed (choose one)
- Happy Garden Tea or mint, chamomile, or vervain tea
- 20 drops reishi mushroom extract in water

I think anyone can understand and appreciate this approach. It is simple: Eat less, and separate your protein and starch meals so they do not trouble digestion. Use diluted fruit beverages and coconut oil to gradually reduce your craving for sweets. Use reishi mushroom extract to enhance energy and willpower.

Making these changes all at once will seem daunting; therefore, make them gradually. The first week, take chlorophyll capsules and a handful of dried seaweed after meals. The second week, add coconut oil or bee pollen after meals. The third week. dilute beverages using half water and half fruit or vegetable juice. Then try to keep the ratio of two fruits to eight vegetables during the day. Enjoy experimenting with Asian superfoods such as shiitake mushrooms and balsam pear bitter melon tea. Try a teaspoon of chyawanprash on toast instead of chocolate during the day.

Foods for Fast-Action Weight Loss

Now that you understand the principles and have learned how to put together daily meals, let's take a look at some of the details. Let's face it: Some food choices are simply better than others, in terms of both calories and nutrition. The good news is that some of the best choices are also the most delicious.

A great pleasure in our Asian-inspired diet is the abundant use of fresh tropical fruits. You might combine fresh pineapple, papaya, mango, and grated coconut or coconut milk. They are cleansing, digestive, and very nourishing. Asian superfoods, such as an East Indian cherry called amla, are dried, powdered, and used as potent detoxifying medicines. Try to add some of the following cleansing foods and juices between meals, or eat them occasionally *instead* of a meal. (Those marked with a star [★] are Asian superfoods.) Be sure to remove any trace of pesticides by following my fruit and vegetable washing recommendations on page 30.

Many of the following foods are laxative or diuretic. You can reduce temporary side effects such as cramping or gas by drinking a cup of hot licorice tea or adding the following spices to hot water: raw ginger, mint leaves, or cardamom powder. Another useful remedy to keep in your pocket is Carbo veg 30C, homeopathic charcoal recommended for indigestion, bloating, and cramping. Wait at least 15 minutes after eating, and never mix a homeopathic remedy with food, beverage, or toothpaste. Melt three small white pills under the tongue, or add a dose to water and sip it between meals.

★HINGVASHTAKA POWDER, a pungent combination of spices including asafoetida, originating from India, is available in East Indian groceries or online. Hingvashtaka powder resolves abdominal bloating and indigestion. To start the day with a bang, I add a pinch of this highly digestive powder to my morning cup of hot green tea. For a tummy-slimming treatment, you might add hingvashtaka powder to fruit juices, raw fruit dishes, or reconstituted fruit (see recipes below).

★ASAFOETIDA (HING) is a powerful deep-acting stimulant cleanser, carminative for gas and bloating, and antiseptic anthelmintic (destroys parasites, bacteria, yeast, and worms). It is often used when cooking legumes and gas-producing foods, but it's too bitter to spice fruit dishes. Add a pinch to your soups and stews, tea, spicy popcorn, or vegetable juices. It is recommended for indigestion, flatulence, abdominal distention, colic pain, constipation, and palpitations. Asafoetida, similar to garlic but stronger smelling, eliminates fat and poisons resulting from eating meat and junk food. Keep it in a sealed jar in your kitchen, and use its pungent odor to chase evil spirits.

Now let's take a close-up look at many of the foods that will help keep you slim.

★Aloe Vera

The aloe we find in American health food stores comes mainly from Texas and Mexico. China is the largest producer of aloe in Asia. When American manufactures realize they can get fine-quality aloe that meets the required standards at a lower price, aloe drinks will flood the market. Until then, you will have to mix them up at home. Aloe is mild-tasting, soothing, cleansing, alkaline, and slightly laxative. And it reduces appetite. Aloe juice and gel are important foods for people who are overweight and those who have diabetes. Add up to ¼ cup of either to juices made from half fruit or vegetable juice and half water or seltzer.

Apples

Apples are a major antimucus fruit. Mucus, weak digestion, and water retention underlie cellulite; therefore, many antimucus foods are also anticellulite foods. Apples, an alkaline food useful for cleansing, contain pectin, which helps eliminate excess water in the intestines and acts as a stimulant for peristaltic movement. That makes them middle-slimming. Apples contain 50 percent more vitamin A than oranges do.

Give breakfast a special zing by combining peeled apple slices with two Asian superfoods: ⅛ teaspoon of hingvashtaka powder and 1 teaspoon of coconut oil. This makes a highly purifying dish. If coconut oil is too rich for you, substitute olive or grapeseed oil.

Apricots

Apricots are quite laxative and alkaline. They contain cobalt, which is necessary for anemic conditions. Dried apricot has six times more sugar than fresh fruit does. To reduce the sugar content, I bring dried apricots to a boil in water, let them soak for at least 1 hour or overnight, then strain off the water. I season reconstituted apricots with cardamom and cinnamon powder and store them in a ceramic jar. For a middle-slimming dish, I substitute ⅛ teaspoon hingvashtaka powder and 1 tablespoon water. Spiced apricots make a nice dessert alone or a pleasant meal when served with 2 ounces of raw goat cheese or goat or sheep feta.

Asparagus

A diuretic wonder food, asparagus contains useful hormones and reduces water retention. ★Shatavari, the East Indian form, is popularly called "wife with a thousand husbands" because it rejuvenates the female sexuality and fertility. In Chinese markets, shatavari is called *tian men dong* and used for dry mouth and rasping cough. It is sometimes used for thirst in diabetes. Our American asparagus is more diuretic, and therefore more slimming, compared with the moistening Asian tonics. If you do not like the malodorous urine resulting from eating cooked asparagus, eat it raw in salads.

Barley Water

Cooked barley is an antimucus grain. Even more cleansing is fermented barley water. Wash ¼ cup of dried barley in some water, adding 1 teaspoon of apple cider vinegar to wash off dust. Put the rinsed barley into a gallon of spring water, and let it ferment for a day or two. Drink 1 cup before meals or in the afternoon as a laxative beverage that improves digestive flora. Replace the water as you use it. You can stop the fermentation process by keeping barley water in the refrigerator. I like to ferment my barley water along with slices of raw ginger, using up to 2 tablespoons or enough to make a brew as strong as ginger beer. You might sweeten it as needed with ½ teaspoon of raw honey, maple syrup, or stevia powder. Step up cleansing and reduce impacted matter in the colon by adding ½ teaspoon hingvashtaka powder per gallon of barley water.

★Bitter Melon

Bitter melon (*Momordica charantia* L.), known as balsam pear, kugua, or laigua in Chinese, as well as many other names throughout India and the tropics, is loved for its bitter taste and cleansing, slimming properties. Chinese bitter melon looks like a light-colored cucumber, about 5 to 8 inches long, that has deep, long grooves. The East Indian variety is smaller with many lumps and bumps. It contains protein, calcium, phosphorus, iron, carotene, pectin, and vitamins B_1, B_2, and C. Its cooling effects are felt by the heart, liver, and lungs.

Bitter melon is used mainly for diabetes, weight loss, and heatstroke and to neutralize and eliminate poisons. It clears the complexion and brightens the eyes. Some people in India juice a ripe bitter melon and drink 1 ounce in the morning to reduce cholesterol, hypertension, and internal heat conditions resulting from the climate or fever illnesses. Bitter melon is antiviral and well known to the HIV natural foods community.

Most people find this vegetable too bitter as a raw juice, but cooks from Asia and the West Indies slice and sauté it with garlic and a dab of black bean paste. It can be added to soups or meat dishes to enhance the flavor or increase their slimming benefits. Cherry Grain Balsam Pear Tea (or another bitter melon tea) is mild-tasting and refreshing. You can find it at most stores in American Chinatowns and online at www.asiachi.com. Steep it as you would a regular tea, or add a handful of the dried sliced bitter melon to soups.

Carrot

Carrots, a popular fasting food, are high in vitamin A and roughage. Dr. Bernard Jensen's favorite fresh juice was carrot, which he said cleaned everything out of his body that should not be there. He sometimes combined carrot juice with raw goat milk from his goat farm in California. Carrots can be juiced with parsley, celery, watercress, endive, dandelion, or romaine lettuce. A pound of carrots has 48,000 IU of vitamin A with only 179 calories, 4.8 grams of protein, and 1.2 grams of fat. Add powdered hingvashtaka or asafoetida for faster cleansing action.

★ Cherries and Amla

The large black cherries, sometimes called bing cherries, are an excellent liver and gallbladder cleanser, useful for gout. You might fast on them along with spring water for a day so swollen joints look and feel cooler. You can sweeten foods with black cherry concentrate from the health food store. Add some to your morning hot tea. Cherries are high in iron and act as a laxative food. One pound yields 1.6 milligrams of iron. Dr. Jensen recommends cherries for their high alkaline content because they rid the body of toxic waste. In his book *Foods That Heal,* he writes that cherries have a wonderful effect on the glandular system. Cherries can be mixed with other fruits and proteins but with neither starch nor dairy foods.

An East Indian cherry called amla is the best food source of vitamin C, yielding 3,000 milligrams per fruit. Amla or amalaki powder (*Emblica officinalis*) is a nutritive, rejuvenating, laxative, astringent herb that improves bruises, hemorrhoids, anemia, diabetes, gout, gastritis, colitis, hepatitis, constipation, liver or spleen weakness leading to a spare tire, and general debility. Some people drink amla tea for hair loss, weak fingernails, bleeding gums, and digestive inflammation or burning. To purify the body, use no more than ⅛ teaspoon of amla powder per cup of hot water the first time because it may cause diarrhea.

★ Chlorella

Chlorella (*Chlorella pyrenoidosa*, *Chlorella vulgaris*), a unicellular green algae that grows in still, fresh water or on soil or tree bark, is the most common food supplement taken in Japan, where it is added to tea, soup, milk, juice, noodles, yogurt, and other foods.

Chlorella has a complex protein that helps heal damaged tissues. It is said to help rid the body of heavy metals, support liver function, and enhance the immune system to reduce the development and spread of cancer. Abundant medical research has been done on chlorella, but it is best to think of it as one of the purest, most potent foods on earth. The following information comes primarily from the article "Chlorella: A Natural Wonder Food" by Joseph Mercola, MD, found at www.mercola.com.

Some studies suggest chlorella may be useful for lowering blood pressure in people who have hypertension. Chlorella (8 grams per day) can detoxify persons affected with cadmium poisoning. Chlorella prolongs survival times in persons afflicted with various forms of cancer, including breast cancer and leukemia, by boosting the immune response. It facilitates the production of important cancer-fighting substances in the body: granulocyte-macrophage colony-stimulating factor (GM-CSF), interferon gamma, and interleukin-1. It also contains a glycoprotein (named CVS) that inhibits the spread of some forms of cancer.

The first thing you might notice when taking chlorella is better digestion, especially if you have bad breath or constipation. Chlorella causes stomach lactobacilli to multiply at four times the normal rate. It is best to take with meals to provide good digestion and assimilation of nutrients.

For people switching from a junk-food diet to a high-fiber natural foods diet, the possible temporary side effects of chlorella are a strong cleansing reaction with gas, cramping, constipation, or diarrhea. For this reason, it is a good idea to start with less than the suggested amount, and gradually increase up to the recommended dose in 1 to 2 weeks. Very sensitive individuals may want to start with as little as a single 450-milligram capsule per day. A person cannot take too much chlorella, because it is naturally detoxifying. However, there is an individual comfort level that determines how much chlorella to take per day. The usual dose is up to 5 to 8 grams a day. To overcome temporary digestive discomfort, I recommend adding an herbal remedy such as Quiet Digestion pills made by Health Concerns or a cup of hot ginger and licorice tea.

It is supposed to take approximately 3 to 6 months for chlorella to begin to remove heavy metals from the blood, depending on the amount of chlorella taken. A person can take as much as 15 to 20 grams per day, depending on the level of heavy metals that are present.

There are three algae and two cereal grasses that are commonly available. The algae are chlorella, spirulina, and blue-green algae (aphanizomenon flos-aquae). The grasses are wheatgrass and barley grass. While all five products are excellent sources of nutrients, some experts believe chlorella is the most valuable of all the green food supplements. Chlorella contains the highest chlorophyll content of any known plant. It has five to 10 times that of spirulina, wheatgrass, and barley grass and is higher in chlorophyll than blue-green algae.

Chlorella and the other algae are abundant in beta-carotene, which is known to prevent cancer. The protein content of the algae is significantly higher than in the cereal grasses. Chlorella is about 60 percent protein; spirulina, 73 percent; blue-green algae, 56 percent; barley grass, 14 percent; and wheatgrass, 18 percent.

★Coconut

One of the pleasures of a tropical diet is fresh coconut from the tree. Fortunately, we can buy pure organic virgin coconut oil in health food stores. It stops your sugar and carb cravings in their tracks. The recommended dose is up to 1 tablespoon of the oil after meals, but that is too difficult to digest or too laxative for some people. Start with ½ teaspoon if you do not need a moistening laxative. You will notice smoother, better-looking skin and hair almost immediately. If coconut is too rich for you or causes nausea or a bloated feeling, avoid it.

If you live in the South, open-air markets sell green coconuts for their juice. In southern India, people often fast with the juice for 1 to 2 weeks before beginning acupuncture or other treatments. It is nourishing enough to sustain health while being very cleansing.

Brown coconuts are a different variety. Their watery liquid is not the milk, which is made by liquefying the white meat inside. The milk made from a brown coconut compares with mother's breast milk in its chemical balance. A complete protein, coconut contains potassium, magnesium, phosphorus, and chlorine. Somewhat laxative, coconut meat is a good bodybuilder for strong bones and teeth. Enjoy the white meat with fruits and vegetables or as a snack by itself. Coconut is 70 percent fat and can be grated onto a salad.

Choose a brown coconut by shaking it. If you hear no water splashing inside, it is spoiled. The dark spots, or "eyes," on one end should not be moldy. Puncture one of the eyes with a knife and place the coconut on top of a glass to catch the juice. I always drink it, although it is not as nourishing as the meat. To open it, I hold the coconut in my left hand and hit it with a hammer in my right hand. Tap very firmly in a vertical line from the eye end to the other end, then horizontally all around the bottom side until it cracks. The shell will come away easily when cut if you first heat the coconut in a 350°F oven for 30 minutes.

Coconut and palm oils got bad press during the 1950s because it was thought they increased cholesterol. Now we know that not all saturated fats are bad. Researchers know that weight loss associated with coconut oil is due to the length of its fatty acid chains. Coconut oil contains medium chain fatty acids, or medium chain triglycerides (MCTs), which are different from the long chain fatty acids or triglycerides (LCTs) found in other plant-based oils used to make most vegetable oils. LCTs are stored in the body as fat, while MCTs are burned for energy.

Coconut oil is nature's richest source of MCTs that increase metabolic rates and lead to weight loss. MCTs promote thermogenesis, which increases the body's metabolism, producing energy. People in the animal feed business know that if you feed animals vegetable oils, they put on weight, whereas if you feed them coconut oil, they become very lean with smooth, shiny coats. According to research found at a number of Web sites, including www.coconutdiet.com, "Increasing MCTs replaces LCTs and reduces fat storage in the body. A diet containing MCT is more effective for weight loss than a low-fat diet." One human study cited found that "MCT-containing meals caused an average 12 percent increase in basal metabolic rate, as compared with a 4 percent increase with the LCT-containing meal." The authors of the study concluded that replacing dietary fats with MCTs could "over long periods of time produce weight loss even in the absence of reduced [caloric] intake."

Outside of a human mother's breast milk, coconut oil is nature's most abundant source of lauric acid and MCTs. Lauric acid is antiviral. Research is cited at www.coconutdiet.com among other sites regarding using coconut for HIV and herpes. Virgin coconut oil is also recommended for ridding the body of parasites such as giardia and worms. It can be used in cooking, on salads, or taken by the teaspoon with meals in place of a dessert. For our use, taking 1 teaspoon of organic virgin coconut oil with meals reduces sweets and carbohydrate hunger and makes you feel full and satisfied. Since it increases metabolism and stimulates a lazy thyroid, it helps burn fat into muscle. Most people notice that adding coconut oil to the diet makes their clothes fit better. However, coconut oil is not a magic bullet for melting pounds. Some people cannot lose weight until they cut all polyunsaturated fats from their diet, and many women who take birth control pills report that they actually gain weight if they use coconut oil.

Garden Greens Juice

You can make this fresh juice in the afternoon or evening with the greens you might ordinarily throw away. The recipe is offered in honor of my friend, James Peter Martin, vegan chef, artist, and naturalist philosopher. A New York native, James made his fortune designing and decorating elaborate wedding gowns with lace and pearls. His parents both died of Hodgkin's lymphoma. When at age 40 he was diagnosed with his parents' disease, he gave up his income and his cigarettes, coffee, and three-piece suit and moved to a farm, where he ate raw fruits and vegetables and romped in the grass—he even ate the grass—with his two beloved dogs. Years later, when I met James in his vegan restaurant on Miami Beach, he was slim, youthful, and cancer-free. I have lost track of the whereabouts of this untamed spirit, but I am sure he is basking somewhere on a sunny beach, drinking fresh green juices.

You do not need a juicer to make this healthful juice, which contains plenty of useful vitamins and minerals. Many sprouts and leafy greens do not juice well, so use a blender instead and add water to make a distilled juice. Use a total of two handfuls of several kinds of chopped leafy greens along with about 3 cups of water. Blend this mixture at high speed for 3 minutes, then let it stand, covered, in your blender for 2 hours to let the sediment settle. Strain the liquid through cheesecloth or a clean linen towel. If necessary, sweeten the strained liquid with pineapple juice.

Choose from any of the following greens: alfalfa sprouts, anise, beet or turnip greens, bok choy, Brussels sprouts, cabbage, celery greens, carrot tops, red radish tops, chaparral, chives, endive, coriander (cilantro) leaves, dandelion, escarole, kale, mint, parsley, sage, Swiss chard, thyme, watercress, and wheatgrass. Make sure the greens are clean and fresh. Spice the juice with a sprinkling of cayenne or raw ginger as needed.

Alfalfa contains calcium, magnesium, iron, potassium, and trace elements needed to build health. It purifies the body and makes body fluids more alkaline, which is important for preventing illness. Dandelion reduces acidity from the digestive tract and the blood. For that reason, it reduces complexion blemishes, cysts, and stones. Watercress and endive are excellent for slimming but taste bitter. Red radish tops are high in iron. Beet greens contain potassium, magnesium, iodine, and iron. Raw or lightly steamed, they make a great liver and gallbladder rejuvenator.

Members of the cabbage family, including Brussels sprouts and bok choy, heal stomach ulcers and purify the body because of their potassium and sulphur content. They also are gas-forming.

Raw juices may give you intestinal grumbling, cramps, or diarrhea if you drink too much too soon. Start with 1 or 2 tablespoons with or between meals and gradually work up to ¼ cup, then 1 cup or more a day. Never begin the day with a green or raw juice. It requires too much digestive power and may result in a headache in the afternoon. Start the day with a glass of hot water or hot green tea.

Grape

A grape diet is delicious and cleansing for the liver, kidney, and bowel. Grapes soothe the nervous system, which makes them a good food for nervous snackers. Grapes are one of the oldest fruits in the world. Grape seeds have been found in mummy cases in 3,000-year-old Egyptian tombs. The low incidence of cancer in winegrowing regions of France may be attributed to the high percentage of grapes in the daily diet. Grapes have a high magnesium and potassium content. Dark grapes are high in iron. Try to get grapes that have seeds, such as Concord, Fresno Beauty, red, and Muscat varieties. Grape skins and chewed seeds are healthy bulk but should be avoided by people with colitis or ulcers. You can blend sweet grapes with citrus or pineapple juice to suit your taste. Used with whey, soy milk, and a raw egg, grape juice is a blood tonic.

To wash away tummy fat and skin blemishes, 1 day a week eat nothing but a pound of grapes every 3 hours along with an 8-ounce glass of water. Have no more than 4 pounds of grapes a day. Dr. Jensen recommended a 5- to 10-day grape diet along with daily enemas for eliminating long-term problems associated with excess catarrh.

Orange

Orange was first mentioned in a 500 BC text edited by Confucius. The sour orange naranga got its name from Sanskrit in about AD 100. It came into the Mediterranean basin long before the fall of the Roman Empire. Seedless oranges appeared in a Chinese horticultural book by Han Yen-Chi in AD 1178. There were 27 varieties then; now more than 200 varieties are grown in the United States.

Oranges are more than a source of vitamin C. They, like all citrus fruits, are particularly valuable in elimination diets because they are alkaline-reacting. A body-acid condition resulting from a high-protein diet can be neutralized and eliminated by the alkaline mineral elements in fruits and vegetables. For acidosis, drink orange juice or eat oranges after meals. In cases of stomach acid deficiency, start the meal with a peeled orange or a glass of orange juice. Orange makes a good fasting diet for people who cannot stop work and rest in bed.

★Pineapple and Papaya

Fresh pineapple and papaya are delightful for breakfast. They are especially useful for people with catarrh problems such as asthma. Both fruits contain valuable digestive enzymes. If you cannot take time to eat but need to improve digestion or heal a sprain or a broken bone, have a handful of papaya enzyme tablets (papain)—about 200 milligrams per tablet—several times a day with a glass of water. Papain reduces inflammation and acid impurities that delay healing.

★Soy milk

Most people buy soy milk in the supermarket because it is convenient and inexpensive. However, Chinese and Japanese people enjoy making mild, fresh soy milk, yogurt, and cheese at home. Soy milk is a complete protein that nourishes, beautifies, and energizes weight loss. Reducing animal protein reduces cholesterol, fat, and calcium loss, thereby protecting us from arthritis, heart trouble, and cancer.

MAKES 2 QUARTS | SOAKING TIME: 4 HOURS; COOKING TIME: 45 MINUTES
  2 cups dried organic soybeans
  5 cups boiled water

In a large jar, soak the soybeans in boiled water for 4 hours or overnight in cold water. The beans will double in size to give you from 4 to

5 cups of soaked beans. Discard the soaking water and, in a blender, combine 1 cup of beans and 1 cup of boiling water. Blend at high speed to make a fine slurry. Repeat for all the beans, and put the whipped beans in a large plastic or glass pitcher.

Meanwhile, in a 2-gallon heavy-bottomed pot, bring 10 cups of water to a boil. Pour the beans into the boiling water and bring to a boil, stirring occasionally with a long wooden spoon. Watch the pot carefully. As soon as it comes to a boil, turn the heat to a slow simmer to prevent it from boiling over. Remove the top foam with a spoon and simmer for 45 minutes, stirring occasionally. Cooking breaks down the acids that make bean proteins digestible.

After cooking the soy milk for 45 minutes, turn off the heat and replace the lid to let it steam until cool enough to pour through a sieve into container(s). Season the milk as needed with up to 1 teaspoon of salt substitute. I enjoy soy milk unsweetened, but most people add stevia powder, maple syrup, vanilla, or carob powder. It can be stored in the refrigerator for 4 to 5 days or frozen.

Watermelon and Watercress

Watermelon, a source of potassium, is the queen of diuretic, slimming foods. In Asia, ★a watermelon fast is recommended for slimming and reducing water retention, mucus congestion, and poisons. (Chinese doctors recommend watermelon for dampness conditions characterized by swelling, slow digestion, and lethargy.) Make a fruit salad, arranging slices of watermelon, celery, daikon radish, and cucumber sprinkled with a dash of cayenne pepper. Add a garnish of watercress, Dr. Jensen's favorite slimming food. Watercress, a very alkaline food, contains sulfur, potassium, and water, which make it healing for the liver and glands. It reduces catarrh and purifies the blood.

In the following chapter, you will learn about seaweeds, vegetables that protect the Earth's blood—the oceans—and purify our blood and strengthen our bones and organs. Sea minerals maintain an alkaline condition in the body that protects against fatigue, illness, and overweight. You don't have to be over 40 to enjoy them.

Chapter 10

After 40

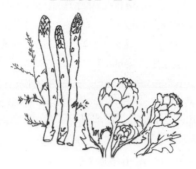

After 40, life intensifies. Baby boomers today are putting kids through college, working independently at home, or assuming executive duties that include travel. Any financial advisor will tell you that Americans have a negative savings rate: They live full-out and do not save money. As a consequence, they must stay active, slim, healthy, and attractive in order to work. Many people choose to work well past retirement age. They may be involved in a second or third marriage or actively seeking one.

At 40, smart women plan ahead, using herbs to make menopause easier. Some hope to become pregnant after years of following a career. Keeping a healthy weight improves all these possibilities.

After 40, what was attractive baby fat in your twenties and voluptuous curves in your thirties now hovers somewhere between pudginess and flab. It becomes increasingly difficult to keep weight off when metabolism is sluggish and hormone balance challenged. Health experts advise exercising more and eating less. That looks fine on paper, but, like rearranging the closets or raking the yard, it is usually left until tomorrow. You will find that herbs offer surprising ways to boost metabolism to meet your growing needs.

The Baseline Diet limits calories and facilitates wise food

combinations. It is simple and sparse, leaving room for flexibility: The hard part of dieting is done. On a typical day, you might have fruit, yogurt or cheese, toast, and tea for breakfast; a hard-cooked egg and celery at midmorning; a big salad or tofu for lunch; a bowl of spicy popcorn or a handful of nuts during the afternoon; and a small, wisely prepared dinner. The rest of the time, juices diluted with water, slimming teas, a healthy mushroom beverage, Rejuvelac, or other cleansing beverages will keep digestion working smoothly. When metabolism is slow or digestion difficult, the rule is this: Increase cleansing.

There are a number of strategies for both men and women over 40 to cleanse their bodies of toxins, keep their weight down and energy levels up, and ensure that their hormones are functioning as they should.

Eat Less and Enjoy More

Eating small portions is a psychological challenge for Americans in love with supersizing and bargains. French chef Pierre Checci, formerly with the New England Culinary Institute who now teaches at Kendall College in Chicago, lost over 125 pounds during 1 year by reducing the size of his meals. Pierre says, "Americans are overweight because they fill their plates with mountains of foods they never taste. They mix appetizers, large entrées, desserts, everything all together. Their plates overflow, but they do not spend time to savor their foods. If something tastes wonderful, all you need is a little to be satisfied. A small dish of pasta with well-seasoned vegetables and a nice sauce, or a small piece of meat nicely prepared along with a big healthy salad, are enough for a meal. For dessert, one bite of the best-quality bitter chocolate is perfection."

I agree and add that we always overeat when diet foods are boring. I compared menus recommended for the over-40 age group, ranging from those on official government Web sites to private doctor- or athlete-generated diet Web sites, and found dull, flavorless prison foods. Take two examples: Who would really want to combine pasta, canned tuna, and cheese as a main dish? How healthy does a snack of two slices of buttered white bread with tea or coffee sound? These meals may hit the calorie target, but they remain sticky and monotonous! Worse, they reduce digestive *qi* because they encourage sluggish digestion and parasites. There are better choices you can make.

THINK SMALL. To really enjoy eating small meals, eat the way most Asians do: Choose plenty of colorful, tasty, crisp fresh produce served with small portions of cooked foods seasoned with stimulating, pungent spices.

DRINK LOTS OF TEA. Iced or hot; served with fresh lemon, milk, cane sugar, maple syrup, stevia powder, mint leaves, fresh ginger, or spices; whipped into smoothies or added to soups, stews, and baking—nothing alters the health-giving benefits of wonderfully digestive, fat-reducing tea! It decreases the absorption of fats in the digestive tract. It helps prevent cancer, heart trouble, and stroke. Tea, a diuretic, also reduces cellulite.

CONSIDER A DIURETIC. Mature people with a sedentary lifestyle or certain illnesses may develop urinary complaints. How do you, someone over 40, know whether you need a diuretic? You cannot always tell by looking at your body. The easiest way to know is with Asian diagnosis: If your urine is no more frequent than two times daily; looks medium to dark yellow, orange, or greenish; appears thick or clouded; or contains streaks or has a lumpy or sandy appearance, you need to drink more water and take purifying diuretic herbs and foods as I recommend in this book. Urine should be clear, have no unusual odor or oily appearance, and be no darker than clear to a very pale yellow.

You can know how much of a diuretic is enough by observing your urine. The easier, lighter, and more frequent the flow, the less likely you are to develop prostate or urinary discomforts. A useful diuretic for men ages 40 and over is Kai Kit Wan (Prostate Gland Pills). Recommended teas in this chapter help to normalize urinary functions.

STAY HYDRATED. The frequency of urination depends only in part on your use of diet foods and teas. It is ideal to drink enough water or tea to reduce weight and impurities without overstimulating the kidneys. One of the best ways to stay hydrated and to reduce illness, pain, and overweight is by drinking cooked broccoli water.

TAKE NUTRIENTS FOR INSULIN CONTROL. Another thing to consider is your waistline and refined sugar intake. Diet authorities suggest that people over 40 develop an oversensitive pancreas that pumps too much insulin into the bloodstream. Certainly years of low-vitality carbohydrates such as white bread, potatoes, pasta, and processed foods overwork the pancreas. You can tell if yours is overworked by observing yourself and habits. Do you have extra weight and fat at the waistline? Bears tend to eat sweets and have a spare tire. If you crave breads, sweets, refined sugars, and overprocessed foods in gen-

---

ARE SEXUAL TONIC HERBS RIGHT FOR YOU?

Are heating and drying herbs suited for your weight loss program? The answer lies inside your tongue. Traditional Chinese medicine (TCM) doctors believe that the people best suited to this approach have dampness (*she*), indicated by water retention; a sluggish digestion and slow elimination; and excess internal cold (*han*), indicated by weakness, chills, low energy, and poor enthusiasm. People with this set of symptoms also have a tongue that looks pale, oversize, puffy, and wet. Put a checkmark by any of the following items that apply to you.

___ A large, puffy, pale tongue
___ Water retention (edema)
___ Low enthusiasm
___ Lethargy

If you responded positively, you may benefit from heating and drying herbs and foods. For the overweight person who feels weak and depressed from a slow metabolism, a drying, heating diet acts like a hot stove under a pot of water. But it is not the best for everyone. If you often feel hot, dry, and thirsty, this approach will not work for you. It is important to note these differences because using the

---

eral—foods that weaken the pancreas—you have a weakened pancreas. In other words, unless we consciously work to correct the situation, we'll always eat to maintain our digestive imbalances.

A daily dose of 600 milligrams of alpha lipoic acid, 20 milligrams of vanadium, and 100 milligrams or more of vitamin E are supposed to absorb excess insulin.

TAKE A WALK. When and how you eat affects digestion and, therefore, weight loss. A meal followed by a nap puts on weight. If you walk to a café or to the park, eat a small lunch without dessert, and walk back to the office, you have given yourself a miniworkout that maintains a steady, fast metabolism.

---

wrong sorts of foods and herbs causes side effects. Let me explain.

One problem for mature overweight people is that diet doctors and supplement manufacturers totally ignore the relationship between sexuality and weight loss. They recommend the same sort of weight loss stimulants for everyone, regardless of age, health, and sex. However, for most people over 40, smokers, and people who use acne drugs or drying allergy medicines, a heating, drying diet including cayenne pepper or certain concentrated health food store supplements will eventually lead to dehydration and, therefore, dryness and burning pain during sex. It is fine to have well-defined muscles and "washboard abs." However, to create that look, it's necessary to reduce fluid content. But no woman wants to feel burning pain during sex. And no man hopes for reduced semen or eventual prostate inflammation.

Concentrated energy supplements, unless they are combined with cooling, moistening herbs, may interfere with normal hormonal changes and body fluids. This chapter offers a balanced approach to slimming, energizing foods and herbs suitable for peri- and post-menopausal women, who have reduced estrogen and sexual fluids, as well as for mature men, who have reduced testosterone and sexual fluids such as semen and prostate fluid.

STASH HEALTHY SNACKS. The worst temptation for self-employed people is noshing. Have slimming snacks ready. I do not mean a low-fat cookie or a diet cola: Try sliced celery, raisins, prunes or watermelon, and spiced tea. Use slimming foods that are already part of your healthy diet.

Distance your computer from the refrigerator. Schedule exercise breaks. It will improve your circulation and reduce computer injuries.

Weight Loss and Sexuality

To keep weight off, we have to reverse the fundamentally weakening effects of aging. From an Asian medical perspective, we must consider our hormones and sexuality. Why would anyone use hormonal herbs for slimming? There are many benefits gained from Asian herbal sexual tonics. Traditional Chinese medicine (TCM) considers sexual potency to be an attitude, as well as a physical capacity. Increasing sexual vitality with herbs enhances joie de vivre, creativity, and drive at any age. It increases courage, optimism, and a willingness to remain attractive and slim.

Have you noticed how castrated male cats and roosters grow fat? Men over 40 tend to have reduced testosterone. Consequently, they develop fat, rounded curves, breasts, weak legs, and sexual dysfunctions. Less testosterone in men means less muscle mass, and a loss of lean tissue causes the metabolism to decline.

Chinese doctors believe that for both men and women, maintaining sexual vitality and a healthy weight are equally dependent upon kidney fire (a function of adrenal energy). According to TCM practitioner Henry C. Lu, PhD, the more kidney fire we have, the less body fat we develop. In *Chinese System of Food Cures*, he writes, "To be slim is to be sexy. A fat fellow will not have a strong sexual capacity, and a fellow with a strong sexual capacity will not be fat; nature does not mix sex with obesity. The burning fire of the kidneys [the testes] will keep burning fat and steaming water out of the body, keeping the body free of obesity."

Women, according to Dr. Lu, have less kidney fire than men and therefore gain weight and retain water easier. We think overweight and cellulite have something to do with the decline in estrogen production, not our lack of fire. In fact, some of us are hot stuff with testosterone to spare. But other women need to light a match under their hormones to promote fertility and libido and, consequently, to reduce edema. Healthy sensuality reinforces exercise and weight loss. Many overweight people shyly avoid exercise in public. Stimulating herbal tonics recharge our carefree enthusiasm in a positive, creative direction and also give us the will to exercise.

Recharge Your Hormones

Chinese herbal doctors believe that an overweight person's enemies are body fat and water. For weight loss, they recommend herbs to "enhance kidney fire" and eliminate excess water. Herbs that reduce body fluids and edema are astringent, diuretic, and diaphoretic. Astringent herbs absorb excess water retention and might be used for diarrhea or asthma. Diuretic herbs increase urination, and diaphoretic herbs increase sweating. All of these are said to burn off excess fat and water in the body. Imagine drinking a tea that simultaneously dries fluids, increases urine and bowel movements, and makes you perspire. Fat cells would become reduced in size, though not in number, because they lacked fluid.

Some adaptogenic herbs such as Chinese ginseng stimulate fat-burning qi energy. We will learn about the ginsengs in Chapter 11.

Reverse Aging to Reduce Fat

The following teas provide a gradual, therapeutic approach to weight loss and enhanced sexuality suited to the baby boomer–plus generation. Used as directed, they cause no unpleasant side effects. If they become too laxative over time, reduce the recommended dosage.

These gentle teas can be used long term by either sex to quicken metabolism, reduce back and leg pains, build muscle mass, and improve sexuality. They are not aphrodisiacs. They do not increase sexual desire but ensure strength, endurance, and hormone balance.

They are profoundly rejuvenating. People who drink them regularly report they feel stronger, more optimistic, and more capable of exercise. Do not wait to become a senior to benefit from them.

EPIMEDIUM AND LYCIUM TEA: Epimedium leaf (*yin yang hao*) and lycium fruit tea (also known as *gou qi zi*, goji berries, and matrimony vine berries) gradually and safely treat sexual dysfunction; back and leg pain; and urinary incontinence resulting from illness, debility, and aging. It is a good tea for dieters because it corrects weakness, vulnerability, and low enthusiasm as it improves vitality and inner calm. This tea is useful for all the energy types. Epimedium, an adrenal tonic, contains a precursor to testosterone. Lycium fruit, moistening and blood-enhancing, is sometimes recommended for dry eyes and blurry vision. This herbal combination is useful for nourishing bone marrow and reversing chronic exhaustion.

Simmer one handful of each herb in 1 quart of water for 15 minutes, and drink 1 to 3 cups daily between meals. Continue as long as you need to strengthen muscles and the lower back and to rejuvenate internal organs.

ANEMARRHENA AND CISTANCHE TEA: Anemarrhena and cistanche tea is useful for hot flashes, constipation, anxiety, weakness, and chronic back and leg pains. *Anemarrhena asphodeloides radix (zhi zi)*, which treats fever, irritability, thirst, rapid pulse, and dry cough, can be successfully combined with *Cistanche salsa (rou cong rong)*, which treats impotence and urinary incontinence, as well as pain and weakness in the lower back and knees. Zhi zi cools the body. Rou cong rong gently stimulates energy without overheating. The two herbs together make a rejuvenating, slightly laxative tea that can be used to deepen shallow nervous breathing and ease lower back tension. This calming, slimming beverage is suitable for menopausal discomforts such as night sweats, chronic fevers from AIDS, or constipation from dryness, a common problem for the elderly.

Simmer a handful of each herb in 1 quart of water for 30 minutes and drink 1 cup in the afternoon for a soothing, refreshing beverage.

Weight Loss, Aging, and Health Challenges

After surgery, childbirth, emotional upset, or illness, some people develop urinary incontinence and/or stress-related diarrhea. That makes weight loss difficult because many slimming foods and teas are laxative and diuretic. If elimination is a problem, schedule toilet time appropriately, and use herbs and foods that suit your energy needs. If you cannot tolerate diuretic or laxative foods, emphasize herbal treatments that increase sweating. Otherwise, here are foods and herbs that can gently help you to lose excess water.

ADZUKI BEANS can be served with meals or cooked with raw garlic in lots of water to make a puree or soup stock. To make a slimming sweet: Cook a thick paste of adzuki beans, using less water than usual. Sweeten it with stevia powder and 1 teaspoon of virgin coconut or grapeseed oil. Form a handful of adzuki paste into a ball and roll it in powdered walnuts.

CORN SILK TEA is diuretic and helps lower blood sugar for people with diabetes. Make a corn silk decoction by simmering corn silk in water for 15 to 20 minutes; it can be added to tea or coffee.

PEARL BARLEY (Job's tears) reduces mucus and increases diuretic action. Fix Job's tears as a side dish, or simmer a handful in water for 30 minutes and pour it over green tea.

WAX GOURD PEEL OR WINTER MELON SLICES can be cooked in soups.

SOYBEANS AND GARLIC should be cooked until soft. One recipe, too strong for most people, calls for two parts soybeans to one part garlic. However, you can cook soybeans with adzuki beans and flavor with garlic. Eat a ½-cup serving of soybeans with meals. Whole soy products provide genistein, a healthy plant estrogen that replaces unhealthy estrogenic compounds from the body.

FAVA BEANS are an astringent food that reduces diarrhea and bloating. One Chinese medical recipe recommends grinding fava beans (*Vicia faba L.*; in Chinese: *can dou*) into a powder. Add 1 tablespoon of the powder to warm water sweetened with a little stevia three times daily. The bean can be cooked in its shell along with garlic and water.

Another recipe calls for fava beans simmered with pumpkin or winter melon skin and served as a soup. Fava beans are diuretic.

POPCORN. I prefer to absorb excess water and slim my waistline with a bowl of spicy popcorn (page 258). This recipe is astringent.

Herbs for PMS, Fertility, Libido, and Weight Loss

When you have PMS, do you eat everything in sight, especially cookies, chocolate, and bread? Do you develop abdominal and breast swelling, cramps, depression, blinding headaches, or irritable bowel syndrome? It is not because you are eating too many calories; your hormones are acting up.

You might starve yourself until you resemble a bean sprout, but that would not improve premenstrual bingeing, weeping, or fits of temper. Hormone-balancing herbs help you maintain a sensible diet. Herbal formulas that treat PMS discomforts are best recommended by herbalists. Consult a professional for the best advice for your needs. Generally, however, Chinese doctors believe that edema and fat are signs of weakness of the spleen/pancreas. Herbal tonics that strengthen the spleen/pancreas also treat PMS, emotional upset, and weight loss problems. The following are useful examples.

BUPLEURUM AND PEONY FORMULA. One useful formula for PMS bingeing is bupleurum and peony (Woman's Balance by Health Concerns), pills recommended for abdominal bloating, menstrual irregularities, PMS and menopausal distress, frustration, depression, liverish headaches, and hepatitis.

Herbs are a much safer way to reduce PMS stress than blocking stress hormones with a chemical drug. You may need those hormones later! Any drug that blocks natural hormone production may have harmful side effects. The herbs used in Woman's Balance that protect the pancreas include cypress buds, which enhance circulation, and citrus rind, which reduces bloating. Poria (*fu ling*) is diuretic. Atractylodes (*bai zhu*) and ginger reduce abdominal bloating and edema. There are many variations of this basic digestive formula, such as Xiao Yao Wan for prevention of indigestion, chest pain, and breast discomfort.

When Asian herbs are unavailable, you can substitute kitchen herbs and spices. For example, ones that enhance blood circulation include cinnamon and myrrh. Because they are warming, they should be avoided during fevers and inflammatory pains. Herbs and spices commonly used as diuretics include parsley, mint, and coriander seed and leaf. Those used to calm spasms and aid digestion include fennel seed, mint, licorice root, dill, lemongrass, and bay leaf.

Avoid overly sharp spices such as ginger, pepper, and cayenne during PMS or menstruation because they can aggravate inflammatory pain. Cinnamon, because it enhances circulation, can increase menstrual flow.

TCM Diagnosis: Examples of Internal Hot and Cold

Overweight is only part of a bigger picture. Traditional Asian herbal doctors, using tongue and pulse diagnosis, determine the underlying causes of overweight so they may choose cooling and/or warming foods that specifically enhance our energy and metabolism. Herbs that normalize hormones and affect menstruation and menopause reduce nervous eating habits, anxiety, and depression. You may not give up chocolate completely or join a gym after taking an herbal fertility tonic, but you may feel like Superwoman.

Here are two examples of problems addressed with hormone-regulating tonics and their impact on weight loss.

Chronic Inflammation

Janet, a high school teacher who weighed just over 200 pounds, had hot flashes long before 50. Her husband smoked, and they quarreled about it. At PMS time she yelled, slammed doors, and got terrible headaches. She ate large quantities of health foods and used diet colas and cookies to perk up her energy. At 42, she was told by her doctor that she had diabetes. She consulted me about hair loss, chronic stress headaches, and depression. Using the Baseline Diet for 3 months, drinking 1 quart daily of bitter

A PMS TEA OR ANTI-BINGEING TEA
FOR EITHER SEX

Anyone can use an aromatic tea when it contains digestive herbs that correct bloating, water retention, and normal abdominal pain. Simmer the appropriate herbs listed below in 2 cups of water for up to 20 minutes. Strain the brew and drink it warm between meals. The herbs and spices are commonly found in your kitchen but are based on Chinese herbal pills recommended for PMS and related addictions. The following chart will help you to choose your best herbal teas for PMS bloating and bingeing. Combine several of the following nice-tasting herbs known for comfort.

HERB/SPICE	AMOUNT	EFFECTS
Mint	½ c fresh or 1 Tbsp dried	Relaxes smooth muscle for reducing spasm pain
Orange peel	½ tsp	Reduces bloating
Lemongrass	1 Tbsp sliced or 1 tsp powdered	Relaxing, reduces pain
Valerian	1 capsule (up to 50 mg) or 10 drops of extract	Relaxing, eases uterine pain and insomnia

melon tea sweetened with stevia and using *Gymnema sylvestre* capsules, Janet saw many improvements—her blood sugar became normal, she lost nearly 50 pounds, and she was well on her way to a new life.

Overweight people with chronic inflammatory problems develop nervous headaches, insomnia, hot flashes, fevers and thirst, nervousness, anxiety, and anger. They may develop diabetes from a pancreas weakened by processed foods. The TCM diagnosis for their condition (internal heat and dampness) includes a swollen, red tongue; a thick gray or yellow tongue coating; spots and dark areas on the tongue; irregular appetite; abdominal bloating; and bad breath. The solution is to cool the heat and get water flowing with cooling, bitter green and yellow vegetables and diuretic and laxative herbs such as dandelion and nettle.

BITTER MELON TEA—sold by various names including Cherry Grain Balsam Pear Tea—improves diabetes, reduces high blood pressure, and works as a laxative.

MUNG BEANS AND SPROUTS detoxify and slim the body.

CHINESE HERBS that promote female fertility and reduce inflammatory symptoms include Fertile Garden, made by Health Concerns. Women who work, smoke, or otherwise live under stressful conditions often develop irregular periods. Stress makes them age prematurely. Fertile Garden's formula includes two great Ayurvedic herbs useful for both men and women: shatavari (wild asparagus), which is moistening and rejuvenating for sexuality; and ashwagandha, which tones muscles, reduces stress, and calms the spirit.

In India, shatavari is given to improve fertility and enhance beauty. It moistens the skin and hair. It also increases mucus congestion and, for that reason, should be used with ashwagandha. Ashwagandha is used for weakness, fatigue, and impotence and to shorten labor time for pregnant women.

Shatavari and ashwagandha are available as powders and pills in East Indian food shops, by mail order, and online. They are both safe for long-term use as rejuvenating tonics. If you make a tea, add ¼ teaspoon of each herbal powder to 1 cup of water or milk twice daily between meals.

If you gain weight during PMS or go on carbohydrate binges, you may need a blood-enriching, balancing tonic such as those described above. If you feel pale and washed out after your period, dieting is not enough to maintain health. In addition, each time you have a troubled period, your diet will fly to the winds. Most women, especially those who smoke or take medications, have to face the problems of blood and energy deficiency before they can lose weight and keep it off.

Chronic Weakness and Chills

Margorie stayed in bed much of the day reading, and at night, an insomniac, she did crossword puzzles. She always ate a big breakfast of ham and eggs, coffee with bitter chocolate, toast and jelly—and then went back to bed. She spent a fortune to learn from doctors at an exclusive sleep clinic that she was a night person. We in Asian medicine recognize that people with challenged adrenal energy (low kidney qi) often stay awake at night, unable to rest and refurbish vitality.

Margorie had never completely recovered from a difficult surgery and hospital infections that occurred 5 years earlier. The surgery had resulted in months of infections and antibiotics. Now nothing was wrong with her medically, except that she felt drained. Her feet were always cold. Her lower back and legs felt cool and moist to the touch. Her urine was pale and sparse, and her entire body was bloated with water. Her periods were sparse and finally stopped too early. She was chronically weak, and allergies sent her to bed for 2 weeks each year. She normally weighed about 180 pounds, but lying in bed during allergy season, she gained additional weight from water retention. Her only relief for her allergies was to fly to the Caribbean, where the trees did not aggravate her symptoms.

Margorie loved rich foods, desserts, and fine wines. After switching from cow dairy to feta made with sheep milk, she lost her runny nose and eye allergy symptoms. Being able to breathe and see again improved her mood.

Gradually, we incorporated the Baseline Diet, adding more vegetables weekly. She could not tolerate soy products, so we used organic eggs, chicken, and fish. She lost no weight for several months but looked and felt young and optimistic. Her waist and dress size became smaller, though she lost only a few pounds. Her energy picked up, and she spent more time awake during the day. She reduced meal portions and wine and lost 15 pounds. Then she hit a plateau that lasted for 2 months. Following my herbal advice, her periods came back, and she lost another 40 pounds.

Margorie made her best progress and lost the most weight after we used a warming, stimulating, hormone-balancing Chinese herbal formula for her and a testosterone-increasing one for her overweight husband. It was like a second honeymoon. They planned activities and vacations together and treated each other with renewed affection.

People who have internal coldness and weakness, like Margorie and her husband, typically have chronic chills, rheumatism and numbness, lethargy, depression, and low immunity. Their TCM diagnosis includes a swollen pale tongue, scallops at the edges of the tongue, excess saliva or chronic nausea, irregular appetite, and abdominal bloating. The solution for them is to warm digestion and burn off excess water.

PUNGENT SPICES increase sweating, and diuretic teas increase urination. Asian cuisine offers scintillating hot Thai, Indian, Chinese, Vietnamese, and Korean spices and cleansing green tea. The safest, easiest pungent flavors that promote sweating and support digestive qi for daily use are cinnamon and fresh ginger added to tea.

WARMING FOODS AND HERBS that increase kidney fire enhance sexuality. For Margorie, I recommended Maternal Herbal pills from Health Concerns, which combine morinda, epimedium, and ginseng to increase libido and promote fertility for women who tend to have chills, an aching lower back, and a lower sex drive. They are women who have a late or slow, sparse period. They feel weak, tired, and depressed. They may eat a cake or cry until the period arrives.

A warming, energizing formula such as Maternal Herbal, which contains testosterone-increasing herbs that are not overly drying, supports qi vitality along with the spleen and stomach. It stimulates vitality and warms the digestive and sexual area. Maternal Herbal should be avoided by women who have hot flashes, chronic thirst, dry mouth and throat, a red tongue, fast pulse, or other signs of internal heat.

Metabolism Boosters for Weight Loss

If you can remember reading about Dick and Jane in the first grade, you grew up eating the basic food groups consisting of animal proteins, starches, fruits, vegetables, legumes, and milk for meals. The combination was designed to fatten Americans after the Depression and World War II. You certainly ate an appetizer, entrée, and dessert at meals. Eating like that, however, gave Dick heart trouble at 45 and Jane cancer at 55.

It's time to think outside the refrigerator and eat light, healthy

Asian foods. Think of a normal meal as a mini-meal or snack: multi-grain crackers, goat cheese, a few olives, and tea; or spicy popcorn and a salad; or dried seaweed, sprout bread, and tea; or steamed broccoli in a lemon sauce sprinkled with dried seaweed flakes on whole grain pasta.

Sea vegetables are wonderful additions to your daily diet no matter what your age. But they are especially nice, crunchy, slimming snacks while sitting at a computer, driving to work, or onboard a cruise ship.

Sea vegetables are virtually fat-free, low in calories, and one of the richest sources of minerals in the vegetable kingdom. Seawater and human blood contain many of the same minerals in very similar concentrations. Sea vegetables contain high amounts of calcium and phosphorus and are extremely high in magnesium, iron, iodine, and sodium. For example, ¼ cup of cooked hijiki contains over half the calcium found in a cup of milk and more iron than in an egg. It also contains vitamins A, B_1, C and E, as well as protein and carbohydrates.

One of seaweed's most important health benefits is its ability to remove radioactive strontium and other heavy metals from the body. Whole brown seaweeds (not granulated) such as kelp contain alginic acid, which binds with the toxins in the intestines, rendering them indigestible, and carries them out of the system.

Among the most common culinary seaweeds available in the United States are the following:

ALARIA, harvested in Maine, is similar to Japanese wakame biologically and nutritionally. Alaria is a rich source of minerals, including calcium and iodine, as well as vitamin K and the B vitamins. It has a black or dark green color. With a more wild, yet delicate taste than cultivated wakame, alaria needs to be cooked longer when used in miso soup.

WAKAME, collected in the cold waters off the island of Hokaido, Japan, is a good source of protein, iron, calcium, sodium, and other minerals and vitamins.

BLADDERWRACK (whole leaf or milled), common to cold northern oceans worldwide, is a sea vegetable that herbalists and supplement makers use for weight loss aid and thyroid stimulation. Bladderwrack is a source of fucoidan, a polysaccharide known to scavenge heavy metals and radioisotopes throughout the body. It is normally available as a whole leaf, coarse cut, or in powder form.

DULSE has a soft, chewy texture, distinctive taste, and a rich red color. Enjoy dulse as a snack or a colorful salad ingredient. It is tasty in soups and zesty when toasted. Dulse flakes and smoked dulse are also sometimes available.

HIJIKI, found primarily in the Far East, contains the most calcium of any of the sea vegetables—1,400 milligrams per 100 grams dry weight (compared with milk with 100 milligrams per 100 grams dry weight). In its natural state it is very tough; after harvesting, it is dried, steamed, and dried some more. When cooked, it rehydrates and expands to about five times its dry volume. If you have never tried hijiki, you are in for a treat. Its delicious, satisfying flavor is a favorite in Japanese restaurants.

KELP from Maine is a thinner and more tender variety than Japanese kombu, and it has a light brown to dark green color and similar nutritional benefits. It is used like kombu in soup stocks, and it can be pan-fried for chips or stir-fried with carrots, and so forth.

KOMBU, according to an informational Web site on Japanese foods (http://ampuku.sharepoint.bcentral.com) is valued for its abundance of minerals that stimulate hair growth; protect bones; soften hard lumps and tumors, especially in fibrocystic breast disease, and speed recovery from radiation treatments. It is rich in polysaccharides known for their anticancer properties and their ability to inhibit the growth of tumors. Its iodine content is used to activate an underactive thyroid and, as such, is often a component of weight loss formulas. It can be cooked with beans to enhance digestion.

LAVER a purple/black, wild North Atlantic cousin to nori, has been enjoyed in the British Isles for centuries. Dry roasting brings out a nutty, salty flavor. Crumble dry-roasted laver over popcorn, soups, and grains. In Scotland and Wales, soaked laver is mixed with fat and rolled oats and fried into a breakfast bread.

NORI (Chinese and Japanese) comes in pressed sheets because raw whole nori is rare. Larch Hanson at Maine Seaweed Company in Steuben, Maine, sells whole nori, which can be toasted and crumbled over foods. He says Maine nori is one third protein. (See additional information about his company at www.alcasoft.com/seaweed.) According to experts at http://ampuku.sharepoint.bcentral.com, Japanese nori seaweed is high in fiber, vitamins, protein, and minerals. Nori provides calcium and iron and contains other important trace minerals. It is traditionally eaten in Japan to strengthen the circulatory system and help lower cholesterol. In addition, nori has been noted to play a large part in the remission of lupus.

SEA LETTUCE, the "salad greens" of the sea vegetables, is a leafy, vibrant dark green, with a distinctive flavor and aroma. This sea vegetable is good raw, it but tends to have a slight bitter taste when cooked, unless added to other ingredients. Sea lettuce is used worldwide in soups and roasted for garnishes.

You can find sources for these seaweeds in the Natural Products and Information Resource Guide on page 348.

Menopause and Overweight

Women may develop hormone or menstrual irregularities at any age. Menopausal discomforts and fibroids are often associated with overweight. Hormone-balancing herbs reduce many discomforts of peri- and postmenopausal women, such as anxiety, nervous snacking and food addictions, fits of anger, insomnia, digestive bloating, cellulite, and rapid weight gain. No serious, long-term approach to weight loss can avoid addressing these issues.

Mature beauty, in the full meaning of the word, may have less to do with fertility than with caring. However, to ensure healthy weight loss along with vitality, grace, physical endurance, and freedom from chronic pain, we need a natural hormone boost. The most important contraindications for using hormonal herbs are active cancers. If that is an issue for you, avoid tang kuei, licorice, tofu, red clover, and yucca because they are estrogenic.

Among my weight loss clients, I have noticed that menopause

intensifies food addictions aggravated by anxiety and inflammation. Because chronic stress, smoking, and overly acidic high-protein diets are inflammatory and aging, many women develop uncomfortable symptoms long before menopause happens. They feel both hot and cold—agitated and overheated and, at the same time, weak and drained. A complicated imbalance requires cooling, moistening rejuvenating herbs that reduce stress and stimulating tonics that correct the underlying weakness.

THREE IMMORTALS: An herbal formula that I often recommend for women who have perimenopausal and menopausal overweight and addictions is Three Immortals (Er Xian Tang) made by Health Concerns. It treats hot flashes, night sweats, migraines, irritability, palpitations, depression, insomnia, back pain, constipation, and lowered sex drive. It cools excess liver fire that causes dizziness and headaches and warms and supports weakened adrenal energy in order to improve sexuality. Several of its herbs, including epimedium and morinda, supply testosterone. Eclipta supports the liver. Anemarrhena, philodendron, and lycium fruit reduce fever and hot flashes. Three Immortals is especially balancing for Dragons or women who smoke; they easily develop menopausal symptoms.

If you prefer, you may substitute the following mild-acting tea. It is useful for anyone troubled by chronic illness, weakness, constipation, and inflammatory pains. In 2 cups of water, simmer for 2 minutes then steep for 10 minutes: ½ cup of fresh blueberries, 1 tablespoon of fresh mint, and the contents of 1 skullcap capsule (up to 200 milligrams). It is laxative, therefore, start with no more than 1 cup between meals.

Rejuvenating Herbs for Weight Loss

Youth is fresh and juicy. The safest ways to reduce aging are with the following moistening Asian herbal tonics. You can feel younger, look better, and crave fewer fattening foods. Shilajit and American ginseng are both refreshing *and* beautifying.

SHILAJIT CAPSULES made from bitumen (a soft coal product

full of rejuvenating minerals) are sold in East Indian food and herb markets. They rejuvenate the body to reverse aging. Shilajit is useful for both men and women in treating reduced sexual fluids, dry skin and hair, insomnia, stress, and anxiety-related addictions—especially for sugar, stimulants, and drugs. For women, it's great for alleviating vaginal dryness. A good way to use shilajit is to take one or two capsules before bed on an empty stomach.

AMERICAN GINSENG TEA is moistening for dry skin. It increases saliva and reduces sweet-tooth addictions.

Both shilajit and American ginseng can improve menopausal problems of stress, dehydration, anxiety, and premature aging and are useful for treating diabetes.

HAPPY GARDEN TEA, made by Yin/Yang Sisters, available at www.eastearthherb.com, contains soothing herbs that ease troubled digestion, sleep, and women's hormonal issues. You can make a pleasant-tasting instant beverage by adding the powdered herbs to hot water.

Moistening, rejuvenating herbs help replace the inner tranquillity and beauty lost with age, emotional stress, smoking, and illness. Hormone-balancing tonics cannot stop aging, but they enhance comfort, support metabolism, and increase endurance. They help reduce fatigue, weight loss apathy, and cellulite. In that way, they support self-esteem and may improve loving relationships, which are the supreme healer and a formidable inspiration for slenderizing.

Part 4

Your Weight Loss Lifestyle

Enjoy the good life: body treatments, restaurants, and celebrations!

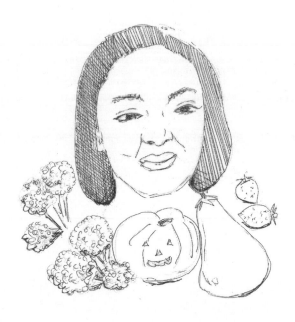

Chapter 11

Be a Winner!

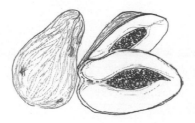

Exercise is any movement that enables you to lose weight. In this chapter, we'll focus on slimming movements for nonathletes, swimming for nonswimmers, and comfortable ways to lose weight for intellectual boomers and bedridden, elderly, pregnant, or injured people.

Why invest in expensive equipment, chic gym wear, or personal trainers if you have no time or energy to work out? Without some type of movement for at least ½ hour daily, however, weight loss is nearly impossible, joints become brittle, and muscles atrophy.

Walk Your Way to Weight Loss

The simplest way to tone metabolism, deepen breath, and firm muscles is walking. Strolling around the block or climbing stairs burns calories. Walking is less percussive than running or jogging and, therefore, causes fewer injuries. Walking in a natural environment worked wonders for one Vermont couple I know.

He, a federal court judge, was called upon to hear a particularly disturbing murder case. Afterward, to clear his mind, he and his wife, a public school principal, walked the Long Trail nearly the entire length of the state in 17 days. They felt like explorers, camped out all the way, and ate what they could carry. Whole grains were their fuel: Amy boiled brown rice, made whole grain noodles with sun-dried tomatoes, and salad. She lost 10 pounds and he, 15. They look radiant and feel great. The trip was so enjoyable they have decided to make it a yearly excursion.

As simple as it can be to exercise daily, we all come up with excuses to avoid it. If you avoid movement because of arthritis pain, ask friend Tiger for dietary and herbal advice (see Chapter 5). If you are too weak or heavy to move, brother Dragon can recommend foods and remedies (Chapter 6). If you have no time to move, Papa Bear will laugh and tell you another funny story. His diet advice is in Chapter 7. Everyone can move *some* part of their anatomy.

Thank You, Esther!

Swimming is the perfect exercise for postmenopausal women, the elderly, injured people, overweight people, and everyone else. Floating relaxes tension, and swimming improves circulation and grace while it protects fragile joints. In the 1945 movie *Thrill of a Romance,* Van Johnson learned how to swim from America's beautiful mermaid, Esther Williams. And watching that movie, so did I. A swimming champion at age 15, Esther dropped out of college to prepare for the 1940 Olympics and, lucky for us, was discovered by a talent scout while swimming with Billy Rose's Aquacade. In her movies, she glides in the water like an angel and makes every move look easy. Here, step-by-step, is how I dropped my fear of water and started to swim (after age 50).

GET WET, STAY WARM. The hard part is getting wet. I do not recommend jumping in feet first like a kid might. It is rude to fellow swimmers and accustoms you to being a sloppy swimmer. If the water is cold, wear a long dance leotard. After being in a cold pool, drink a cup of hot ginger or cinnamon tea or take a hot shower to warm up.

EASE IN GENTLY. To begin floating, dangle your legs up to the knees, then slip into the water up to your waist—usually 4 feet deep. Walk around to feel the water's resistance. Later, it will hold you afloat.

GET SOME SUPPORT. When you are comfortable, put your

elbows up over the edge of the pool so that you are supported, and allow your legs and hips to float. You are ready for the next step.

FLOAT IN SAFETY. Find an area of the pool shallow enough to stand. Take a round lifesaver that looks like a doughnut or a foam toy used for floating and place it under your chin and on your chest. Slowly float around the pool with your head completely out of the water, while holding the lifesaver.

PROTECT SENSITIVE AREAS. You will make tremendous progress if you wear a nose clamp to keep water out of your nose and goggles to protect your eyes. I use a snorkel with goggles and a mouthpiece, so I breathe underwater like a fish. That way I can stay in the pool much longer and practice my strokes to look like Esther. I highly recommend a snorkel for anyone who has had whiplash or another neck injury or surgery.

LOOK FOR SWIM BARGAINS. The best bargain in New York is the city's recreation centers, where you can exercise and swim for $35 a year with a regular membership—only $10 for seniors. You might be able to find a similar bargain near you. Check your local YMCA and at www.ymca.net for locations. Many YMCAs around the globe honor your membership, so you can swim when on vacation.

Floor Dancing

If you want to firm and sculpt the tummy, thighs, and hips; feel centered and elegant; balance your posture; and lose fat, floor ballet is your thing. I hate exercise tapes in which a straight-legged girl barks like a sergeant, "Okay! Now do this!"

Instead, relax and listen to the soothing voice of Peter Martins, ballet master in chief of the New York City Ballet, on the *New York City Ballet Workout* video and DVD, available online at www. amazon.com. If you have ever watched, enthralled by sleek, muscular dancers, this exercise tape gives you a taste of their daily workout. Feel artistic and graceful while becoming fit.

Do not be inhibited by ballet. I skip ahead in the tape, often avoiding the athletic warmup exercises, and focus on the tummy-shrinking bar exercises, done lying flat on the floor. They strengthen and shape abdominal, lower back, thigh, and leg muscles to improve your stance, walk, and posture. You improve alignment and agility but avoid injury and fatigue—no need to jump or spin until your glasses fall off. Plus, you can listen to classical music and that wonderful baritone voice.

If ballet is not your thing, take a tip from the Radio City Rockettes: It is not how fast or high you kick but how often that counts. (Several of the athletic Rockette dancers are massage therapists and use energy-enhancing herbs from this chapter on a daily basis.) You, too, can be a Rockette—kick yourself into shape with their video *The Radio City Rockettes Kick into Fitness*, available at www.amazon. com. It's a scream. If your muscles feel not quite up to the challenge, take ashwagandha powder or capsules, the East Indian ginseng that builds muscle strength and endurance and heals nerve injuries. Every time I mention exercise of any kind, especially dancing, Papa Bear tells me, "Bears don't dance." Fortunately, there are many alternatives; see for yourself.

Animal Form Exercises

During the Han Dynasty, a famous Chinese doctor named Hua Tuo, known as the father of surgery, lived from AD 110 to 207. He developed physical exercises that resemble the postures and movements of five animals. The five animal forms (*wu qing xi*) are a forerunner of today's *qigong*—physical culture used to promote longevity. Hua Tuo believed the body has an innate need for activity that we should not ignore. With careful healing movements and breathing, we gain energy and enhance blood circulation, which prevents illness, fatigue, and overweight.

Hua Tuo's animal forms are popular in China with health-conscious people and martial artists because they build agility, strength, and mental focus. They also prevent chronic pain and a flabby body. I have adapted them here for nonexercisers and non–martial artists to enhance digestion and weight loss. The simple postures help you communicate with your totem, the animal spirit that expresses your personality.

Movements for Dragons

Are you a fire-breathing Dragon who lacks steam to get off the couch? Your exercises can be done lying flat. They tone metabolism and focus your attention for targeted weight loss. Breathing evenly and smoothly also helps to focus the mind. Apply one drop of essential oil of bergamot orange or grapefruit under your nose to make breathing a pleasure.

Lie on a bed or the floor with a pillow placed under your head and feet. Breathe deeply and slowly while listening to a symphony or concerto; Dragons think big. Slowly lift your head and feet off the pillows 1 inch and hold the position for a count of 10. Count with the music, of course. Relax, continue to breathe, and lower your head and feet. Repeat making a jackknife by lifting both ends of your body. One to 3 inches off the pillow is sufficient to tone your abdominal muscles as you hold the position and breathe in a relaxed manner.

Lie flat on your stomach, and do the same movement in reverse. Several times, lift your head and shoulders and feet off the pillows to the count of 5, then 10. Slowly release and rest. A 10-minute workout is enough to engage and strengthen your abdomen and lower back. This exercise is excellent for preventing abdominal bloating, back injuries, fatigue, and sluggish digestion.

Movements for Bears

Are you a honey Bear who loves sweets? Your sweet tooth makes you drowsy, which may cost a fortune in the stock market and lead to bad eating habits. Bear exercises slim your waistline and, thus, protect digestion and circulation. Remember to take hawthorn berry capsules along with your green tea, and put one drop of essential oil of juniper berry under your nose.

While at your computer, every time you save your work to a disk or your documents—hopefully, every 30 minutes to 1 hour—get up and walk a few steps or stretch over as far as possible toward the floor. Seated, inhale, and as you exhale, bend forward until your chest touches your thighs. Inhale on the way up, and slowly repeat this movement several times.

Sit with your feet flat on the floor straight in front of you, shoulder-width apart. Without twisting your hips, inhale, and as you exhale, twist your upper body to hold one side of your chair. Hold for a few seconds and breathe normally. Release and return to center. Repeat this chair stretch to the opposite side.

Movements for Cranes

Are you an elegant Crane trapped in a swan's body? Swans glide in water but waddle on land. Crane exercises gradually develop your balance, agility, grace, and fitness. You may feel more balanced by putting a drop of essential oil of lavender under your nose.

Stand with your feet together and arms at your sides. Inhale slowly into your lower abdomen for a few minutes. Stretch your back and neck gently as though your head were floating. Move your hands in front of your chest and bring them together with palms facing in a prayer position. Let your shoulders drop. That aligns your internal organs and brings oxygen to renew them. Stay in that position, if possible facing the sun, until you feel warm and relaxed.

Drop your hands in front of you with palms together. Inhale as you lift your arms to the sides and overhead. They are your wings. At the top of your reach overhead, stretch upward slightly, and very slowly bring your arms in a circle down to your sides as you exhale. After you do this a few times, you will feel like you are flying and will get into a nice comfortable rhythm. Inhale going up, and exhale while bringing arms down. Happy landings!

Movements for Tigers

Do you feel, think, and act like a Tiger? Your feline bones, joints, and muscles need healthy proteins and natural sodium foods such as okra and celery for a graceful gait, lightning speed, and a powerful leap. You may need the power and persistence of a sleek cat but feel weak as a kitten. Tiger movements are slow, graceful, and confident, like a big cat slinking into the deep woods. They ensure proper calcium absorption and lend support to your muscles and joints. Swimming is perfect for cats; so is this special walk.

Stand beside a chair and hold on to the top with your left hand. You are going to lift your leg and arm on one side, then the other. Inhale into the lower abdomen a few times to feel your balance. Put your weight onto your left leg. Inhale, and very slowly lift your right leg and arm at the same time. There is no need to lift them high; a few inches will do. The important thing is to coordinate your movements so that both arm and leg move slowly together. Inhale going up, and exhale going down. Claw the air and growl if you like.

Switch sides and repeat this until you feel confident and graceful. Eventually, you can let go of the chair and move forward. When you do the Tiger Walk, keep your balance centered in your abdomen as you move with the arm and leg of one side at a time.

Get a Little Traction

Is there a better way for people with neck or spine injuries or post-menopausal women with fragile joints to exercise for weight loss? Yes, indeed. The ultimate nonexercise is traction. It stretches your spine and neck, allowing them to find their natural healthy shape as you quietly lie on your back. Poor posture, computer work, neck and back injuries, and aging tend to make support muscles weak, so the neck and spine shorten or bulge into painful curves. In some cases, disks may compress the spinal cord, causing pain and numbness.

The spine deteriorates if it loses its natural shape. That often results from whiplash. With injury or aging, rich lubricating fluids are less able to penetrate the joints, causing nutritional loss and premature aging. When the spine is properly shaped, fluid drawn into the joints promotes spinal balance and joint wearability. Chronic discomfort greatly reduces our ability and desire to exercise.

Sitting for hours crunches the belly, as well as the spine. The more you sit, the more you feel and look out of shape. Sitting is tiring and slows metabolism. If you are weak or overweight or have injuries that prevent exercise, consider using a neck and back stretcher—a traction device—as a way to interrupt work for a health break. It saves wear and tear in the long run.

A home traction device safely realigns the natural curve of the neck and spine to overcome discomfort and poor posture. It allows the spine to breathe and joints to be lubricated by spinal fluids. All you have to do is lie on a pump traction device and adjust it to your needs. It stretches and limbers your spine. That sort of traction feels especially comforting after a long car ride, using a computer, playing sports, or following any activity that jars or tenses the neck or spine.

You can shop online at health and medical Web sites to find traction and spine trainer devices. Look for the best price. I found the Low Back Elliptical Rocker Posture Pump at www.arc4life.com because I was already pleased with their neck traction device, the Posture Pump 1000.

As you pump the adjustable expanding air cells with air and the traction elongates the spine, you'll notice a warm, relaxed feeling through the neck and back. Check with your chiropractor or physical therapist before using any traction device, because it may increase certain injuries. It is not advised for people with severe rheumatoid arthritis or infections with serious inflammation.

Avoid Pain and Fatigue

My brother Eric is a competitive athlete and doctor of chiropractic, and I, through hard knocks, have acquired valuable herbal information useful for accident-prone dance- or athlete-wannabes. Once, in the desert sunshine of New Mexico, a wasp stung my horse. He bucked and shot across the field, leaving me bent over a fence with a few injuries. Eric was there to help me heal. He has patients who avoid riding, field sports, dance, or any movement because of chronic pain. This chapter shares what we have both learned from caring for ourselves and others.

HOMEOPATHIC ARNICA MONTANA 30C is ideal if you are nonactive. A natural remedy for pain, swelling, and bruising, it may well suit your needs. Because it enhances circulation, homeopathic Arnica works well for people who physically tire easily and those who, following a massage or walk, feel as though they've been beaten. Taken before or after exercise, the remedy allows you to enjoy movement and intensifies its healing benefits. Melt three pills under your tongue or in a little water between meals, and let the healing process begin.

MAGNETS are another pain remedy and natural exerciser that can be used while reading in bed, watching the TV news, working at your computer, or driving to a supermarket. Homedics makes TheraP magnets to wear around your wrist to relieve carpal tunnel syndrome or around your waist and knees for weight loss. They are intended for reducing back and knee pain and injury. However, enhancing blood circulation tends to soothe muscle spasms and improve posture. Wearing a magnet belt increases local sweating and reduces tiredness. Wearing magnets in the knee area stimulates important acupressure points used for slimming. Do not become dependent on magnets. Vary their use; for example, wear them every second day. When magnets are worn constantly, muscles do not tone as quickly as if you use them for an hour a day.

Note: It's fine to ratchet up your workout to assure weight loss. But before you enter a gym or begin running or any vigorous workout routine, make sure to check with a chiropractor or other health professional trained to review your x-rays and let you know about injuries that may impede your progress. Do not wait until pain or paralysis indicates a structural problem.

Fuel for the Workout

Bodybuilders and athletes use adaptogenic herbs such as ginseng to increase endurance during gym workouts and exercise. I wondered if the same herbs could help my overweight clients lose pounds. The answer was a qualified yes—as long as the herbs were used along with the Baseline Diet (or Comprehensive Diet in Chapter 9) and regular exercise.

Adaptogenic herbs are not weight loss herbs in the same sense as green tea. They do not reduce fat intake or absorption, but they allow the athlete or nonathlete to work harder and longer at exercise. What counts most for weight loss is eating less and exercising more. Among my clients and friends, the most popular choice among herbal energy tonics was, of course, a sweet, tasty liquid extract called Active Herbal Formula made by Zand. It contains eleuthero (Siberian) ginseng root, astragalus root, American ginseng root, ginkgo leaf, codonopsis root, fo-ti root (*Polygonum multiflorum*), and licorice root. It is almost sweet enough to be a dessert. It is contraindicated for anyone who has high blood pressure or kidney disease. There's one more negative: I found one summer that its pleasing aroma, as it comes through the skin, attracts mosquitoes, who love a sweet flavor.

Eric, a former light-heavyweight Mr. New Mexico, works out at the gym as his busy schedule permits and uses adaptogenic herbs, including Chinese and raw tienchi ginsengs for energy and muscle tone and ling zhi (*Ganoderma lucidum)* mushroom for joint comfort and endurance. I have talked to women boxers, runners, tennis pros, golfers, and hikers who agree: Stamina without muscle aches or tremors is what counts for smooth performance on the playing court or the dance floor.

Stamina is also needed for weight loss. Adaptogenic herbal tonics increase willpower as much as endurance. Everyone is encouraged by good results. If you have tried dieting, exercising, or diet pills without results, you need an energy boost to lose weight. Otherwise, low vitality and low spirits will probably send you back to the pastry shop!

Muscles, because they support posture, balance, and internal organs, require nourishment and support from herbs. Chinese herbs that build vitality offer exceptionally good results for anyone who wants a slim, athletic body. Energy-boosting herbs help prevent injury and fatigue. Some speed metabolism to keep weight off.

In your local health food store, around the world, and on the Internet, you will find Asian herbal combinations, including various ginsengs, astragalus, and other adaptogenic tonics. A number of highly successful American manufacturers of herbal supplements have been founded by American acupuncturists. McZand and East Earth Trade Winds products are backed by American research done at clinics associated with their companies.

Once for an article I was writing, I e-mailed Michel Czehatowski, founder of East Earth Trade Winds in Redding, California, with an herbal question. He answered from China, where he was completing advanced studies in acupuncture. Among energy-enhancing products, he recommends Dragon 'Seng, a combination of ginseng and powerful tonic herbs designed to be used daily.

More recently, when I asked Czehatowski about herbs he recommended for weight loss, he listed Get Svelte instant beverage by Yin/Yang Sisters, Bojenmi Tea, and Panta Tea (gynostemma). He said that most of his clients had no time or interest in changing their diet and used a daily slimming tea to speed digestion. The teas he mentioned all ease digestion. Bojenmi, because it contains hawthorn berry, also improves circulation and heart comfort.

Chinese tonic herbs, which enhance the functioning of internal organs, do not offer exactly the same results for everyone. People vary. A lot also depends on how herbs are combined and used. If adding energy and endurance herbs makes you feel temporarily off center or spacey, your digestion may be weak. Especially in the beginning, I recommend using a digestive remedy with meals. One good remedy is

---

CHINESE HERBAL INSPIRATION

Chinese energy-boosting herbs improve performance, endurance, grace, and freedom from pain, partly because they enable you to deal with stress. Some of the most popular tonics are several forms of ginseng, astragalus, epimedium, and lycium fruit. Although they can be used separately as pills or teas or cooked in soup, their best results are in herbal combinations. For example, Chinese (*ren shen*), American (*si yang seng*), and Siberian (*ciwijia*) ginsengs can be combined to strengthen muscles, increase circulation, and improve glucose management. For maximum performance, other adaptogenic herbs such as *Schizandra chinensis* (*wu wei zi*) or *Astragalus membrana-ceous* (*huang qi*) can be added, which reduce energy loss from strain and excess sweating.

Vitality Combination—which contains poria, ginger, atractylodes, and paeonia—made by Sanjiu (999), one of China's largest herb manufacturers. It is distributed by East Earth Trade Winds. Poria and atractylodes slenderize, and ginger builds energy.

The Ginsengs: Power Up Your Workouts

Adaptogenic herbs, such as ginseng, enable us to overcome extreme climate, pollution, fatigue, or nervous tension. If you use adaptogens to energize your workouts on a regular basis, take a dose during midmorning and midafternoon, as well as half an hour before your workout. Avoid all tonic herbs, especially ginseng, if you catch a cold or flu.

CHINESE GINSENG (red ginseng, Panax ginseng, and *ren shen*), the best-known adaptogen, is considered warming: It stimulates metabolism, energy, and resistance to cold weather. It reverses chronic fatigue, weakness, low blood pressure, weak sexuality, and poor memory.

Use it only if you have a pale tongue and chronic chills. Avoid it if you have a dry red tongue, thirst, nervousness, headache, or fever. To warm the body and build resistance, you might eat a small cooked root with meals once daily or drink the tea anytime to speed digestion of proteins and carbs. Many ginseng pills, extracts, and combinations are available.

Dosage of Chinese ginseng depends on your level of fatigue, blood pressure, size, and, for women, menopausal factors. Start with the smallest recommended dose and watch for these signs of overdose: thirst, dizziness or headache, insomnia, crankiness, and reduced body fluids (dark urine, reduced semen, or vaginal dryness). You can balance the heating and drying effects of Chinese ginseng by combining it with cooling, moistening American ginseng.

AMERICAN GINSENG (white ginseng, quinquefolium, *si yang seng*) reverses dryness. It replenishes saliva and reduces thirst. American ginseng acts as a stimulant for people burned out from stress, sugar and salt addictions, excess sweating, or chronic fever conditions.

Singers have told me that American ginseng tea helps them to sing long performances without throat irritations. Several of my clients, college students who practically lived on coffee and doughnuts, have said that American ginseng reduced their sugar cravings. If you have a dry, red tongue, drink American ginseng tea all day, especially at the gym. To refresh your breath, melt some instant American ginseng tea in your mouth.

NEUTRAL GINSENG (codonopsis, *dang shen*), neither warming nor cooling, speeds metabolism and turns fat into muscle. Andrew Gaeddert, founder of Health Concerns and author of several books, including *Healing Digestive Disorders*, recommends for muscle weakness codonopsis along with Chinese ginseng and astragalus, an energy- and immune-boosting herb. When I called him at his Get Well Clinic in Oakland, California, he reported that he had treated some 15 athletes, including several triathletes and a world record–holding runner. Their chronic fatigue and endurance problems improved dramatically within 2 to 4 weeks with a combination of astragalus, Siberian ginseng (Eleuthero ginseng), *Ganoderma lucidum*, and codonopsis.

GANODERMA. Acupuncturists including Janet Zand, OMD, LAc, founder of McZand Herbal Inc., recommend ganoderma (*ling zhi*) for recovery after painful workouts. She has treated many athletes, including medal-winning American and Canadian Olympic runners and swimmers. Her clients reported that after a tough workout, they felt physically spent. Within 1 week after using a combination of 350 milligrams of highly concentrated (10:1) ganoderma extract combined with a smaller amount of cordyceps and 100 milligrams of Siberian ginseng, each four times daily, the athletes had no problems with recovery and could do two consecutive workouts.

Ganoderma is best suited for cardiovascular enrichment. Here's another way to take it: Buy the dry mushroom from a Chinese herb shop, and have the herbalist chop it into pieces or make a powder. Simmer a handful in a slow cooker of water for 6 hours. Or you can simply take 6 to 10 capsules daily between meals. Whether you work out in a gym, dance, swim, or rock in your traction back exerciser, using Chinese adaptogenic herbs enhances energy, willpower, and weight loss.

Learn from Martial Artists

Weight loss is not a problem faced exclusively by out of shape people. Most of my clients have been women, so I tend to think of them first. However, *all* athletes and bodybuilders—both men and women—strive to lose fat, stay fit, and gain endurance. Recently, I joined an online martial arts community with members throughout the world. The forums have weight loss advice from members, much of which could be summed up as: Tough it out. Burn more calories than you consume.

Their fortitude is inspiring, but that approach works for a short while, not as a lifestyle. J. is an example taken from the martial arts Web site. He is a 30-year-old man weighing over 300 pounds who practices Tiger Claw Kung Fu, a martial art that, when played full out, aims to disable acupuncture meridians. He lost 20 pounds in 2 months and wrote: "There are no real magic pills that don't bear unpleasant and unhealthy side effects, and the low-carb deal leaves a person without enough energy to really work out hard. My diet involves discipline and dedication, keeping your fat low, your calories low (like under 1,200 a day), and eliminating junk food and fast food completely from your diet. No special rewards, no quick pick-me-ups with a Snickers bar. No pop. No caffeine. No snacks. Never, ever. No fast food if you are running late; I'd rather starve. And don't just drink lots of water, drink *only* water. If you wouldn't put arsenic in your body, don't put alcohol in your body. If you wouldn't put cocaine in your body, then don't put a Taco Bell steak chalupa into your body. If you really want to lose weight, then get yourself ready for months of suffering and sacrifice. Soon, the suffering turns to joy and the sacrifice turns to reward."

His diet is even more sparse than the Baseline Diet, which recommends herbs for energy, slimming teas, and an occasional healthy sweet. The months of suffering approach will not work over the long haul. Why not enjoy tasty, slimming, healthy meals as a lifestyle instead? There is no need to hit your head against a wall.

Another bit of advice from the same site was also interesting but a lot more realistic. It feels good to agree with someone with a background so different from mine. Dan, age 33, a graduate teacher and coach working on his PhD, specializes in muscle physiology and bio-mechanics. He is doing research on neuromuscular, mechanical, and metabolic adaptations to exercise. He wrote about timing meals in relationship to gym workouts: "Eating healthier and more natural is definitely a good thing to do. Eating a high-carb, high-vegetable, moderate-protein, and low-fat diet would definitely reflect the eating patterns of the Eastern countries. I have been in Korea, Japan, and Thailand. You never see fat Asians until they get on the lower-carb, low-vegetable, high-protein, and higher-fat diet when they move to a Western country or to a larger city in their own country.

"The bottom line is this: You can eat as natural and healthy as you want, and if you eat more calories than you burn, you are still going to get fat. It eventually comes down to energy balance. Track your calories, eat a few hundred less every day than you burn, and you will lose a pound or two a week. If you maintain your resistance exercise while you are trying to lose fat, you can minimize your mus-cular loss and decreases in bone density. Any faster than that, and you can have problems."

I end this chapter with an encouraging e-mail from one of my women weight loss clients, certainly a winner. Melanie writes: "I think I'm a prime example of someone who absolutely *hates* to exer-cise . . . and I have proven to myself (I hate to admit) that exercise *is absolutely required* along with diet to lose weight. My job is physical. I take the stairs, I walk around the store, and walk after lunch. Another thing that I am really strict about was this—never, ever eat before going to bed. When my activity went up at work, I lost 13 pounds in 3 weeks, then another pound over a week. I've broken through 180, and am looking forward to 170, 160, 150, 140!!! My clothes fit better, my waist is coming back, my hips aren't as round, my arms are more toned (they still wave after I'm finished waving, but that'll take care of itself with a little more work). My opinion of myself is much improved, and I'm just looking forward to seeing my body again. The way I remember and love it!"

What a cheery mood—from daily exercise at work!

Chapter 12

Eating Out

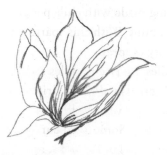

Come fly with me and be my guest at Asian restaurants in North America and the Far East. This is a virtual trip; no need to pack a bag, but bring a hearty appetite. We will sample exotic and familiar dishes that stimulate weight loss. Americans have grown too accustomed to fast foods lacking savor and charm. Let's find haunts where conversation naturally turns to good eating. The keys to Asian cuisines for healthy weight loss are fresh ingredients, delicious herbs and spices, and lots of tea.

Thai Taste

Flavors used to make sumptuous dishes from Thailand are hot, sweet, and sour. Thai sauces have depth from contrasting seasonings. A typical peanut dipping sauce used for barbecued chicken or beef contains more than peanuts. The recipe for 1½ cups of peanut sauce calls for teaspoon masaman curry paste, 2 tablespoons each fish sauce and peanut butter, 3 tablespoons each ground paprika and garlic powder, 2 cups coconut milk, and 4 tablespoons crushed toasted peanuts, all simmered for 15 minutes.

American Thai restaurants, like others in North America, temper their scorching ingredients to suit our tastes. In New York, my local favorites are Royal Siam on 8th Avenue and Pongyal on West 23rd Street in Chelsea. To remain slim in such a tempting atmosphere, order a salad and a small entrée or two appetizers. *Sum tum* salad is made with grated raw cabbage, cherry tomatoes, crushed peanuts, and a spicy dressing. It makes a nice appetizer or light meal anytime. Thai salads, appropriately called *yum,* have thinly sliced grilled chicken or beef served on lettuce with a savory dressing made with chile pepper, sugar, vinegar, minced red onion, and fresh mint. With this sparkling sauce, you are satisfied eating a small quantity of meat.

Singapore noodles are rice noodles stir-fried with vegetables and curry powder and garnished with dried chiles. You might enjoy chicken or beef satay, in which thin strips of barbecued meat are dipped into peanut sauce. Some Thai curries are made with pineapple to improve digestion. Thailand's cooks, and Asian restaurants in general, serve small portions and exciting, piquant flavors blended to speed digestion. Let's go to the place where Thai cooking began.

Visiting Bangkok

We are in Bangkok. It is a hot night, and we have decided to have a late meal. In the Riverside section of old Bangkok, where taxi boats transport passengers and rice barges drift along the canal against a backdrop of glittering temples, we pass by the gorgeous Grand Palace and Wat Pra Kaeo (the Temple of the Emerald Buddha), which present an overwhelming display of colors, images, and architecture. Inside the temple grounds, a huge golden stupa contains relics of the Buddha. We jump on a Sky Train that links the entire city and arrive in Bangkok's new shopping and entertainment center at Sukhumvit.

Lemongrass, located at 5/1 Soi 24 Sukhumvit Road, is a garden restaurant in a traditional Thai wooden house. Small palm trees sway in the yard. Ornate music wafts through the air. Greeting the beautiful, smiling server dressed in brightly colored silk, we put our hands together in prayer position in front of the chest and say, "*Soo-waht—DEE—ke.*" Settling into cushioned chairs, we feel at home in the tropical atmosphere. The menu is slightly more expensive than at other local places, with main dishes at about 200 baht, just under $5 in US dollars.

Everyone in Thailand loves green papaya salad. Street vendors sell it from pushcarts. In a country that loves to eat and serves some of the best Asian foods available, green papaya salad is a slimming light meal. Green papaya is more astringent, cleansing, and digestive than ripe papaya. On top of thinly grated green papaya are sprinkled dried shrimp powder and a hot, tangy sauce. The recipe calls for ¼ pound of shredded papaya with some shredded carrot as a garnish, two crushed garlic cloves, four ground dried chile peppers, three 7-inch-long string beans cut into 1-inch pieces, three sliced cherry tomatoes, 2 tablespoons fish sauce, 1½ tablespoons lime juice, and 1 tablespoon each palm sugar, tamarind juice, crushed peanuts, and dried shrimp powder. We tell the chef to make it mild.

At Bangkok's outdoor food markets, you point to a fish you want fried or steamed. Vendors make a steaming bowl of soup filled with your choice of sliced pork, beef, sprouts, vegetables, and rice noodles.

Thai curries are made with very hot chili paste and sweet coconut milk. They are more inflammatory than fattening. To cool your palate, suck the juice from a slice or two of fresh lemon. You might be tempted to order an iced drink in Asia, but refrain. Water is never sterilized before it's frozen.

After finishing a bowl of egg noodles with chicken in a curry sauce (a mere 80 baht, or $1.92), we decide to stroll down to one of Anna's Cafés at Two Pacific Place, 142 Sukhumvit, for dessert. Anna's restaurants are named for Anna Harriette Leonowens, the English governess to the children of King Rama IV of Thailand, also known as King Mongkut. We remember Yul Brynner's brusque manners and bald pate in *The King and I*. King Mongkut is revered as one of the 19th century's great Asian statesman, who protected his people from colonial rule. Anna and her toddler son arrived aboard the steamer Choa Praya in March 1862. The rest is a Hollywood musical.

Perusing the dessert menu, we find the usual chocolate mud cake and cheesecake along with Thai specialties such as *kluay tod* (slices of banana fried in a rich sauce and served with vanilla ice cream).

Watching our diet, we decide instead to share a coconut ice cream with water lily seeds (50 baht, or $1.25). Eating in Thailand is a bargain. The lovely sites and friendly people, however, will cost you your heart. Next stop: Japan.

A Long Life on the Fast Track

Japanese people are the longest-lived on the planet—not because they sit and contemplate life. Women, who typically run the family budget, may stay at home or work—just as American women do. Diet, not stress, is the important health factor. Japanese cuisine is light, subtly flavorful, and elegantly served. The great appeal of Japanese cuisine is the patient care given to details when preparing and serving quality ingredients. A wise old Japanese MD internist also trained in Japanese kenpo herbal medicine told me that Japanese people who serve the traditional foods and perform the tea ceremony at home live the longest.

There are always two cuisines in Asia: a simple one for home use and an elaborate one in restaurants. Japanese office personnel and professionals often work late into the evening and may have a long ride home. It is not surprising that their popular dishes—fish rolls, sushi, sashimi, soups, and steamed dishes (*mushimono*)—can be eaten standing at a counter or running for a bus. At home, you are likely to have a big bowl of steamed rice served with a few bites of a steamed fish or a meat dish. Often, the meal contains a whole soy food such as edamame (green soybeans in the pod) served with a salad and a glass of iced sake.

The excellent longevity of Japanese people is attributed to their high-fiber, low-calorie diet of fresh fruits, vegetables, and fish; seaweed soups; whole soy foods such as tofu, edamame, and nato (fermented soybeans) added to noodles; and lots of matcha green tea. Okinawans, who often live to be over 100, use turmeric (the spice) and drink tea made with grated turmeric root, a known cancer fighter. Daily, they fix slimming bitter melon sautéed or added to soups or meats (see recipe on page 127). Try baked eel, a dish you will find only in Japanese restaurants. It is sweet and tender served sliced on rice or fixed as sushi or sashimi. Cooked eel provides our best natural food source of vitamin D.

Green matcha tea from Japan is made by whipping finely ground tea powder with a whisk brush while adding hot water. It has a bright, light green color; a sparkling clear quality; and an ethereal aroma and flavor. In Japanese cuisine, the rule is elaborately presented small portions prepared and served in a prescribed order. An example is *chawan mushi,* an egg custard made with shrimp and sliced shiitake mushrooms. Opening the custard steaming dish, you find a meal that resembles a miniature sculpture. The ingredients are added in a traditional order (chicken, shrimp, fish cake, and mushrooms), from heavy to light, as you might arrange a floral setting. The warm custard is garnished with spinach and lemon peel. The dish, though complicated, will neither trouble the digestion nor add pounds if you dine slowly with a happy group of friends. That, too, is a Japanese custom.

A large businessman's breakfast served at the New Otani Hotel and Garden in Los Angeles's Little Tokyo district includes a tray of small dishes: sliced melon, orange juice, miso soup, pickled and steamed vegetables, seasoned spinach, tofu garnished with scallion and radish, a bowl of white rice, a dish of broiled fish, and a poached egg dipped in soy sauce, accompanied by Japanese green tea. The portions are small, rich, and varied enough to last all day. To lose weight, politely call the server and apologize very humbly, saying that you have been called to a meeting. Have the meal boxed up, then enjoy the tasty portions throughout the rest of the day.

After resting a day on the beach, drinking green coconut juice and eating watermelon to slenderize, we are ready to fly again. We have savored Thailand's sweet, pungent flavors and Japan's subtle bitter greens and mild steamed dishes. Now we will sample China's array of local cuisines.

Secret Chinatown

Most Americans have a favorite Chinese restaurant. The Chinese have fed us, made our china and table linens, and clothed us since the

California gold rush in the 1850s. You miss something special if you order only your usual favorites at Chinese restaurants. China's regional cuisines vary greatly.

Cantonese dishes from South China feature mild-flavored seafoods and jasmine tea. In Guangzhou and Shanghai, shellfish from shrimp and crab to snails are prepared to perfection. Rubbery, tasteless cooked snake is served as a local delicacy and a medicine for rheumatism.

The Bund is Shanghai's boardwalk on Nánjing Dong Lù, where the European quarter entertained movie stars and royalty during the 1920s and 1930s. Noël Coward lived at the Peace Hotel (Héping Fàndiàn), a charming monstrosity of Chinese deco at Nánjing Dong Lù #20. People who come to China to eat pumpkin ravioli and olive bread can find it at M on the Bund, located at #5 on the Bund. The view of the Huángpu River from their balcony during summer is rated as the best in town. However, the food across the street at #3 on the Bund is better and less expensive.

In southern China, I have enjoyed eating and chatting with the people at open-air restaurants, in huge dim sum parlors, and while traveling by train. The (third class) train provides hot water so that passengers can brew their own tea. In poor regions of Szechuan, Yunnan, and Hunan, the *vin du pays* is pork, white rice, and few vegetables. Soups are oily noodles. Meat dishes are made less fattening by adding hot peppers. Yunnan Tuocha tea reduces fat and cholesterol. In northern China, you also find noodle soups or fattening Mongolian twice-fried beef. Digestive pu-erh red tea helps settle the stomach and prevent bloating and overweight.

America's Chinatowns

In San Francisco's Chinatown, restaurants swirl around Kearny Street and Grant Avenue. Tourists happily mill through the streets as Chinese families practice tai chi in Portsmouth Square. At the corner of 919 Kearny Street and Washington is House of Nanking. The aroma of toasted garlic and green onion pancakes beckons. The prices are moderate, the portions are generous, the food is rich and delicious, and the service is always quick. You can find chicken with Tsingtao

Beer sauce, sole with garlic sauce, or sizzling scallops and Nanking-stuffed mushrooms.

An insider's spot is the ABC Cafe at 650 Jackson Street. ABC is slang for American-born Chinese. They offer heaping bowls of congee, a rice porridge that in China is served for breakfast. In San Francisco, Chinese locals order it with vegetables, meat, congealed duck blood cubes (to enhance blood supply on days when you feel weak and woozy), shrimp, or fried dough sticks. Close your eyes and imagine you are in Hong Kong. The cooks banter in Cantonese as they wield cleavers behind a glass window.

In Manhattan's Chinatown, Eighteen Arhans, a tiny pristine Buddhist temple restaurant located at 227 Centre Street near Grand Street, is operated by Jingshe, a Buddhist nun, and Nancy the cook. The restaurant has two wooden tables, a lunch counter, and statues of various Chinese deities, including the Chinese god of tea, and a painting of Kuan Yin, the Chinese bodhisattva of compassion. Their ginger tea with honey is a must. The restaurant owners are featured in my DVD, *Asian Health Secret*s, which introduces New York Chinatown's herb shops, street foods, and local color. (It's available at www.amazon.com.)

Chinese temple cooking is slimming because it is vegetarian; uses fresh ginger and garlic; and features noodles, tofu, gluten, vegetables, soups, and rice dishes in a charming, intimate atmosphere. Down the street at 214 Centre Street in the heart of Manhattan's Chinatown, you will find another Buddhist temple. If you visit on a Sunday morning at 10:30, you can bow along with the large congregation and repeat the many names of Buddha during the ceremony. Do not pass up the vegetarian lunch cooked by nuns that follows in the large basement kitchen. Chinese temples from New York and Seattle to Hong Kong serve their guests healthy vegetarian meals for a small contribution.

Middle America has Chinese restaurant chains, some with buffets. In Rutland, Vermont, we like the Panda Pavilion in a mall at 283 Route 4 East. They serve slimming seasonal vegetables, such as asparagus. An appetizer large enough to be a main dish is chicken *soong,* made with minced chicken, vegetables, and pine nuts and served on lettuce leaves.

Many American Chinese restaurants feature a health food section on their menu, including steamed dishes. Steamed chicken, seafoods, or vegetables along with a light sauce served on the side cuts calories. Many up-to-date Chinese restaurants now serve brown rice, which is lucky, because the fried rice dishes always contain MSG (monosodium glutamate). If you ask the server for red tea (*hong cha*), you may get the one served in the kitchen. It may be a dark fragrant oolong or semisweet Po Ni (called *bo lay* in Cantonese), which is more digestive than jasmine tea. Everyone will be delighted that you speak Chinese.

Vietnamese Fare: Fresh and Minty

Vietnamese cuisine is slimming because it tends to be less oily than Chinese cooking and hot and spicy like Thai cooking. Vegetables and grilled meats often come with sweet, hot dipping sauces; spongy white rice noodles; fresh sprouts; and lots of fresh mint leaves. Summer rolls are delicious appetizers made by wrapping chopped lettuce, sprouts, grated carrots, and boiled shrimp in thin rice rolls. Dipped in a sweet vinegar dipping sauce, they make a light, healthy snack.

If you want a big bowl of mixed seafood soup simmered in a light vegetable broth or a soup made with very thinly sliced beef brisket served with mung sprouts and Chinese basil, or duck and medicinal Chinese herbs, Vietnamese restaurants are for you. They are reasonably priced and offer large portions.

If you love Vietnamese cuisine, you will never go hungry, especially in Southern California. Orange County has thousands of great Vietnamese restaurants, especially in the Little Saigon section of Westminster and in Garden Grove. For help in locating Vietnamese restaurants, visit the Web site www.saigoninfo.com and go to the English language section.

Visiting Mother India

Agni, the god of fire, gave birth to Indian cuisine. Any Ayurvedic digestive or weight loss powder or pill contains fat-burning hot, salty, bitter, and sour spices. Overly sweet and oily flavors are omitted because they retard digestion and circulation. Hot, pungent flavors stimulate acids that dissolve fat, while bitter and sour flavors drain toxins, inflammation, and fat from the body. Stimulating hot, pungent Indian ingredients include chilies, black pepper, pippali (a dried, long black pepper), clove, ginger, cinnamon, and asafoetida. Black salt is added as a digestive stimulant. Cooling bitter flavors include cumin, coriander, and turmeric. Astringent sour flavors include lemon, lime, and tamarind paste, made from laxative tamarind tree pods. Semisweet ingredients include green cardamom pods or the ripe seeds and fennel seeds. Curries and masalas vary from region to region, but they all contain both hot and bitter cooling spices.

Choose sweet, bitter, sour, and hot flavors to enhance each other the way a painter might juxtapose red and green to intensify contrasting colors. Overweight, illness, and aging overtake the person who fails to uses flavors wisely. Hot, pungent, acidic foods break down fat and poisons. Bitter and sour alkaline foods eliminate them. We need hot, bitter, and sour in the right proportions. Observe your tongue: If it is very red, you need cooling (bitter) green tea, amla, cumin, dill, coriander, and fennel. If it is pale, you can use hot hingvashtaka, ginger, and pepper, and hot and sweet cardamom and clove.

At home in India, you normally have freshly made chapatis—whole wheat flour crepes made with sunflower oil, water, and ghee (clarified butter)—vegetables stir-fried in a little oil with a pinch of cumin and mustard seeds, and spiced tea made by adding cardamom pods, fennel seeds, and other spices and milk to black tea.

The farther south you travel in India, the hotter dishes become. We are going to break in our tastebuds gradually by taking mint or chlorophyll capsules with meals. Another way to balance overly hot dishes is to follow them with yogurt.

India is a great place to be vegetarian. Fresh ingredients easily spoil in a hot climate. Fats and oils become rancid and develop an odor. To stay safe and slim in Indian restaurants, eat fruit you can peel, boiled rice and dal (lentil sauce), cooked vegetable dishes, and tea. Avoid the tempting oily sweets. To cool your burning palate after a meal, have yogurt or lassi, a drink made with yogurt and fruit or salt and ice water. Better yet, make it yourself without adding water.

Needless to say, Indian restaurants in Europe and North America are less spicy than those in India. If you are in Chicago, you might enjoy the quiet elegance of Tiffin, located at 2536 West Devon Avenue. The ceilings are painted with blue clouds. The authentic menu features tandoori king prawns and chicken tikka masala (chicken in a tomato-cream sauce) for about $10. Start the meal with vegetable *samosas* (fried dumplings), traditionally served with a red-hot onion dipping sauce and a cooling tamarind dipping sauce. The menu includes a large selection of vegetarian items, as well as desserts such as *gulab jamun* (fried cheese balls doused in honey.) To keep your waistline, you might have such a dessert with an afternoon tea, not following a big meal.

At less expensive Udupi Palace, nearby at 2543 West Devon Avenue, start off the meal with the *sambar vada* (fried lentil doughnuts) or *aloo bonda* (lentil dumplings topped with onion and potato). *Malabar adai* are pancakes made with mixed lentils and vegetables. *Pesarattu* is a moong dahl and rice crepe topped with onion and chilies. Remember, follow rich, hot, and spicy meals with a big salad instead of a fattening creamy dessert to balance the meal's flavors and energetic effects.

Tibetan Momo Land

You are in for a treat if you have never dined at a Tibetan restaurant. You can find one just about anywhere by consulting the official Web site of the Tibetan government: www.tibet.com. I had my first *momos* (meat- or cheese-filled boiled dumplings) in Lhasa during the summer of 1985 in the shadow of the Potala Palace. Today, we can enjoy vegan, vegetarian, and meat dishes in Tibetan restaurants from New York to Europe, Australia and beyond, while relaxing in a serene atmosphere graced by photos of the Potala and the winning smile of HH the Dalai Lama. Bloomington, Indiana, has a large Tibetan community and several fine restaurants.

Anyetsang's Little Tibet, located at 415 East 4th Street (North Grant Street) in Bloomington's university district, customizes some dishes. There are several kinds of dumplings on the menu. Traditional Tibetan dishes are made with buckwheat *tsampa*, a Tibetan staple; noodles and vegetables tend to be heavier than in other Asian cuisines. It is not surprising. Tibet's altitude is over 12,000 feet, so the foods are intended to nourish and ground the inhabitants. That is why Tibetan tea contains whipped butter and salt. Oily, rich flavors are grounding, nourishing, rejuvenating, and fattening. *Momos* are meant not to be slimming but to prevent winds on the high Tibetan plateau from blowing away its inhabitants. You may love them on cold, miserable days, when you need comfort food. *Kham amdo thukpa* is a stew made with thick noodles.

The best Tibetan tea for weight loss is Sorig Bad-Kan Tea, available online at www.tibetan-medicine.org. It restores healthy digestion and stimulates energy. It is a warming, invigorating morning tea that helps you work and play outdoors in cold weather. If you have a pale tongue and slow metabolism or chronic wheezing asthma, you can enjoy it anytime.

In New York, at Tsampa, located at 212 East 9th Street, you will find a lighter shiitake pancake, with scallion, garlic, and ginger served with an apple-walnut sauce. The tsampa plate has brown rice, chickpeas, steamed tofu, broccoli, kale, and hijiki seaweed with a peanut sauce. *Tse gyathuk nopa* is a baked noodle dish with garlic and ginger topped with vegetables. When visiting Indian or Tibetan restaurants, expect things to slow down to Himalayan time. Let your work-and-worry mind drift away to a rainbow land. Tasty, filling dishes and a cozy atmosphere make Tibetan restaurants an unexpected blessing. You are likely to meet world travelers and Tibetan monks among fellow diners. When you visit, greet the staff in Tibetan: *"Tashi delek!"* means hello and good luck.

Chapter 13

Holiday Fitness

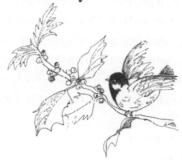

The holidays are a great time to show off your slimmer figure. Because they are numerous throughout the year, holidays can either ruin or improve your waistline and general health. In Chapter 2, we covered the parameters for safe cleansing fasts with juices that jump-start weight loss. Because most people have neither the time nor the desire to fast during holidays, this chapter contains a few simple tricks that enable you to reduce while celebrating.

A slimming snack of fresh fruit between meals speeds digestion and begins detoxification. A pot of tea reduces fat absorption in the gut throughout the entire day. A big dose of B vitamins taken before drinking, a dose of homeopathic Nux vomica 30C melted in your mouth ½ hour after drinking, and stimulating an acupressure point or two can prevent a hangover.

We will cover ways to make the holidays pain and gain free. There are special advantages for slimming between feasts. For one thing, a cleansing food may ease tension and make meeting old friends easier. Like a Tiger, ever on the ready for self-improvement, make holiday celebrations weight loss opportunities.

Birthdays and Weddings

These happy occasions have no season and can involve anything from a piece of cake and a cup of coffee to days of elaborate feasting. To prevent digestive problems or recover from rich eating, simplify your diet completely with soup. Avoid starches, especially bread and cookies, as well as animal proteins. A day or two of vegetable soup, accompanied by complete rest, can serve as a simple fast either before or after holiday indulgence. A simple vegetable soup contains ingredients that can speed the metabolism and reduce edema because it requires more energy for digestion than the calories that it provides. The soup's digestion burns calories, and its diuretic and laxative effects reduce water in the body. Here is an example of how that works.

Anka, a bride in her twenties, once asked for my recipe for a pre-wedding soup so she could lose 8 to 10 pounds and fit into her tight lace dress. A fashion model, Anka was accustomed to extreme measures. Her favorite meal at that time was a salad, 1 ounce of steak tartare, and a fruit-filled candy bar! Anka was so young that her weight problem might be called baby fat. A cleansing, alkaline vegetable soup did her a lot of good because she smoked cigarettes and ate unwisely most of the time.

To make the soup, Anka used the peelings of five white baking potatoes and a bunch of carrot tops. She also chopped one-quarter of a green cabbage, several ripe tomatoes, one carrot to sweeten the brew, a large yellow onion, some yellow squash, and a handful of okra. She cleaned her refrigerator of leftover vegetables and simmered all of this at low heat for 1 hour.

She ate the soup, mildly seasoned with paprika, throughout the day and evening. After 3 days of consuming vegetable soup and water and watching Marx Brothers movies, Anka lost 9 pounds. She said the brothers' exuberance was inspiring. She quickly regained strength, looked stunning in her gown, and kept extra weight off for at least 2 months. With occasional soup fasts and Marx Brothers movies, I understand the marriage is still going strong.

The Fourth of July and Fries

The Fourth brings picnics and barbecues with chips, hot dogs, fries, and other fatty treats. There are a number of things you can do to get you through this hot and greasy season.

TRY LECITHIN. To protect the liver and keep weight off, increase your intake of lecithin. If you normally use 1,000 milligrams daily of soy lecithin, up the dose to 3,000, or one capsule with each meal.

ENCOURAGE THE RIGHT BACTERIA. You may also need to increase acidophilus to populate the colon with friendly bacteria. Candida yeast increases from stress, summer heat, travel, and our use of antibiotics, as well as from illness and pregnancy. (Remember during any time of recovery to balance the colon with useful bacteria from acidophilus and yogurt, adding ¼ teaspoon of turmeric powder.)

BE KIND TO YOUR LIVER. You can also increase your chlorophyll intake to protect your liver. Essential fatty acids from evening primrose oil are liver protective and anti-inflammatory for common summer problems such as headaches, rashes, and acid dyspepsia.

ENJOY THOSE SUMMER TOMATOES. Another useful food is cooked tomato, which balances the pH of the colon. When you cook tomato paste or stewed tomatoes or use a prepared pasta sauce, add the following stimulating herbs: oregano, a natural antibiotic; parsley, a gentle diuretic; a pinch of rosemary, a stimulant to support heart and adrenal energy; and a bay leaf to soothe digestive spasms.

FORGET THE SODA. Give adults and kids carbonated drinks made of half seltzer and half apple or mango juice, which are liver cleansing.

SUPPORT YOUR DIGESTION. To prevent indigestion and jaundice after eating fried foods and rancid fats, take a dose (three pills each) of the following homeopathic tissue salts: homeopathic Nat sulph 6X and Kali mur 6X. Your liver, complexion, and disposition will benefit.

Thanksgiving Sweets

We love a big traditional Thanksgiving dinner with friends and family. Ours is vegetarian. The trimmings are actually the healthiest part of the meal—take extra helpings.

ENJOY CRANBERRIES. Unsweetened cranberry purifies the urinary tract. My favorite cranberry recipe is made with 1 pound of raw ground cranberries, ¼ cup of orange juice and some grated orange rind, and ½ cup of raw walnuts. Wash the fruit and grind it with the juice and nuts in a blender. Spice as needed with a dash of clove powder.

MAKE SUGLARLESS PIES. Sugarless pumpkin pie provides essential vitamins, including A, B complex, and C, and minerals that improve digestion and clear the complexion. Pumpkin is high in potassium and sodium and has a moderately low carbohydrate content. You can sweeten pies by adding ½ teaspoon of nonfattening stevia powder.

FOLLOW THE MEAL WITH HOMEOPATHY. Homeopathic Carbo veg 30C (homeopathic charcoal) settles the stomach and absorbs intestinal gas when taken 20 minutes after a big meal. Always use homeopathic remedies between meals and 20 minutes after drinking coffee. Otherwise, regular and decaffeinated coffee cancel the remedy.

Christmas, Hanukkah, and Hangovers

Some of our most cherished holidays call for merriment with friends. And those celebrations often involve alcohol. Be kind to yourself and your friends. Always provide alternatives to alcohol, and if you must imbibe, do so wisely. Here are some tips to see you through.

SERVE NONALCOHOLIC EGGNOG. A nourishing, low-fat eggnog is made with ½ cup of low-fat soy milk, ¼ cup of water, and the juice of ½ organic lemon or 2 tablespoons of key lime juice. Season it to taste with a dash of nutmeg and up to 1 teaspoon of vanilla extract.

REACH FOR THE B'S. To avoid a hangover, take two to three B-complex vitamin pills before celebrating. You should be getting between 50 and 100 milligrams total of vitamin B_1 (thiamin), B_2 (riboflavin), B_3 (niacin), and B_6.

FOLLOW UP WITH HOMEOPATHY. After drinking, if you feel hung over or stuffed in the sinuses and generally out of sorts from overindulging, take a dose of homeopathic Nux vomica 30C. Made from a bitter nut, it clears your senses—but will not necessarily improve your driving. If you're under the influence of alcohol, do not drive home, even after using Nux vomica.

TRY ACUPRESSURE. If all else fails, you can massage several acupuncture points to ease your hangover. (I do not recommend using needles unless you are a trained, experienced acupuncturist.) Place a dab of essential oil of sandalwood on the third eye, between the eyebrows, to cool the entire body. If you don't travel with essential oils, place your pointer finger between the brows for several minutes as you inhale and exhale slowly. Then press both temples with your fingers.

Press downward over the center of your abdomen with the palms of your hands. You are bringing excess painful energy down toward your navel. With the first three fingertips of one hand—thumb, pointer, and middle fingertips—slide past the thumb of the opposite hand about 1 inch past the wrist. You can find this acupuncture point another way. Place your palms together as though in prayer. Turn your right hand around counterclockwise to make an X with the thumbs. The point— the luo point of the lung acupuncture meridian—is where the pointer finger of one hand touches the opposite arm. (See the drawing.) This point, when vigorously stimulated with massage on each arm, helps settle the stomach and reduces headache, dizziness, and nausea.

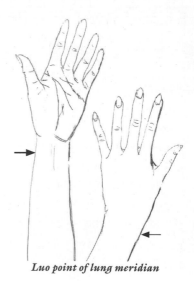

Luo point of lung meridian

WEIGHT LOSS LIQUOR

Eastern Europeans, Italians, and Asians have a long history of herbal liquors used for family beverages and medicines. Here is one of my Hungarian family recipes for digestive bitters. It's ready in 2 to 3 weeks, so you will need to make it well ahead of time in order to have some on hand for the holidays. Bitters are often used to enhance appetite and ease digestion. Our liquor combines digestive garden herbs for a kick to the metabolism. You can vary your recipe according to your tastes. Gentian root is very bitter and can increase appetite when overused.

MAKES 1 LITER | PREPARATION TIME: 2 TO 3 WEEKS

- 1 teaspoon dried shredded orange peel
- ¼ cup fresh mint
- ⅛ cup fresh tarragon leaves
- ⅛ cup hawthorn berries
- 1–2 teaspoons sliced gentian root
- 2 tablespoons grated fresh ginger
- 1 tablespoon juniper berries
- 1 teaspoon sliced betel nut

Steep the herbs in a sealed bottle of gin away from heat and light for 2 to 3 weeks. The longer you leave it, the stronger it tastes. Add anywhere from 20 drops to half a shot glass (no more) of this bitter/sweet digestive liquor to orange or grapefruit juice.

To chase a hangover, mix 1 raw egg, a dash of Tabasco sauce, and ½ shot of this liquor. This is called a Prairie Oyster. The recipe was featured in the 1972 movie *Cabaret* when Liza Minnelli taught Michael York how to eliminate a hangover. The albumin (a protein) in raw egg white absorbs the alcohol.

Lately, people have become concerned about salmonella when eating raw eggs. The best solution is to use health food store powdered egg protein or to use only organic egg yolk. Do not consume raw egg white. Albumin binds with heavy metals keeping them in the body long enough to cause trouble.

Another useful point for dizziness, nausea, and headache from weakness and drinking is Stomach 36, in front of and to the outside of each kneecap. (See the drawing.)

Ramadan, Fasts, and Feasts

Ramadan, the ninth month of the Muslim calendar, is a time when Muslims concentrate more on their faith and less on normal life. They don't eat or drink during daylight hours. Smoking and sexual relations are for-

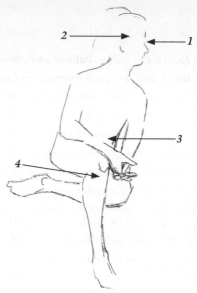

(1) Place sandalwood on the third eye; (2) Press the temples; (3) Press downward on the abdomen to the navel; (4) Massage acupressure point Stomach 36.

bidden during fasting. At the end of the day, the fast is broken with prayer and a meal called the *iftar*. Religious fasting, meals skipped for any reason, or long-term irregular eating habits usually cause fatigue, spaciness, and chronic indigestion. To take full advantage of any such opportunity to mentally and physically heal yourself, you have to know how to fast and especially how to break the fast. See page 330 for details.

An American friend who visited North Africa during Ramadan told me how much he enjoyed the nightly festivities, including elaborate feasts held in family homes: "It was so hot in Marrakech, we slept all day and celebrated at night, and we loved it."

Islam means "submission or obedience to God." Muslims cannot eat pork, and other meats must be *halal* (allowed), which means they are slaughtered in a way that gives the least pain, and "in the name of God" is recited before it is killed. Muslims cannot drink alcohol or gamble. They are required to be kind to strangers. I witnessed this in a local health food store when my friend quickly recited something in

Arabic and ate a slice of pizza. I asked him what was required during Ramadan, and he told me, "You cannot lie."

He continued, "The good that is acquired through the fast can be destroyed by the telling of a lie, slander, denouncing someone behind his back, cursing, or being greedy." To this list of sins, I would add that thinking mean thoughts, breaking the fast suddenly, or eating unhealthy foods will also destroy the benefit of the celebration, whether it is Ramadan or your personal cleansing routine.

When the Ramadan fast ends (the first day of the month of Shaw-wal), it is celebrated for 3 days in a holiday called Id-al-Fitr—the Feast of Fast Breaking. Gifts are exchanged. Friends and family gather to pray and to share large meals.

Fasting Herbs

If you interrupt your daily routine with a fast—no matter what the season—you had better use digestive remedies to maintain your energy, mental focus, and blood sugar balance. If you eat wonderfully rich Arabic or other spicy foods at night, the best digestive remedy is strong mint tea, which relaxes digestive spasms. Her is a recipe I learned from a Tunisian friend while I attended college in Paris: Boil water with sugar added—you can use stevia powder instead. Crush a handful of fresh mint leaves, and pour the boiling water over them. Add extra mint leaves for appearance. Let it steep for at least 5 minutes, so the mint reaches its full, rich flavor.

If you have difficult digestion with bloating or nausea, you might add sliced raw ginger while steeping the tea. A dash of cardamom powder is a nice addition for added energy and spicy flavor. For excess mucus congestion, add a twist of dried orange peel.

New Year's, East and West

For New Year's, Michael and I traditionally avoid the huge crowd that gathers at Times Square. We stay home with our cats and enjoy a romantic candlelit meal, such as baked fish, steamed asparagus, salad, and champagne.

In China and in Asian communities throughout the world, the Lunar New Year is also called Spring Festival. New Year's Day, which usually falls at the end of January or in early February, is the first day of the first month in the lunar calendar. During the Lunar New Year, Chinese people greet each other with "Xin Nian Hao"—or "Guo Nian Hao"—Happy New Year. "Gong Xi Fa Cai"—or "Gung Hay Fat Choy"—is used in Cantonese-speaking regions, such as Guangdong province and Hong Kong. The direct translation of "Gong Xi Fa Cai" is "Wishing You Good Fortune!" or "A Happy and Prosperous New Year!"

For a week before the New Year, Chinese mothers clean house, pay debts, contact old friends, shop for new clothes, and decorate their home with traditional paper hangings that are blessings for health, luck, and happiness. On New Year's Eve, the family gets together to usher in the New Year, which they hope will be rich, happy, and successful. The Spring Festival is the most important holiday in China. It lasts 15 days, from New Year's to Yuan Xiao Festival or Lantern Festival. In the countryside, people decorate their windows with *chuanghua* (window flowers), large paper-cut forms. Most chuanghua are red lucky symbols, such as children holding fishes or flowers or animals from the Chinese zodiac.

On New Year's Eve, families spend the night watching the year go out, chatting or playing card games, watching TV, and nibbling sweets and nuts. The children set off firecrackers you can hear pop throughout the night. To celebrate Yuan Xiao, the end of the Spring Festival, Chinese people make small round dumplings of sticky rice containing sweet fillings. *Yuan* means "round one" and *xiao* means "overnight." Here is a Chinese New Year recipe modified to reduce calories.

LOW-FAT DUMPLINGS (VEGETABLE ROLLS)

Normally, all family members sit together to make dumplings (jiaozi) on New Year's Eve, while chatting or watching TV. Steamed jiaozi are eaten on the first day of the new year. Our dumplings can be kept in the refrigerator overnight or cooked immediately. The traditional dumpling has a heavy dough wrapper, but we will cut calories by using lettuce leaves. Therefore, we have to steam the dumplings, not boil them. Instead of pork, we will use diced vegetables and pine nuts. The result is a light, crispy vegetable roll that melts in your mouth and begins your New Year's weight loss resolutions.

MAKES 20 SMALL VEGETABLE ROLLS | PREPARATION TIME: 40 MINUTES

 5   *hard-cooked eggs, mashed into a paste*
 1   *teaspoon low-sodium soy sauce*
 ½   *cup finely chopped celery*
 ½   *cup finely chopped carrots*
 1   *scallion, chopped in very small pieces*
 2   *teaspoons ginger, peeled and chopped to very small pieces*
 ¼   *cup pine nuts*
 ⅛   *teaspoon Chinese five-spice powder: mixed powdered anise pepper,*
     star anise, fennel, cloves, and cinnamon (called wu xiang fen
     at Chinese supermarkets)
 20 *romaine lettuce leaves*

To prepare the filling, mix the egg with the soy sauce and enough water to make a thick paste. Add the celery, carrots, scallion, ginger, nuts, and five-spice powder and blend well.

Separate the lettuce leaves. To reduce dirt and pesticides, soak them for 10 minutes in warm water, adding 1 tablespoon of vinegar. Rinse with clean water. If they are soft and pliable, you can fill and roll them up to make dumplings. Otherwise, steam them very lightly for less than 1 minute to make them pliable.

To fill the dumpling, spoon a heaping tablespoon of filling onto 1 lettuce leaf at the thick end. You may need to slice the thick stem about 1″ so that you can roll up the filling—thick end to the tip of the leaf. Stick the ends of the dumpling inside to make a firm lettuce roll.

Place the lettuce rolls side by side into a bamboo or metal steamer. If you do not have one, place the dumplings in a covered pot to which you have added no more than ⅛" of water. Steam the dumplings for less than a minute to warm them. Overcooking makes them soggy. They should be moist yet crisp.

The best way to serve dumplings or vegetable rolls is with a special sauce. Mix together 4 tablespoons light soy sauce; 2 tablespoons Chinese wine vinegar; 1 tablespoon chopped scallion; 1 teaspoon peeled, chopped ginger; 1 teaspoon finely chopped garlic; and 1 teaspoon Chinese sesame oil. Dumplings can be stored uncooked in zip-top bags in the freezer.

For information about Chinese New Year and to order New Year's red and gold paper decorations, red cards in which to offer money gifts to relatives, and traditional bright red clothing, as well as to find recipes, see www.chinasprout.com. The old year is done; the new one begun. Make it your best with foods that naturally enhance kindness and all your fine, beautiful qualities.

Chinese Pills for Digestion and Breathing Comfort

If this year has caused anger and frustration, why not take the opportunity to use liver-cleansing herbs? Your spring will be easier and more effective if you prepare now and use digestive herbs again in March. I have several suggestions, depending on your particular needs.

XIAO YAO WAN (pills) is a balanced digestive formula from Chinese medicine that contains ginger, mint, three blood-enhancing herbs, bupleurum, and diuretic *fu ling*. Together, the herbs assure digestive comfort and blood sugar balance, especially useful for hypoglycemic spaciness or depression.

LUNG TAN XIE GAN WAN (pills) is useful for anger, constipation, headache, hyperthyroid conditions, vaginal discharge, and herpes. The dose varies from 5 to 10 pills, three times daily or as needed. This herbal formula has been used in high doses in Chinese hospitals to calm angry or violent patients. The main ingredient is 20 percent gentian, the same ingredient used in most Italian after-dinner digestive bitters.

HUANG LIEN (COPTIS) is recommended for headaches, dizziness, dry cough, stomach ulcers, and liver inflammation leading to hot flashes, irritability, or skin blemishes. It is a very safe, mild, detoxifying herb used in China for infantile fever and convulsions and for older people to reduce a brain enzyme linked to Alzheimer's. Used alone, coptis does not improve memory, but because it reduces excess acid, it is slightly calming. The recommended dose is four pills twice daily. Coptis can be taken long term as needed.

HOMEOPATHIC REMEDIES are especially useful in autumn and winter—good times to fight mucus buildup, which can increase fat, cellulite, and many conditions made worse from mucus impurities, such as asthma, congestive heart problems, arthritic stiffness, fibroids, high blood pressure, chronic fatigue, and depression.

If you have thick mucus, difficulty breathing, and sadness and usually withdraw into a corner to bemoan your troubles, homeopathic Pulsatilla 30C taken once or twice daily between meals, as needed, will lift your energy and mood as it improves breathing. A stronger, deeper treatment is best done under the guidance of a professional homeopath. Some remedies reach the origins of illness, which often involve sluggish conditions or irregular digestion and elimination that lead to toxicity. For example, if you have wet mucus, excess malodorous saliva, sore throat or bad breath, sour-smelling perspiration, or dizziness or headache and tend to have a hot temper, homeopathic Mercury (Mercurius solubilis 6X) is sometimes taken once or twice daily to detoxify the body from long-term problems. It is cooling and dries excess malodorous discharges. After a day or two, or when you have finished with homeopathic mercury, it is often followed by a dose of homeopathic Sulphur 6X.

Now let's take a look at some tips and techniques that will help you though *any* holiday.

Smoking and Winter Holiday Blues

Smokers need special help during the holidays. An autumn or winter cold easily turns to pneumonia, depending on the age and health of the smoker. Holidays can be depressing or lonely for anyone. But because smokers feel extra pain, congestion, and pressure in the lungs, they feel holidays and other miseries more acutely. Some people complain of feeling grief in their chest. They stuff their sorrow with rich foods, drinks, and smoking. But that only makes things worse. Many times, using herbs to ease breathing will give us a new outlook.

CHING FEI YI HUO PIEN is a cleansing Chinese herbal pill that cools lung inflammation and clears sticky thick phlegm, dry cough, sore throat, oral and nasal sores, toothache, and constipation. It contains skullcap, gardenia, *Rheum officinalis*, peucedanum, sophora, trichosanthes, platycodon, and anemarrhena. Skullcap cools and cleanses the liver, anemarrhena reduces fever, and the other herbs clear phlegm. The recommended dose is four pills twice daily between meals. You know you have used enough when you can breathe easier, your complexion has cleared, and your dark mood has lifted.

If this or similar herbal combinations for cooling and cleansing the lungs are not available, you can cook tremella white fungus or use *lo han kuo* instant beverage as a sweetener for teas and foods. Lo han kuo, a round hollow brown-colored pod the size of a tennis ball that is available in Chinese supermarkets, is very sweet when cracked open and cooked for 10 minutes or more in water. Both tremella and lo han kuo are cooling and refreshing for the lungs. So are asparagus, oatmeal, and flax seeds when cooked to make a soft gel.

REMEDIES FOR BALANCING AND CLEANSING benefit people who overeat and drink and smoke. Those are emotional needs, not related to hysical hunger, and best treated with balancing, cleansing remedies that support rejuvenation. The autumn and winter holidays present a fine opportunity for personal rebirth. We must nurture vitality and beauty with foods and herbs that purify body and mind.

They include bitter digestive herbs such as mint, pungent digestive herbs such as ginger, and bitter laxative foods such as rhubarb.

UNSWEETENED PIES made with apple/rhubarb, strawberry/rhubarb, berries, cherries, and prunes are delightful ways to harmonize family gatherings.

HUANG LIEN (COPTIS) AND CHING FEI YI HUO PIEN PILLS help ease hot flashes, chronic fevers, smoker's cough, high blood pressure, headaches, complexion blemishes, and chronic overweight that can interfere with your celebrations. If you have no time to fast but have these inflammatory problems, or if, for any reason, you need to cleanse the liver, lungs, and skin, take a nightly dose of coptis or Ching Fei Yi Huo Pien pills. They feel deeply cooling and refreshing, and they reduce complexion problems, holiday anxiety, and the drying effects of radiator heat.

Oats Are for Beautiful Creatures

The best foods to eat any time nervousness and fatigue leave you drained are antistress foods that increase vitality and support sexuality—our fountain of youth. These include dried figs and cooked oatmeal with raisins and powdered goat whey. Oats make a good meal for horses and other beautiful creatures that are large and powerful, that have a refined sensibility, tired muscles, and sensitive nerves. Oatmeal is a brain, nerve, and sex food for humans. Use it freely during convalescence, mental and physical exhaustion, and inflammatory joint conditions. It is an everyday remedy for Tigers because it provides valuable vitamins and minerals.

Nutritionist Bernard Jensen, PhD, wrote in *Foods That Heal*, "There is nothing better for impotence than slowly cooked oatmeal, raw egg yolk, iron, phosphorus, and sleep." Foods rich in phosphorus include wheat bran, pumpkin and sunflower seeds, prunes, apricots, and raisins. For a natural source of iron, sweeten beverages with black cherry concentrate. Here is my favorite recipe for old-fashioned oat cakes, a nourishing, fortifying snack. Have them anytime with tea.

OAT CAKES

Oat cakes are high-fiber munchies that leave you feeling fully satisfied and gradually reduce cholesterol. (For low-fat oat and other recipes, see www.fatfree.com and www.quakeroats.com.) If you are in a hurry but want a tasty hot breakfast or afternoon tea snack, just add ½ cup of quick-cooking oat flakes to a corn muffin mix. Otherwise, here is a basic recipe. I have omitted sugar and honey, but you may use ½ teaspoon of stevia powder to sweeten it, especially if you have diabetes.

MAKES 14 TO 15 | PREPARATION TIME: 15 MINUTES

> *2¼ cups all-purpose flour, oat flour, or soy flour*
> *1 cup quick rolled oats, uncooked*
> *1 teaspoon baking powder*
> *½ teaspoon baking soda*
> *2 tablespoons powdered goat whey*
> *3 tablespoons canola oil*
> *1½ cups low-fat milk (or water), with 4 teaspoons lemon juice*
> *½ cup raisins or chopped dried apricots or 1 tablespoon grated orange*
>   *or lemon peel (optional)*

Preheat the oven to 450°F.

In a large bowl, combine the flour, oats, baking powder, baking soda, and whey. Mix them well. Mix in the oil with a fork, a few drops at a time, until the mixture resembles coarse crumbs. Add the milk or water all at once. Stir with a fork until the dry ingredients are moistened. Add the raisins, apricots, or orange or lemon peel (if using). (Do not overmix.)

Drop the stiff dough by ¼-cup portions 2" apart on ungreased cookie sheets. Bake them for 10 to 12 minutes, or until they are light golden brown. Serve them warm. You can quick freeze them in zip-top freezer bags.

Snacks That Reduce Edema

When hours of travel or holiday stress increase your water weight, keep antiedema safeguards handy, including some of the following sour foods, green foods, berries, and powdered whey. They are useful for reducing PMS pudginess or for the week before the dance. They are safe enough to eat daily.

SOUR FOODS drain excess water from the cells. They include grapefruit, a fine source of sodium, potassium, and calcium useful for reducing body fat, cooling acidic conditions such as blemishes, and relieving catarrhal conditions such as sinus congestion and digestive bloating.

Naturally fermented sauerkraut, made without sugar, is a weight loss food that contains useful minerals and is laxative. Sauerkraut is also high in chromium. Eat some with brunch or during the afternoon between meals to increase dietary fiber and wash through the digestive tract. Have a lunch of ½ cup of naturally fermented sauerkraut and a baked potato garnished with 1 teaspoon of grapeseed or canola oil, dried oregano leaves, black pepper, turmeric powder, and lots of fresh parsley. People with very weak digestion can steam sauerkraut lightly and flavor it with cumin powder or paprika.

ALKALINE FOODS help to detoxify the body. My nutritionist friend Rita Miller, who heads a weight loss clinic for the United States Air Force in Panama City, Florida, sent me a nutritionist's joke that explains the origin of sin: "In the beginning, God created the Heavens and the Earth and populated the Earth with broccoli, cauliflower, and spinach, green, yellow, and red vegetables of all kinds, so Man and Woman would live long and healthy lives." As the joke continues, God created the potato and Satan created potato chips. God created yogurt to keep the figure fair, but Satan brought forth white flour from the wheat and sugar from the cane and combined them. Woman went from size 6 to size 14 . . . and so on. You see the point.

Rita's clients are military personnel too out of shape to be deployed abroad. They have desk jobs and eat junk foods like most Americans and, therefore, cannot pass a performance test that requires running a mile and other measures of minimum fitness. Rita finds that most people lose weight, reduce unhealthy cholesterol, and regulate blood sugar problems with a diet rich in fresh fruits, vegetables, and whole grains. Rita lost weight and felt perky for the annual Air Force Base Swing Dance using the Bear Diet.

Our best alkaline foods are easy to find and use. Beet greens, broccoli, and zucchini provide potassium. In addition, beet greens in salad or lightly steamed provide magnesium, iodine, and iron. Beet greens are nice for PMS water retention because iodine is necessary both for normal thyroid function and sexual hormone production. Women lacking iodine often develop irregular periods and water retention. Beet greens are mildly cleansing.

Broccoli, a famous anticancer food, is high in vitamins A and C and low in calories. When eaten with protein, broccoli becomes a brain food, helping to drive amino acids to the brain. It is a useful food for young brides and others who have trouble staying with a diet or remembering what they ate. One American president, who famously disliked broccoli, was fond of saying that the better part of his job was showing up. Broccoli may not improve performance, but because all greens make the body alkaline, broccoli allows us to show up for work with a clear complexion, sweet breath, and calm disposition.

Celery, cooked chayote, dried chervil tea or raw chervil in salads, spinach, Swiss chard, and watercress are greens that provide important minerals for healthy slimming. Watercress is best for rapid weight loss because it stimulates and detoxifies the liver and makes body fluids alkaline. Add fresh watercress to vegetable juices and eat it by the bunch. It is high in sulfur and potassium to ensure a radiant complexion as you lose weight.

Seaweeds such as dulse, nori, and green kelp are salty-tasting. They are much better for weight loss and health than salted nuts or chips or fried foods of any kind. Have up to ½ cup of dried seaweed daily if you want to stimulate weight loss. Bladderwrack (*Fucus vesiculosis*) works the fastest to tone the thyroid, but its taste can be unpleasant. Some people find it too stimulating. Start with delicious dulse and nori, then add toasted green kelp. Experiment with them in cooking and as snacks.

CLEANSING FRUITS can give you a laxative whoosh for breakfast. Try a handful of laxative prunes, 1 cup of fresh blueberries, a ripe persimmon, or an 8-ounce can of pumpkin pie filling. Get rid of the previous night's heavy meal with a cleansing ripe fruit and a pot of hot green tea. If digestion is weak or you tend to have headaches, avoid raw foods first thing in the morning, and add fresh ginger to your tea.

A slimming beverage contains few calories and burns calories for digestion. A low-calorie meal in a glass is made by adding a scoop of health food store protein powder to half water and half pineapple, apple, or mango juice. If you have candida yeast infection, use vegetable juice instead.

POWDERED GOAT WHEY helps keep the colon healthy. If rich foods irritate your stomach or cause constipation, be sure to get your whey. Table salt and salted nuts increase edema, but natural high-sodium foods, including very ripe citrus fruits, okra, celery, and powdered goat whey, eliminate toxins and increase useful intestinal flora. Raw okra and celery can be added to salads. Powdered goat whey can be added to warm water, juice, or low-fat yogurt to reduce stomach acidity and constipation. It is nice and soothing for bedtime.

The predominant mineral useful to the stomach is sodium, an electrolyte critical for digestion and a vital component for building blood and preventing intestinal putrefaction. Disorders of the stomach and lymphatic and glandular imbalances can often be traced to inadequate sodium reserves. Goat milk's minerals are balanced for optimal absorption. They include calcium, vitamin A, B complex vitamins, choline, and as much potassium and nearly twice the vitamin D as cow's milk. Powdered goat whey added to warm water or juice daily reduces joint aches and digestive discomforts.

Fifty percent of the body's sodium is found within the bones. Sodium keeps calcium in solution along with potassium to prevent bone spurs and arthritis. Goat milk is an excellent food for anyone who suffers from chronic constipation, gastrointestinal diseases, and joint stiffness. People who are allergic to casein, the protein in cow's milk, often can safely use goat products, which contain a different protein. With enhanced digestion, you can enjoy any season.

Our gourmet journey has, for now, come to a close. But your adventures in Asian cuisine and culture are only beginning. Good health, happiness, and long life to you!

Conclusion

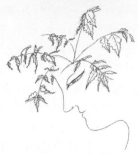

This book, Web sites including www.asianhealthsecrets.com, and discussion groups resulting from them have created a worldwide family. Nothing is more endearing than sharing weight loss challenges, successes, and recipes with those who understand you best. Tigers, Dragons, Bears, and Cranes around the world have helped each other to achieve lasting health and beauty.

The Baseline Diet, individualized menus, reviews of Asian restaurants serving slimming dishes, and natural remedies for emotional support allow anyone to live life to the fullest by remaining slim. During holidays and family celebrations, my readers know ways to remain calm and centered without relying upon former addictions. Some readers came to realize their emotional relationship to foods—their food karma—and were able to improve their needs for comfort and approval and their appearance. Other readers simply followed my diet and exercise advice and lost weight.

I predict that this book, which stresses safe, time-tested Asian health foods, will lead the way to an improved relationship between consumers and the health food industry. An educated public demands a sophisticated, global marketplace, not gimmicks and dangerous fads.

Statistical weight loss studies rarely determine success with personal health and well-being. Even the best, most carefully controlled diet study involving many participants fails to address *individual* addictions, digestive *qi*, and food karma. Testing does not change your tastes, your emotional cravings, or your habits. Only you can improve your life. However, on the path of gaining energy to lose weight, you can take charge of your diet with the help of your totem. Your animal nature craves health and happiness even while you may be afraid, sick, or disappointed. Learning positive ways to behave like a Tiger, Dragon, Bear, or Crane can reshape your figure and save your life.

It is the way of all plants to flourish. My New York garden is at the General Theological Seminary in my Chelsea neighborhood. Each spring its canvas is awash with pink, purple, and pale yellow tulips. Yellow and white crocuses resemble faces, and the weeping cherry tree shrugs from the weight of its pink flowers. The American elm trees sprout green leaves. Every season brings an opportunity for renewal. During winter, while my New York garden sleeps, I visit the South to anticipate spring's flowering.

Homestead and southward into the Florida Keys form a corner of the tropics where many Asian farmers grow Chinese and East Indian fruits, vegetables, trees, and herbs. One winter, my friends Paul and Craig at the Grove Inn in Homestead gave me a 10-inch-high neem tree. The neem is sacred in India. Yogis chew the bitter bark and brew the dried leaves as a natural antibiotic tea that fights skin rashes, parasites, and tooth decay. Driving north to New York, I sadly watched the leaves wither and fall. Trees do not travel well, but nature strives sometimes against incredible odds to be beautiful. At home, I kept the potted tree on a sunny windowsill, cut back the delicate trunk to 2 inches above the soil, and, at Paul's suggestion, added fresh brewed, cold green tea leaves as a mulch. In several months, fresh leaves sprouted on the neem tree.

You are part of an eternal renewal that lies beyond human understanding. The Tiger in you seeks adventure. The Bear loves the company of friends and delicious meals. The Dragon seeks vitality and inner peace. The Crane in you yearns for the freedom of an open sky and spiritual awakening. Your dawning awaits within you.

Because a family normally has more than one sort of animal energy type, the following are good to keep on hand in the kitchen.

Salt Substitutes

It is best to completely avoid table salt so that you will not stress your kidneys and possibly raise your blood pressure. For my popcorn, I use canola oil, turmeric powder, and asafoetida powder. Turmeric has anticancer and antibiotic properties, and it supports healthy intestinal bacteria. For people who enjoy salty foods, dried sheets of nori seaweed or a handful of dried dulse or toasted green kelp flakes is a tasty, crunchy snack packed with protein.

Sea vegetable flakes can be sprinkled on or into foods When toasting seaweed, set the oven at 200°F and use a glass (non-metal) baking dish. When the seaweed strips are crisp (about 5 minutes), crumble them into a jar or whip them with a blender to make a powder you can use instead of salt.

My current favorite salt substitute is powdered green kelp seaweed. You can order it in bulk from sources in Maine, listed in the Natural Products and Information Resource Guide (page 348). The following salt substitutes also work fine: dulse seaweed powder, basil, cumin, oregano, light soy sauce, and apple cider vinegar.

Seasoning without Salt

Any Asian herbalist knows that spices affect energy as well as digestion. Bay leaf, marjoram, saffron, and especially nutmeg are sedating. Use them with care for anxiety. To avoid danger, never use more than a pinch of nutmeg over the course of a day. Sage, thyme, mustard, chives, curry powder, black pepper, and ginger are stimulating. The latter two increase appetite and acidity; therefore, avoid them if you have ulcers. For inflammatory symptoms such as acid reflux, sprinkle cumin powder or dillweed onto foods or add them to beverages.

Sugar Substitutes

Sugar, honey, and molasses are bugaboos for weight loss. One teaspoon of white sugar contains 16 calories, and 1 teaspoon of brown sugar has 17 calories. One tablespoon of molasses has 55 calories. One tablespoon of honey has 21 calories, and you cannot cook it. Raw honey contains useful enzymes and nutrients, but cooked honey resembles glue in the digestive tract.

For its flavor and convenience, my favorite sugar substitute is vanilla extract. These three sweeteners are especially recommended for people with diabetes.

- ½ teaspoon of stevia herb powder = 4 calories
- 1 teaspoon cinnamon powder = 6 calories
- 1 teaspoon anise powder = 8 calories

Anyone can reduce sugar cravings and improve insulin production to prevent and treat diabetes by supplementing a low-sugar diet with capsules of gymnema (*Gymnema sylvestre*), available from East Indian food shops and online at various Web sites including www.himalayausa.com and www.herbalsalon.com. (Find the mechanism of its action, research data, and traditional information about gymnema and other Ayurvedic herbs at www.himalayanhealthcare.com.)

Breads

Yeast makes both bread and your breadbasket expand. It is best to avoid refined grains and soft breads and cereals. Crunchy and chewy foods are better for you. Most whole grain yeast breads contain from 73 to 78 calories per ounce. One flour tortilla is 159 calories, while one whole wheat tortilla has 73 calories.

If you eat commercially made bread, make sure you can see the grain. German-made whole grain breads contain whole wheat, rye, bran, and natural fermenting agents. In this country, you can find The Baker breads, which I recommend, in most supermarkets.

Whole Soy Products

Tofu is a healthy meat substitute for many people throughout the world. In Japan, where longevity statistics are the best in the world, people eat whole soy products several times daily. They include green soybean pods, cooked soybeans, tofu, tempeh, and natto, fermented soybeans added to noodles or rice.

The Australian government Web site www.betterhealth.vic.gov. au highly recommends two daily servings of whole soy products to promote health and well-being—for example, 500 milliliters (about 2¼ cups) of soy milk per day or 100 grams (about ½ cup) of tofu per day. Eating soybean-based foods may reduce the risk of a range of health problems, including high blood pressure, coronary heart disease, arthritis, and cancers of the breast, colon, prostate, and skin.

Tofu's calories vary according to its density.

- ½ cup firm tofu = 183 calories
- ½ cup silken, firm tofu = 70 calories
- ½ cup silken, soft tofu = 62 calories

Soy is a high-quality protein that contains all the essential amino acids, similar to those found in meat and amaranth seed, a wild green. Tofu or tempeh (made with a calcium coagulant) provide calcium. The soybean is high in fiber and protein, low in saturated fat and cholesterol.

Grains

The grain highest in calories is cooked kasha (buckwheat groats), with a whopping 343 calories per ½ cup. That grain prevented many a Russian from freezing to death during long Siberian winters. Calories give us body heat. Cooling grains contain fewer calories. They include:

- ½ cup cooked millet = 143 calories
- ½ cup brown or white rice = 108 and 103 calories, respectively

- ½ cup cooked barley = 97 calories
- ½ cup cooked oats = 90 calories
- ½ cup cooked couscous = 88 calories

Tea

Robert McCaleb, president of the Herb Research Foundation in Boulder, Colorado (www.herbs.org), has suggested that if Americans drank tea (*Camellia sinensis*) instead of coffee, we could greatly reduce our fat intake. Tea reduces fat absorption in the digestive tract, and its acids speed digestion and elimination. No matter if you drink white, green, red, oolong, or black tea; no matter if you add milk, lemon, or ice, tea has amazing health benefits. Depending on the type and how long it is brewed, 1 cup of tea contains about half as much caffeine as coffee.

Beyond slimming the body and toning metabolism, tea protects regular users against heart trouble and various cancers. Five to 6 cups daily reduces harmful LDL cholesterol and increases good HDL cholesterol. Tea decreases liver cell damage. It contains catechins, specialized acids that help prevent skin, lung, mouth, esophagus, stomach, liver, prostate, breast, and rectal cancers. Flavonoids in tea inhibit oral bacteria that may lead to heart trouble and oral cancer. Tea increases necessary digestive bacteria in the intestine and thereby enhances absorption.

Commercial decaffeinated teas may use harmful chemicals. The best process is called CO_2, or carbon dioxide decaffeinization, which is expensive. An easy way to reduce caffeine in your tea at home is a two-step method.

1. Put dried tea leaves into your tea pot. Add just enough nearly boiling water to cover them. That warms the tea pot. Wait for about 20 to 30 seconds. Pour off the water, which removes any dust from the tea and most of the caffeine.
2. Then add enough water to make 1 cup or mug. Let it steep for about 15 seconds, and pour your tea into your cup.

That way, you awaken the tea's flavor but do not allow the leaves to sit in water for a long time, which increases bitter-tasting tannins that may irritate the stomach. Using this method, you can use the same leaves to make cups of tea all day.

Natural Products and Information Resource Guide

Before you look any further, search in your own backyard for top-quality Asian products available at Wal-Mart stores and online at www.walmart.com, www.vitaminshoppe.com, and www.amazon.com.

AYURVEDIC (EAST INDIAN) HEALTH PRODUCTS

Butala Emporium Inc.
108 East 28th Street
New York, NY 10016
212-684-4447
www.indousplaza.com
e-mail: service@indousplaza.com

Amla, Chyawanprash, herbal powders (churna), pills and capsules, Good Care Slimming Tea, Anti-Obesity Tea

By the Planet, Inc.
5111-A NW 13th Street
Gainesville, FL 32609
888-543-9294
815-301-8667 (fax)
www.bytheplanet.com
e-mail: info@bytheplanet.com

Asian herbs and beauty products; customer service representatives who speak Spanish, Mandarin Chinese, Taiwanese, and German are available for assistance.

Foods of India
121 Lexington Avenue
New York, NY 10016-8122
212-683-4419
212-251-0946 (fax)

Major brands of Ayurvedic herbs, spices, foods; Indian fresh produce, cookware, incense, and books

Indian Herb Care
www.indianherbcare.com

Weight loss products including Abana (HeartCare), Ayurslim capsules, Karela (Bitter Gourd) Medohar Guggulu, Neem capsules, and Shilajit capsules

Yogi Teas
Golden Temple Inc.
2545 Prairie Road
Eugene, OR 97402
800-964-4832
www.yogitea.com

Organic herbal teas

CHINESE HERBS AND TEAS

East Earth Trade Winds
PO Box 493151
Redding, CA 96049-3151
800-258-6878
www.eastearthtrade.com
www.eastearthherb.com

Chinese teas, tea pots, Chinese patent remedies, Long Hay Flat herbs, Yin/ Yang Sisters instant beverages, Reishi+ extract, mushroom products, incense, essential oils, pain-relief products, and books

Health Concerns
8001 Capwell Drive
Oakland, CA 94621
800-233-9355
www.healthconcerns.com
e-mail: herbalist@healthconcerns.com

Health Concerns brand and Chinese patent remedies

Kontakt
Dalasa Handelsgesellschaft mbH
Pfarrplatz 4, A 1190
Wien, Austria
+43-1-3784096
www.charantea.com
e-mail: info@charantea.com

Bitter melon products in Europe

Kowloon Bay Inc.
81 Bowery Street
New York, NY 10013
646-613-9521

Chinese herbs, patent remedies, and foods

Lin Sister Herb Shop
4 Bowery Street
New York, NY 10013
212-962-5417
e-mail: linsisterherb@aol.com

Chinese herbs and patent remedies, Yin/Yang Sisters instant beverages

Long Life Teas
180 Vanderbilt Motor Parkway
Hauppauge, NY 11788
800-848-7331
www.long-life.com

Organic herbal teas

The Maté Factor
119 Third Street
Ithaca, NY 14850
800-656-3668
www.matefactor.com

Yerba maté tea, rooibos chai, organic green tea

Vermont Tea and Trading Company
PO Box 1050
Middlebury, VT 05753
888-ALL-TEAS

Rooibos chai

Wing Hop Fung
727 North Broadway
Los Angeles, CA 90012
800-239-6888
www.asiachi.com
e-mail: info@asiachi.com

Cherry Grain Balsam Pear Tea, Chinese teas, medicinal mushrooms, bulk herbs, patent remedies and liniments

SEAWEEDS

Maine Coast Sea Vegetables
3 Georges Pond Road
Franklin, ME 04634
207-565-2907
207-565-2144 (fax)
www.seaveg.com

A commercial source of certified organic sea vegetables that supplies many American health food stores. Their products include 2-ounce reclosable packages or bulk lots of common seaweeds, seaweed seasonings, chips, and other seaweed snack foods.

Maine Seaweed Co.
P.O. Box 57
Steuben, ME 04680
207-546-2875 (phone/fax)
www.alcasoft.com/seaweed

A small family-owned business on the Maine coast. They hand-harvest and dry Atlantic seaweeds: kelp, alaria, dulse, nori, and bladderwrack. They also sell a Family Pack, a select mix containing over 3 pounds of kelp, alaria, dulse, nori, and digitata, plus recipes and a forager's handbook. They also sell a seaweed fertilizer and offer a chatty newsletter.

THAI COOKING INGREDIENTS

www.citruscentre.co.uk

www.foodsubs.com

www.fourwindsgrowers.com

www.importfood.com

www.templeofthai.com

www.thaifoodandtravel.com

JAPANESE KONNYAKU (AKA SHIRATAKI, KONJAC) NOODLES

www.konjacfoods.com

TIBETAN TEAS AND HEALTH AND BEAUTY PRODUCTS

Tibetan Medical and Astro. Institute
Men-Tsee-Khang Exports
PT 62/5, Kalkaji Extension
New Delhi, India 110019
(91) 011-26214897 / 26436823
(91) 011-26211738 (fax)
www.tibetan-medicine.org
e-mail: Info@tibetan-medicine.org

Sorig Loong Tea for nervous anxiety, Sorig Tripa Tea for inflammation and hypertension, and Sorig Bad-Kan Tea for low energy and weight loss

NUTRITIONAL SUPPLEMENTS AND GARDENING PRODUCTS

Chlorella Europe
PO Box 350
Ramsgate, Kent
CT11 9YP
United Kingdom
+44-0-1843-585064
www.chlorella-europe.com
e-mail: chlorella@europe.com

Fungi Perfecti, LLC
PO Box 7634
Olympia, WA 98507
800-780-9126
www.fungi.com
e-mail: mycomedia@aol.com

Mushroom supplments, books, research, classes, and kits

High Mowing Seeds
813 Brook Road
Wolcott, VT 05680
802-888-1800
802-888-8446 (fax)
www.highmowingseeds.com

Seeds for the garden

Puritan's Pride
800-645-1030
www.puritan.com

Affordable herbs, nutritional supplements, and essential oils

Wal-Mart
www.walmart.com

Affordable herbs, vitamins, and health books

RAW FOODS DIET INFORMATION

Living and Raw Foods
www.living-foods.com

Online community and information

RawFood.com
www.rawfood.com

Books on raw-food diet and related topics and information on retreats

Raw Food Talk: The Raw Food Diet Forum
www.rawfoodtalk.com

Vegan and vegetarian recipes

HOLISTIC HEALTH INFORMATION AND RELATED RESEARCH

Asian Health Secrets
www.asianhealthsecrets.com

Articles on Asian health foods, teas, Asian restaurants with slimming dishes, and lively forums for Tigers, Dragons, Bears, and Cranes

American Botanical Council
www.herbalgram.org

American Dietetic Association
www.eatright.org/public

American Herbal Products Association
www.ahpa.org

ChinaSprout
www.chinasprout.com

Information and resources for families with adopted Chinese children

Dietary Supplement Information Bureau
www.supplementinfo.org

Herb Research Foundation
www.herbs.org

Institute for Traditional Medicine
www.itmonline.org

Chinese herbal research

National Center for Complementary and Alternative Medicine (NCCAM)
www.nccam.nih.gov

National Certification Commission for
Acupuncture and Oriental Medicine
www.NCCAOM.org

Rejuvenation Research
Indexed in PubMed. Subscribe at www.
sens.org
Editor in chief, Aubrey D. N. J. de Grey,
department of genetics, Cambridge
University

An authoritative peer-reviewed journal
that publishes leading work on the imple-
mentation of rejuvenation therapies in
the laboratory, clinic, and relevant basic
research

Index

C

Crane energy type *(cont.)*
    meals for, 228–38
    menus for, 238–43
    Metal element and, 65, 70–71
    movements for, 302
    natural antidepressants, 219–20
    overview, 61, 63–64, 209–10,
        243–44
    questionnaire and, 78
    sprouts for, 229–30
    TCM for, 243
    teas for, 221–23
    tremella for, 227
Cravings. *See also* Addiction
    anti-bingeing tea, <u>286</u>
    current, examining, 9–10
    emotional basis of, 6–7, 10
    of energy types
        Bear, 63, 79, 175–76, 187–88,
            190–91, 192–94
        Crane, 64, 79
        Dragon, 63, 79, 81, 152
        Tiger, 65, 79
    qi's effect on, 9
    for salt, reducing, 152
    solace sought through, 19–20
    for sweets, reducing, 45, 123, 187–88,
        190–91, 192–94
Cumin, 148, 151
Curry, 233–34, 236

D

Dampness, 91–93, 138, 141–42
Dancing, 299–300
Dandelion capsules, 113, 191
Dang shen (codonopsis), 309
Death wish, 71
Dehydration, 52, 90, <u>91</u>, 118, 277
Depression, 10, 14, 18, 219–20
Desserts, 26, 253
Diabetes, 5, 174, 182–89, 254
Digestion
    assessing your qi, 85–86
    balancing foods for, 12, 13
    chewy foods aiding, 5
    Chinese pills for, 333–34
    Digestive Bitters for, 43, 130

emotions and, 69
    qi as energy of, 6
    slowed by desserts, 26
    slowed by naps or baths, <u>255</u>
    supplements for, 25, 43, 213, 325
Diuretic foods, <u>12</u>
Diuretics after 40, 277
Dong quai root, 212
Dragon energy type
    balancing foods for, 150–52
    Bear combined with, 78
    breakfast for, 157
    coffee substitutes for, 149–50
    cravings, 63, 79, 81, 152
    determining, 80–82
    diet overview, 145–46
    emotional eating, 76–77, 144–45
    Fire element and, 66–67
    herbs and supplements for, 152–53
    homeopathic remedies for, 139–44
    illnesses, 61, 63, 77, 80, 137–38,
        171
    meals for, 156–65
    menus for, 166–70
    movements for, 301
    overview, 61, 62–63, 137–39, 171
    questionnaire and, 76–77
    TCM for, 171
    teas for, 146–48
    Water element and, 65, 67–69
Drain Dampness pills, 43–44, 115–16,
        153
Dressings, salad, 46, 124
Drugs, Cranes and, 217–19
Dulse, 29, 116, 253, 291, 339
Dumplings, 332

E

Earth element, 65, 69–70
Ease Plus pills, 107–8
Eating out
    Chinese cuisine, 316–19
    Indian cuisine, 319–21
    Japanese cuisine, 315–16
    Thai cuisine, 312–15
    Tibetan cuisine, 321–22
    Vietnamese cuisine, 319

Eclipta alba, 215
Edema. *See* Water retention
Eggplant, 161–62
Eggs, recipes using, 332
Elements
    Earth, 65, 69–70
    Fire, 66–67
    Metal, 65, 70–71, 211, 238–39
    Water, 65, 67–69
    Wood, 65, 71–73, 105
Emotions
    as basis of cravings, 6–7, 10
    digestion and, 69
    in Dragon energy type, 138–39
    eating due to, 76–77, 139–45,
        175
EndoTrim, 220
Energy. *See* Qi or vitality
Energy types. *See also specific types*
    animal symbols for, 59–61
    cravings associated with, 79
    determining yours, 80–82
    illnesses common to, 79
    not needed for Baseline Diet, 24
    overlap of, 78, 79
    overview, 61–65
    weight loss questionnaire, 73–80
Enoki mushrooms, 153
Epimedium leaf tea, 282
Exercise
    adaptogenic herbs for, 305–9
    animal forms, 300–303
    floor dancing, 299–300
    getting a checkup first, 305
    martial artists' tips for, 310–11
    pain remedies, 304–5
    swimming, 298–99
    traction, 303–4
    walking, 279, 297–98
    for weight loss, 84, 97

F

Face
    beauty treatment, 227–28
    diagnosis from, 85–86, 97
Fasting, 18–19, 52–54, 118, 329–30
Fatigue, 19, 45, 336

Fats and oils
    avoiding for weight loss, 12
    in Baseline Diet, 34–35
    coconut oil, 192, 268–69
    combining foods with, 12, 13
    garlic and parsley oil, 55, 113
    good vs. bad fats, 34–35
    healthy sources for, 5
    heating, dangers of, 35
    omega-3 oils, 180, 220
    storing oils, 35
Fava beans, 283–84
Feed Your Tiger Diet
    foods for fast weight loss, 261–74
    menus, 256–60
    principles of, 252–55
    supplements, 252–54
Fennel, 193
Fenugreek, defatted, 186–87
Fiber, 36–37, 49–50
Fire element, 66–67
Fish, 121, 159
5-HTP (5-hydroxytryptophan),
    219–20
Flavors. *See also specific flavors*
    addiction to, 11
    arthritis or rheumatism and, 118
    associated with Fire element, 66
    balanced combinations, 11–12, 12
    effects of, 4–5, 11
    overview, 10–13
    weight loss and, 96
Floating, 298–99
Floor dancing, 299–300
Folate, 30
Folic acid, 31
Food pyramid (USDA), 93–97
Formic acid for gout, 181
Fourth of July, 325
Fruits. *See also specific kinds*
    balancing milk with, 51
    in Baseline Diet, 25, 30–32
    for Bear energy type, 179
    cleansing, 339–40
    in Feed Your Tiger Diet, 263, 265–66,
        271–72, 274
    increasing daily intake of, 32
    raw food diet, 52

Pumpkin, 150
Pungent foods or flavor. *See also* Spicy
  foods
  for arthritis or rheumatism, 118
  balancing bitter foods with, <u>12</u>
  combining animal protein with, 36
  as digestive, 5
  for Dragon energy type, 150–51
  energetic effects of, 11
  stressing when losing weight, 12
  for weakness and chills, 289

Q

Qigong, <u>8</u>, 61, 300
Qi or vitality
  assessing, 85–90, 97–98
  attending to, 87–88, 97
  cravings affected by, 9
  enhancing, 212, 336
  foods supporting, 213
  sexual vitality, <u>278–79</u>, 280–81
  troubled or stuck, 6, 88, 141–42,
    143–44
Questionnaire, weight loss, 73–80
Quiet Digestion pills, 25, 43

R

Ramadan, 329–30
Ratatouille, 161–62
Raw foods, 37, 52, <u>81</u>, 98, 351
Red yeast rice pills, 180
Rehmannia, 185, 200
Reishi mushrooms
  for Crane energy type, 212, 213
  for edema reduction, 153
  for enhancing vitality, 212
  extract, 37, 254
  for fatigue, 19
  in Feed Your Tiger Diet, 254
  health benefits of, 37
  for joint comfort, 306
  overview, 309
  for Tiger energy type, 113
  Tiger Mushroom Wine, 37
Rejuvelac, 231
Restaurants. *See* Eating out
Rheumatism, treating, 118–19

Rhubarb, 129–30
Rooibos tea, 147, 178, 221–22
Rosemary tea, 149
Royal 1 & One black tea, 178

S

Sage leaf tea, 149
Salads
  dressings, 46, 124
  raw beet in, 37
  recipes, 164–65, 238
  for Tiger energy type, 123–24
Sal ammoniac, 140, 142, 143–44
Salmon, 159
Salt substitutes, 343
Salty foods or flavor, 5, 11, 12, <u>12</u>, 152
Sauces, 127, 163–64, 232–34, 235,
    312, 326
Schizandra berry, 128, <u>307</u>
Sea lettuce, 292
Seaweeds
  in Baseline Diet, 28–29
  for cleansing, 253
  metabolism boosters, 290–92
  overview, 28–29
  for reducing cellulite, 116–17
  for reducing salt cravings, 152
  resource guide, 349–50
  Seaweed Salad, 238
  toasted, 28, 253
  for weight loss, 25, 339
Seeds and nuts, 33
Servings, <u>81</u>, 93–97, 276–77
Sexuality, <u>278–79</u>, 280–81, 284–85
Shatavari, 287
Shiitake mushrooms
  for edema reduction, 153
  in Feed Your Tiger Diet, 254
  Sukiyaki, 163–64
  tea, 44, 45, 147, 212, 254
Shilajit capsules, 188–89, 293–94
Shi or *she*. *See* Dampness
Shirataki noodles, 49–50, 151–52,
    162–63, 164–65, 236–37, 350
Shrimp, 234–37
Siberian ginseng. *See* Ginsengs
Silica, 67
Skin brushing, 55

Tianfang broadleaf tea, 178
Tibetan cuisine, 321–22
Tibetan herbal teas, 55–56, 109, 147, 222, 350
Tienchi ginseng. *See* Ginsengs
Tiger energy type
  arthritis and rheumatism, 118–19
  breakfast for, 123
  cellulite, reducing, 114–17
  cleansing, foods for, 111–13
  coffee substitutes, 110–11
  constipation, 117–18
  cravings, 65, 79
  determining, 80–82
  diet overview, 108–9
  herbs and supplements for, 113, 121–22, 123
  illnesses, 62, 64, 64–65, 79, 80, 104, 135
  meals for, 122–30
  menus for, 130–35
  movements for, 302–3
  nervous eating by, 76, 105–7
  overview, 62, 64–65, 103–6, 135–36
  questionnaire and, 76
  TCM for, 136
  teas for, 109–10
  varicose veins, treating, 117
  withdrawal symptoms in, 107–8
  Wood element and, 65, 71–73, 105
Tofu, 123, 128–29, 236, 345
Tomatoes, 32, 36, 49, 325
Tongue, 53, 89–91, 91, 97, 138, 174, 278
Tonics. *See* Herbs and tonics
Traction, 303–4
Traditional Chinese Medicine (TCM)
  after 40, 285–89
  for chronic inflammation, 285–87
  dampness in, 91–93
  diabetes in, 174, 182–83
  for energy types
    Bear, 182–85, 207
    Crane, 243
    Dragon, 171
    Tiger, 136
  Fire element in, 66
  kidney-yin deficiency in, 184–85
  liver and gallbladder in, 71–72

lung-fire syndrome in, 183
sexuality in, 280–81
spleen/pancreas function in, 88–89
stomach-fire syndrome in, 183
tongue diagnosis in, 89–91
for weakness and chills, 287–89
Trans fats, 35
Tree ear fungi, 47–48, 128–29, 159–60
Tremella, 184, 196, 227
Trigonella foenum-graecum
  (fenugreek), 186–87
Triphala churna, 119
Triphala guggul tonic, 181
Tu Chung tea, 109
Turmeric, 49, 110, 148, 194, 228

U

Urinary incontinence, 277

V

Varicose veins, treating, 117
Vegan diet, 23
Vegetables. *See also* Greens; Salads
  in Baseline Diet, 25, 30–32
  for Bear energy type, 179–80
  fiber sources, 36, 37
  increasing daily intake of, 32
  potato substitutes, 125
  raw food diet, 52
  washing pesticides from, 31
Vervain tea, 149, 178
Vietnamese cuisine, 319
Visualization exercise, 8
Vitality. *See* Qi or vitality
Vitality Combination tonic, 308
Vitamin B-complex pills, 327
Vitamin D, 104, 119–22

W

Waist size, 83
Wakame, 290
Walking, 279, 297–98
Water. *See* Beverages; Teas
Watercress, 150, 274
Water element, 65, 67–69
Watermelon, 274

Water retention
  reducing, 43–44, 152–53, 281,
    283–84, 338–40
  tongue indicating, 90
  troubled qi indicated by, 86, 88
Wax gourd peel, 283
Weakness, 17, 287–89
Weddings, 324
Weight loss
  acupuncture massage for, 220–21
  after 40, 275–85, 289–94
  aging and, 283–84
  Baseline Diet for, 5–6, 24
  chlorella capsules for, 225–27
  clinical observations, 13–15
  commonsense guidelines for, 96–97
  dietary attitudes and, 4
  Dragon challenges for, 138–39
  enjoyment as factor in, 84–85
  exercise for, 84
  fast-action, foods for, 261–74
  health benefits of, 83
  health challenges and, 283–84
  increasing fiber for, 36
  jump-starting, 51–54
  metabolism boosters for, 289–92
  Native American herbs for, 185–88
  questionnaire, 73–80
  rejuvenating herbs for, 293–94
  sexuality and, 280–81

supplements in Baseline Diet, 25
three ways to, 81
tremella for, 227
withdrawal symptoms, 98
Weight management goals, 8–9
Whey, powdered goat, 340
White fungus, 184, 196, 227
White tea, 109, 147, 346–47
Wine, 37, 160–61
Winter melon slices, 283
Withania (ashwagandha), 250, 287
Withdrawal symptoms, 98, 107–8, 111
Woman's Balance formula, 284
Wood element, 65, 71–73, 105
Wu wei tse (schizandra), 128, 307

X

Xiao Yao Wan pills, 243, 284, 333

Y

Yeast infection, 51, 273
Yin and yang, 59, 184–85, 249–50
Yin yang hao tea, 282
Yin/Yang Sisters brand beverages, 110,
  146–47, 222. *See also specific
  drinks*
Yucca, 125